Rehabilitation
Nursing
SECRETS

Rehabilitation Nursing SECRETS

JEANNE FLANNERY, DSN, ARNP, CRRN, CNRN, CCH
Professor, Adult Nursing
School of Nursing
Florida State University
Tallahassee, Florida

SERIES EDITOR
LINDA SCHEETZ, EdD, APRN, BC, CEN
Assistant Professor
College of Nursing
Rutgers, The State University of New Jersey
Rutgers, New Jersey

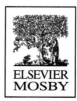

ELSEVIER
MOSBY

ELSEVIER
MOSBY

11830 Westline Industrial Drive
St. Louis, Missouri 63146

Notice

Pharmacology is an ever-changing field. Standard safety precautions must be followed, but as new research and clinical experience broaden our knowledge, changes in treatment and drug therapy may become necessary or appropriate. Readers are advised to check the most current product information provided by the manufacturer of each drug to be administered to verify the recommended dose, the method and duration of administration, and contraindications. It is the responsibility of the licensed health care provider, relying on experience and knowledge of the patient, to determine dosages and the best treatment for each individual patient. Neither the publisher nor the author assumes any liability for any injury and/or damage to persons or property arising from this publication.

International Standard Book Number 0-323-03145-5

Executive Publisher: *Barbara Nelson Cullen*
Editor: *Sandra Clark Brown*
Developmental Editor: *Sophia Oh Gray*
Publishing Services Manager: *John Rogers*
Senior Project Manager: *Cheryl A. Abbott*
Design Project Manager: *Bill Drone*

Printed in the United States of America

Last digit is the print number: 9 8 7 6 5 4 3 2 1

To my mother, Myrtle Louise Stone, RN, who gave her entire life to providing healing care to others. She never met a person that she could not offer guidance or direction to help that individual solve his/her problem. Though she did not call it rehabilitation nursing, her actions instilled in me my commitment to rehabilitation philosophy.

Contributors

SHARON A. ARONOVITCH, PhD, APRN-BC, CWOCN
Assistant Professor
School of Nursing
Florida State University
Tallahassee, Florida
8. Skin Integrity
10. Bowel Elimination
21. Orthopedic Rehabilitation
30. Nursing Management for Wounds

SUSAN R. BULECZA, MSN,CNS, APRN-BC
Skills Lab Coordinator
School of Nursing
Florida State University
Tallahassee, Florida
8. Skin Integrity
11. Bladder Elimination
13. Functional Mobility: ADLS
20. Burn Rehabilitation
25. Spinal Cord Injury Rehabilitation
26. Immune System Disorders Rehabilitation
27. Degenerative Disorders Rehabilitation
28. Neuromuscular and Debilitating Disorders Rehabilitation
32. Pediatric Rehabilitation

LOUISA L. DOWLING, MSN, ARNP
Family Nurse Practitioner
Digestive Diseases Clinic
Tallahassee, Florida
9. Nutrition Care

Sandra H. Faria, DSN, RN
Associate Professor of Nursing
School of Nursing
Florida State University
Tallahassee, Florida

Jeanne Flannery, DSN, ARNP, CRRN, CNRN, CCH
Professor, Adult Nursing
Director, Graduate Program
School of Nursing
Florida State University
Tallahassee, Florida

Sue B. Pugh, MSM, ARNP, CRRN, CNRN
Neurological Clinical Nurse Specialist, Case Manager
Tallahassee Memorial Hospital
Tallahassee, Florida

DENISE A. TUCKER, DSNRN, CCRN
Associate in Nursing
Coordinator of Adult Family
School of Nursing
Florida State University
Tallahassee, Florida
    16. End-Stage Renal Disease Rehabilitation
    17. Kidney Transplant Rehabilitation
    31. Palliative Care and End-of-Life Issues

MARY BETH VICKERS, BSN, MSN CANDIDATE, RN, CLNC
Faculty
School of Nursing
Tallahassee Community College
Tallahassee, Florida
    22. Diabetes Rehabilitation

Preface

It is important for nurses to understand that rehabilitation begins early and is not limited to a rehabilitation facility. Due to the shortened length of stay in acute care facilities and increased acuity of patients, the need for early application of rehabilitation nursing principles has become paramount. Because rehabilitation, as a focus, has essentially been removed from academic nursing curricula, this book is designed to close the gap between academic education and practice. It will serve both the novice nurse and the expert nurse by providing a "what," "why," and "how," approach through a quick question and answer format addressing assessment, monitoring, therapeutic interventions, pathophysiology of common disorders requiring rehabilitation, and client/family education. Additionally, it is grounded in evidence-based practice and includes clinical "pearls" for significant conditions. I hope this book will assist nurses in improving quality of life, providing cost-effective quality care, achieving client satisfaction, and helping clients to reach optimal function in the shortest period.

I would like to thank all the contributors for their time and commitment to providing a practical resource for nurses on rehabilitation strategies. Most especially, I would like to thank Susan R. Bulecza, MSN, RN, CNS, APRN-BC for her dedication, endless hours of research, and commitment to the creation of a comprehensive and unique book.

Jeanne Flannery

Contents

5. Appendixes

Top Secrets

1. Quality is a perception of the individual, based on his/her own philosophy, values system, experiential knowledge, education, family, etc.

2. The rehabilitation goal after spinal cord injury is to optimize functional ability and independence.

3. Immune disorders share the common element of disrupting the body's ability to regulate and protect, which results in chronic disease occurrence and a need for adaptation.

4. Functional assessment guides the rehabilitation professional in evaluating the client's ability to function in a dynamic environment by producing goal-directed behaviors to achieve optimal outcomes as independently as possible.

5. It is thought that sleep allows the central nervous system to evaluate its status and to rebalance its various activities, storing input into memory. Without this time to regroup, disruption in cognition occurs and can result in psychosis.

6. Regardless of the patient's diagnosis, assessment of bowel and bladder elimination must be thorough and ongoing.

7. The rehabilitation nurse has the opportunity to discuss the lifelong impact of transplant during the time the patient has been on dialysis.

8. Cardiac rehabilitation programs focus on increasing cardiac capacity through exercise and educate the population on risk factors such as diet modification, tobacco and alcohol cessation, and management of cardiac drugs.

9. The best energy conservation strategy for the respiratory patient is to use breathing techniques in coordination with movement or activity.

10. Rehabilitation for a burn patient begins the first day of injury.

11. Extent of skin loss and depth of the burn are the main factors that determine the rehabilitative course.

12. Autonomic dysreflexia is always a medical emergency for a spinal cord injured patient.

13. The most common complications following repair of a fracture are DVT, pulmonary emboli, and fat emboli.

14. Wound cultures are only to be obtained from the pink, healthy tissue of a wound after cleansing the wound with normal saline.

15. The nurse must realize that all injuries to the skin, no matter the size or location, affect the patient's quality of life and psychological well-being.

16. By utilizing tools designed specifically for assessing a child's abilities and limitations, the nurse and collaborative partners can collect a wealth of information for use in care planning, resulting in more individualized goals, interventions, and outcomes in pediatric rehabilitation.

17. It is important to address the issues of self-care, education, employment, and independent living early in a child's rehabilitation process in order for maximum independence to be achieved.

18. Family-centered and community-based case management services are a critical service component for children with disabilities.

19. Children with disabilities are at high risk for alterations in feeding and nutrition due to anatomical, developmental, sensory, neuromotor, and/or psychosocial environmental conditions.

20. Good communication between a child's caregiver and health care providers is key to ensuring that the child is given optimal opportunity for motor development without restriction due to unfounded fear of injury.

21. Breast feeding should not be ruled out for a child with cleft lip/palate.

22. How a child with a spinal cord injury reacts to his/her injury is going to depend on the level of physical, emotional, and cognitive development.

23. The American's value system, which is built on individualism, personal freedom, and independent decision-making, is radically different from many other cultures, thus creating a barrier for American nurses to provide culturally competent care.

24. Education about life style change is the most important intervention for patients with end-stage renal disease, including dietary and fluid restrictions, medications, and symptom recognition.

25. Patients with end-stage renal disease will probably require lower doses of medications to achieve therapeutic effects.

26. Patients diagnosed with terminal illness should receive rehabilitation to assist them to live comfortably and to the fullest extent possible.

27. Quality of life must be defined by the individual living it.

28. Complementary modalities have always related to rehabilitation and nursing philosophies; but it was not until after World War II that rehabilitation was allowed into the "accepted" circle of specialties. Because complementary therapies are founded on holistic principles, they still are not accepted by many physicians in the United States.

29. Chronic pain treatment without rehabilitation will not be effective, because the nurse empowers the patient to be in control of his/her pain through education about all relief measures, cause, prevention, coping, measures, and regaining functionality to achieve a better quality of life.

30. Dementia is approaching epidemic proportions in prevalence in America and with the fact that Americans are living longer and 78 million baby-boomers are approaching old age, it can only grow worse without prevention or cure.

31. The art of rehabilitation nursing is finding hope and satisfaction in a small improvement and instilling that positive feeling within patients and families, often in the face of their unrealistic goals.

32. Standardized care plans designed for medical diagnosis cannot guide rehabilitation nurses effectively since they must address multiple complex, chronic, and disabling conditions within one patient.

33. Rehabilitation is not a right for Americans; it is a privilege.

34. Community-based rehabilitation nursing has a focus to prevent disabilities and an expectation to create a partnership with the entire community.

35. It is unlikely the best outcomes can be achieved in the management of patients where the principles and process of rehabilitation are used unless rehabilitation nurses, especially those who are nationally certified, are utilized.

36. The most reliable method for estimating a patient's protein stores is to use a serum pre-albumin level.

37. The basic principle to use when deciding on which nutritional therapy to use is "if the gut works, use it."

38. Hemoglobin A1c provides the best long-term snapshot of glycemic control because it measures the amount of glucose bound to the RBC for most of its lifespan.

39. Stroke survivors represent 75% of all long-term care patients, 60% of rehabilitation patients, and 50% of hospitalized neurological patients.

40. Ateplase (Activase) is the only thrombolytic drug approved by FDA for treatment of stroke; it must be administered within 3 hours of the first symptom; thus, stroke is now called "brain attack."

41. Sleep-related complaints are the second most common reason for elderly physician visits.

42. Polypharmacy (use of many medications, often prescribed by a variety of physicians) is a major problem with older adults; consequences such as toxicity or non-therapeutic effects could be avoided by using a nurse case manager.

43. Rehabilitation nurses need to educate the public to improve the TBI prevention strategies in the United States.

44. Clinical evaluation is paramount to the diagnosis of DAI because microscopic neural damage is not evident on radiological examination.

45. The focus for a patient with TBI on admission to an acute care facility is to prevent secondary and tertiary brain injury.

46. Outpatient and emergency departments should provide careful education regarding long-term sequelae of concussion, rather than just the 24-hour monitoring guidelines.

47. GCS score, based on assessment of arousal, can predict severity of TBI but does not evaluate cognitive functioning; therefore, a patient can achieve the maximum score and yet be far from a normal cognitive level on LOCFAS or other cognitive assessment instruments.

48. Rehabilitation for a patient with TBI begins as soon as ICP is stable in ICU; there is no time to waste in cognitive recovery.

49. Difficulty in developing an independent attitude can often be one of the biggest barriers that the patient, along with rehabilitation team, has to overcome.

50. Although most spinal cord injuries do not result in complete severance of the cord, many become complete injuries from the secondary inflammatory damage that occurs within hours.

Rehabilitation Nursing SECRETS

Section 1

Rehabilitation Nursing Practice Issues

Chapter 1

Definitions, Philosophy, Goals, and Scope

Jeanne Flannery

1. What is the definition of rehabilitation nursing?

Many definitions of rehabilitation nursing exist, and formally the definition revolves around that which the American Nurses' Association and Association of Rehabilitation Nurses (1988) have published: "the diagnosis and treatment of human responses of individuals and groups to actual or potential health problems stemming from altered functional ability and altered lifestyle."

2. What is the priority of rehabilitation nursing?

The priority of rehabilitation nursing is to provide assistance to those who have chronic conditions or disabilities for the purpose of helping them attaining or maintaining the highest level of functioning possible, optimal health and well-being, and effective adaptation to alterations in their lifestyles.

3. What are the present goals of rehabilitation nursing?

Goals consistently focus on prevention of disorders that are chronic, disabling, or developmental. When disorders are not preventable, then the prevention of further disability and complications becomes the focus. The goal always involves promoting independence, maximizing potential, and restoring optimal functioning. Effective patient coping and adaptation are reinforced through the establishment of authentic, therapeutic relationships to enhance the quality of life.

Emphasis is on adaptation, not just recovery. The focus is on abilities, not that which the patient cannot do; rehabilitation nurses accentuate the positive. Accepted fact is that a disability affects the whole family, and all are involved in the rehabilitation process. The goal of rehabilitation nursing is to begin rehabilitation on day one.

4. How does one assess the scope of rehabilitation?

One must examine rehabilitation on three levels to determine its true scope:
1. Personality
   a. The nurse evaluates the patient's motivation.
      - Ability and willingness to mobilize physical and psychological resources

- Ability to cope with the disability
- Commitment to improving

b. The nurse assesses the personality of the patient.
  - Interests (hobbies, athletics)
  - Self-esteem (How do patients feel about themselves?)
  - Achievements (Did the patient work hard in school and on the job?)
  - Recognition (leadership qualities, goal orientation)
  - Introverted/extroverted (learning style, preferences, relationships)
  - Values (work ethic, integrity, independence)
  - Personal strengths

c. The nurse assesses significant others' goals and motivation.
  - Are family and friends supportive?
  - Is there agreement among the support group?
  - Do some of the supporters have long-term commitment?
  - Will some of the supporters work hard when needed?
  - Does the patient accept the supporters and their efforts?

d. The nurse assesses the patient's response to the demands of the rehabilitation environment.
  - Degree of adaptation to the milieu
  - Acceptance of philosophy (patient is not "sick")
  - Acceptance of norms (patient participates in therapy or must leave)
  - Adapts to "tough love" ("I'll show you how and help you, but I will not do it for you.")

2. Social System

  The nurse collaborates with all rehabilitation team members to assess the relationship of the therapeutic milieu and the patient's perception of real-life situations. What tension exists among the subsystems at work in the patient's world?
  - Living space
  - Occupation
  - Family roles and responsibilities
  - Transportation
  - Income
  - Expenses
  - Resources
  - Identified problems and causal model, and changes that are possible

  The team members must look at their interdisciplinary approach based on this holistic assessment.

3. Culture

  This is not the concept of culturally competent care, but a separate basic issue. The nurse assesses how the patient fits within the culture of America.
  - Rehabilitation nurses tend never to abandon the occupational role.
  - Rehabilitation nurses have the right to work and tend to believe that everyone desires to work; therefore rehabilitation nurses want to provide some opportunity for the patients to work who no longer can do the jobs they have always done. (Patients may differ from this basic ethic.)

The team logically defends American values, which contain noble, humanitarian concerns. This premise is assumed to fit all persons.
- Lessening suffering for every person
- Restoring to the fullest extent possible physical, social, and emotional well-being

And finally, rehabilitation nurses consider the basic underlying expectation.
- Rehabilitation nurses expect to resocialize persons with disabilities.
- Rehabilitation nurses want to minimize the degree of disruption that the disability brings into the social system.
- Rehabilitation nurses have moved children with disabilities into mainstream education. No longer are these children sheltered in a special school.
- Rehabilitation nurses are trying to make the interface of the social system in America more seamless for those who have disabilities.
- Progress is constant, and rehabilitation nurses must continue to support this belief with changes such as in the work world, transportation modifications, building structures, recreation devices, home designs, and van redesigns.

5. What is the art of rehabilitation nursing?

The art of rehabilitation nursing is knowing when to listen, when to push, when to hug, when to laugh, when to cry, and how to be honest. The art is the ability to weave the fabric of progress out of many scattered intervention threads with lots of failed tries and a few baby steps forward. The art is finding hope and satisfaction in a small improvement in the face of patients' and families' unrealistic goals and instilling that positive feeling within them.

6. What is culturally competent rehabilitative nursing?

Consideration and respect by the nurse for the patient's beliefs, values, and customs reflects culturally competent care of the disabled person. The nurse assists the person through a culturally different health care system. Americans' beliefs may be much different from those of different ethnicities. For example, in this fast-paced society, a nurse actually can offend a Puerto Rican patient if the nurse does not spend time with the patient just to talk (not just for interventions). Time spent with the patient is rated much more highly than efficiency in providing all the care needed in a short period of time.

7. Who are the members of the rehabilitation team?

The team is composed of the patient, physician, nurse, occupational therapist, physical therapist, speech pathologist, social worker or nurse case manager, vocational counselor, music therapist, recreational therapist, chaplain, and family/significant others. Depending on the type of disorder, the members are selected to meet the specific needs. Others may be added, as required, such as a neuropsychologist, cognitive therapist, or pulmonary technician.

8. Compare the terms *multidisciplinary, interdisciplinary, and transdisciplinary.*

   - *Multidisciplinary*—Decisions are made within the discipline, and roles are within the boundaries of each discipline. Conflicting goals may exist among disciplines. The nurse may be the mediator.
   - *Interdisciplinary*—Decisions are made across disciplines through consensus, and tasks are shared; teamwork requires much communication and collaboration. The nurse may be the coordinator.
   - *Transdisciplinary*—Goals are mutual and decisions transcend disciplines; roles are mutual as well, with ill-defined boundaries; members perform tasks that may be identified with a different discipline when needed. Generally, great appreciation exists among disciplines for one another. If appropriate cross-training is provided, progress toward goals can be seamless, with less duplication of effort. The coordinator varies among disciplines, depending on the patient's primary needs.

9. What is the specialty for a physician who has a practice in rehabilitation?

   The medical rehabilitation specialist is called a physiatrist. This physician has specialized with a residency in medicine or physical medicine. The practice of physiatry tends to be in a rehabilitation facility, rather than an office. The physiatrist may prescribe agents unique to the specialty, such as exercise, heat, massage, biofeedback, electrical stimulation, and diathermy, in addition to usual care.

10. Describe patient-centered models of rehabilitation.

    Patient-centered practice embraces the philosophy of a partnership between patients and providers. The approach considers that which is important to patients and how care is likely to affect them. The age, the type of disorder, the cultural system, and family system can provide the basis for four separate specialist models of services within this model.

11. Describe provider-centered models of rehabilitation.

    Provider-centered models focus on the provider role, such as primary care, case management, nurse-managed care, and independent practice, or consultations, as a system of care.

12. What is the case management model of rehabilitation?

    The case management model of rehabilitation provides service to a population that is identified as high risk and high cost. The patients typically have complex medical needs and require multiple services to provide comprehensive health care. Meeting their needs generates the highest costs. This model of care is coordinated by an advanced practice nurse case manager through precertification screening, referral for appropriate management, education, and discharge planning. This nurse advocates and negotiates for the patient's care over a continuum of services.

13. What are the phases of rehabilitation?

- First, in the disease/organ-impairment phase, the patient faces the limitations resulting from psychological or physical disease or injury that causes impairment of an organ.
- Next, in the person-disability phase, the patient has functional limitations and has lost the ability to carry out self-care and activities of daily living considered normal for an individual.
- Finally, in the society-handicap phase, persons are unable to interact effectively in the environment so that they fulfill the roles normal for them. Although the problem may be societal failure to ensure ease of interaction, society calls the problem a disadvantage or handicap. This perception is external to the persons with disabilities and in opposition to their own perceptions.

14. What has been the trend in changing terminology?

- From biblical times until the 1940s the use of the word *cripple* was accepted. The word conveyed a vision of beggars and elicited the emotion of pity.
- Then came the term *handicap*, which described the burden a person must bear in life, which was considered to place that person at a disadvantage. The term evolved from horse racing, where the jockeys drew lots to learn their starting position at the gate. The lots were placed in a jockey's silk cap for drawing. Certain positions had less of an advantage at the start. Later, to level the competition even further, jockeys were weighed. If some weighed less, they had to place their "hand in the cap" (the jockey's silk cap was used to hold rocks or weights, from which the lighter ones needed to select enough weights to put in their pockets to make them all even). In the current world this term is not viewed as being politically correct to apply to another individual. Patients may be insulted when nurses try to ascribe to them a disadvantage. An excellent example is frequently evident among the deaf. Often the deaf do not choose to have surgery to restore any degree of hearing because they see no disadvantage from their impairment.
- The term *disabled* has replaced handicap, as in designated parking spaces. This term, though with less negative connotation than handicap, still may stir patients to defend themselves. The term implies that the individual is not capable of performing a task or a role. The compensatory strategies that are taught to patients during their rehabilitation often provide different ways to perform the task. For example, though the patient cannot walk, the patient is so capable in the wheelchair that any role the patient decides to fill can be accomplished, even Olympic racing.
- Presently the term *challenged* has been used in a variety of circumstances to sound less intimidating, such as visually challenged rather than blind. To what extent this term will become the norm is yet to be seen.

Generally, a good rule of thumb is to listen to patients describe themselves. Once rehabilitation has been accomplished, patients choose a comfortable way to describe their status. Rehabilitation nurses learn from the patients.

15. What is excess disability?

This term *excess disability* refers to the patient's inability to perform that is greater than the disability usually associated with the impairment. This situation often results from caregivers' fostering dependence by "doing for." Frequently, the family members are trying to be helpful, and their negative influence evolves from their lack of understanding of their role and responsibilities in the patient's rehabilitation.

Another cause for excess disability is the lack of time of staff, or the lack of staff who care for the patient. Allowing patients to do tasks for themselves is time consuming and may not result in the tasks' actually being accomplished so that staff members ultimately must complete the tasks or do them anyway. As a result, patients may not be permitted to try. Over time, disuse increases the impairment and requires more care from the caregiver. The outcome is unsatisfactory for both partners. For this reason, the team determines weekly the amount and types of assistance required while the patient is in acute rehabilitation and, according to progress made, following discharge. The rehabilitation nurse must see that all members of the team are aware of the plan and are following it.

16. Can a disabled person be considered well?

Wellness can be achieved without complete physical or mental well-being through a rehabilitation nurse's actions to reduce limitations. Restoration, maintenance, and promotion of healthy lifestyle interventions enhance wellness. Through rehabilitation adaptation to the impairment can produce a positive view in patients that supports wellness.

17. How does research play a role in rehabilitation nursing?

Documentation of outcomes is necessary to support that the appropriate level of care is being provided. The rehabilitation nurse must be committed to consistent research and validating nursing practice. Nursing outcomes data need to be aggregated, analyzed, and published to support cost savings and positive results. The nurse can create clinical pathways, care maps, and guidelines as standards across the continuum of care. This approach is important in the case management model.

18. When should rehabilitation begin?

Answering this question requires knowing who is being asked.
- If the patient's significant others are posed this question, their unfaltering response will always be "Now!" From their perspective all that can be done must be done, by everyone, instantly, and must continue until their loved one is made whole once again. The response is driven by emotion.
- If the question is posed to health care providers, particularly nurses, and even more especially, rehabilitation nurses, the answer will be, "at the scene," or "on admission." The responsibilities that all nurses have in providing any care are always to prevent complications and to enhance well-being.

Without a rehabilitation focus in care, patients may develop numerous problems, such as deep venous thromboses, contractures, pressure sores, pneumonia, dehydration, or weight loss, all of which not only may extend the hospital length of stay but also may prevent rehabilitation from beginning. . The response is research based.

- From the perspective of the patients, rehabilitation begins when they accept that something is wrong and that a need exists for specialized therapy to improve the situation. The main reason for including this perspective is that the patient is considered to be an active member of the team and must be willing to participate in therapy. The patient is a partner in the design of the rehabilitation program and the setting of goals. Although all the team members can do their part with a patient who is unable to participate because lack of understanding or unwillingness to participate, for any number of reasons, the outcome is not likely to be the desired level of improvement. The whole team may be performing in all aspects possible for a patient who, for example, is comatose, to stimulate response, maintain function, and prevent complications. This is certainly rehabilitation, even though passive. However, the goal is to have the patient ready to begin as soon as the patient can participate actively.

19. How does the term *rehabilitation* differ from *restorative care*?

Rehabilitation and restorative care have considerable overlap; however, restorative care usually is applied to those patients who are not appropriate for formal rehabilitation. They may have little to no potential to improve or already may have reached their optimal level of functioning. Some patients, because of comorbidities, are simply unable to endure the activity of rehabilitation. If, for example, the comatose patient remained comatose after the team had worked intensely for a reasonable period, the patient would be transferred to a facility where restorative care would continue.

Restorative care may not involve qualified therapists providing procedures and techniques; however, nurses provide interventions that promote adaptation and maximize the patient's abilities. Restorative care, like rehabilitation, focuses on that which the patient can do and serves to reduce the level of care needed, promoting a greater degree of independence.

The activities within the scope of rehabilitation nursing include

- Toileting
- Walking and mobility exercises
- Dressing
- Grooming
- Eating
- Swallowing
- Transferring
- Amputation and prosthesis care
- Communication skills
- Specialized self-care skills such as diabetic management, ostomy care, and self-administration of medications
- Supportive care to maintain bodily functions

Key Points

- Transdisciplinary goals are mutual, and decisions transcend disciplines. Members perform tasks when needed that are identified with different disciplines, and a great appreciation exists among disciplines for one another.
- A disabled person can achieve wellness.

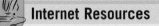

Internet Resources

Association of Rehabilitation Nurses
http://www.rehabnurse.org/

The National Rehabilitation Information Center
http://www.naric.com

Bibliography

1. American Nurses' Association, Association of Rehabilitation Nurses: *Rehabilitation nursing: scope of practice—process and outcome criteria for selected diagnoses,* Kansas City, Mo, 1988, American Nurses' Association.
2. Hargrove SD, Derstine JB: Definition and philosophy of rehabilitation nursing: history and scope including chronicity and disability. In Derstine JB, Hargrove SD, editors: *Comprehensive rehabilitation nursing,* Philadelphia, 2001, WB Saunders.
3. Hoeman SP: History, issues, and trends. In Hoeman SP, editor: *Rehabilitation nursing: process, application, & outcomes,* ed 3, St Louis, 2002, Mosby.

Chapter 2

History, Trends, and Legislation

Jeanne Flannery

1. How did rehabilitation begin?

Rehabilitation truly started with the principles Florence Nightingale used in 1859 to allow patients to do for themselves. See Figure 2-1.

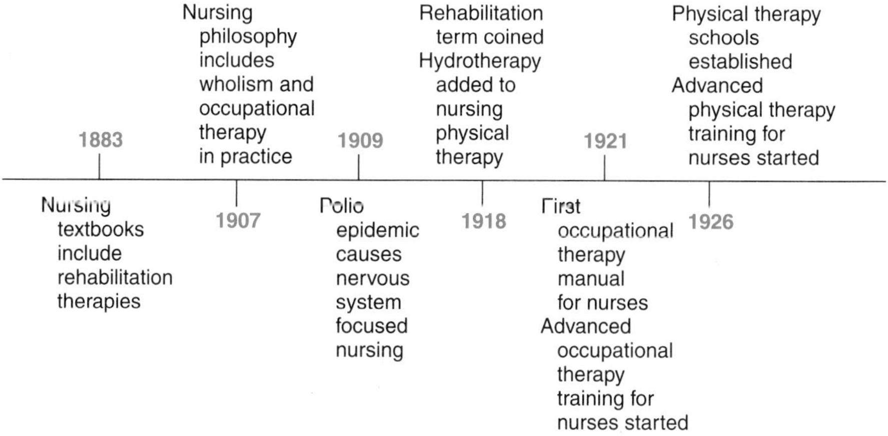

Figure 2-1. Rehabilitation milestones timeline: 1800-1920s.

2. What are the milestones of progress in rehabilitation in the United States from 1800 to the 1920s?

- Following the Civil War, funding was provided for artificial limbs, and nursing schools were started. In 1883 nursing textbooks included therapy with water, electrical stimulation, range of motion, and massage to weakened muscles. Orthopedic and brace care was a nursing focus in New York City for crippled children.
- In 1907 the philosophy of nursing incorporated caring for the whole person. Nurses performed occupational therapy as part of their care.

- In 1909 the first polio epidemic started nursing caring for persons who had nervous system diseases.
- In 1918 World War I ended. "Reconstruction of disabled servicemen" was the initiative the Public Health Service hospitals started. Douglas McMurtrie coined the term *rehabilitation* to replace the phrase "reconstruction of disabled servicemen." Hydrotherapy was added to nursing techniques of physiotherapy. Reeducation of disabled patients was determined to be a necessity.
- In 1921 an occupational therapy manual was written for nurses.
- After the war, interest in rehabilitation waned for a few years, based on the poor outcomes for the veterans. Few interventions existed that could reduce the disability. Few paraplegics survived. Vocational rehabilitation services for civilians in the form of sheltered workshops were started. Veterans were taught to work around their disabilities.
- In 1926 physical therapy schools were established; training took 18 months beyond nursing school. Convalescent care changed from peaceful retreats to skilled care and therapy and return to society. Rehabilitation was determined to begin when acute illness was "cured" or ended.

3. **What are the milestones of progress in rehabilitation in the United States from the 1940s to 1950s?**

See Figure 2-2.
- In 1941 Sr. Kenny revolutionized treatment of polio through the use of hot packs and passive range of motion rather than the previously accepted practice of immobilization in the acute stage. The patient was taught how to participate in muscle reeducation.
- In 1942 World War II was in progress and the armed services were participating actively in reconditioning and rehabilitation programs with hospitalized patients. Early ambulation, work therapy, bed exercises, and graduated exercises reduced hospital length of stay and pneumonia. At the end of the war the Veterans Administration system had no rehabilitation hospitals. Because 90% of the paraplegics from World War I had died within the first year, there had not seemed to be a need. However, of the 2500 paralyzed veterans of World War II, 1780 returned to their homes. With the use of antibiotics and nursing care, a different outcome from that in World War I occurred; therefore the rehabilitation hospitals were established. With rehabilitation, 1500 of these veterans obtained employment.
- In 1943 federal and state rehabilitation programs were established under the Vocational Rehabilitation Act amendment. All aspects of rehabilitation were now available to civilians injured in industrial and motor vehicle accidents. With the opening of many rehabilitation centers and with nursing journals publishing articles, the word *rehabilitation* came into vogue.
- In 1951 the first book on the subject, *Rehabilitation Nursing*, was published. Author Alice Morrissey described the rehabilitation nurse as the coordinator of the work of the rehabilitation team. From this publication the nursing specialty derived its name. The previous incorrect perception by most persons that rehabilitation started after acute and convalescent care was changed to

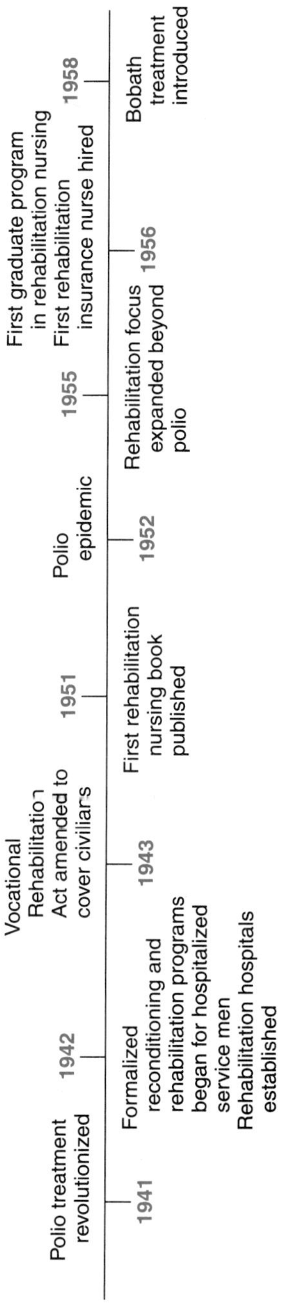

Figure 2-2. Rehabilitation milestones timeline: 1940s-1950s.

beginning as soon as possible. The term *activities of daily living* was coined at Rusk Institute, where Morrissey was nursing supervisor of the Department of Physical Medicine and Rehabilitation at Bellevue Hospital.
- In 1952 another polio epidemic caused hospitalization of 21,769 persons with acute disease. The mortality rate for the bulbar type was 40%.
- In 1955 after Salk introduced the polio vaccine and polio abated, rehabilitation expanded to include head trauma, spinal cord injury, stroke, amputations, cardiac events, arthritis, and other disorders that threatened the patient's independence.
- In 1956 Boston University started the first graduate program in rehabilitation nursing. During this same period, Liberty Mutual Insurance Company (the forerunner of case management) hired the first rehabilitation insurance nurse.
- In 1958 Karl and Berta Bobath introduced their innovative neurodevelopmental treatment approach for stroke, cerebral palsy, and other neurological impairments.

4. **What are the milestones of progress in rehabilitation in the United States from 1960 to 1970?**

See Figure 2-3.

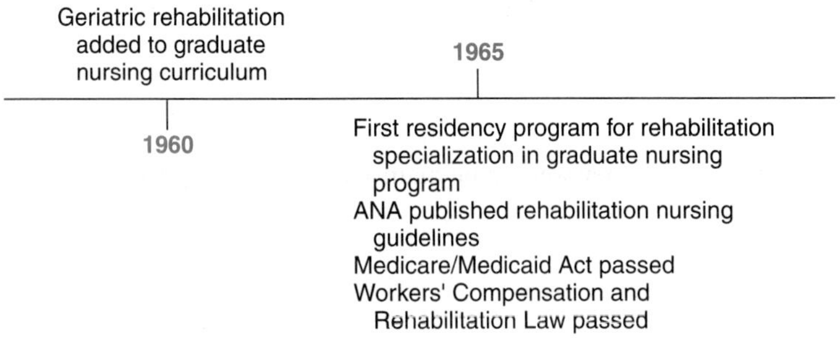

Figure 2-3. Rehabilitation milestones timeline: 1960s.

- In the early 1960s the first rehabilitation insurance nurse, Harriet Lane, developed specialized geriatric rehabilitation content for the Boston University graduate program.
- In 1965 Barbara Madden, who had established regional respiratory centers for polio patients under the National Foundation for Infantile Paralysis, became the director of nursing at Rancho Los Amigos Medical Center. She began the first residency program for rehabilitation specialization for graduate nursing students. The American Nurses' Association published *Guidelines for Practice of Nursing on the Rehabilitation Team: An Answer to a Growing Need;* the government passed Medicare and Medicaid legislation and passed the Workers' Compensation and Rehabilitation Law and Vocational Rehabilitation Act amendments.
- Trauma continued to escalate in a faster-paced society, and with improved technology and research, persons began surviving catastrophic events and

living longer. Once-fatal conditions changed to chronic, disabling conditions. Rehabilitation nurses became pivotal in all levels of care and in all settings. They entered the workplaces and homes, assessing needs and prescribing equipment, and structured modifications and activities. They educated all populations in the standards of best practice, procedures, special programs, and daily care management, including the patients and their caregivers. No longer was rehabilitation seen as having to occur in a specialized hospital.

5. **What are the milestones of progress in rehabilitation in the United States from 1970 to 1980?**

See Figure 2-4.
- In 1972 disabled individuals were provided with coverage under Medicare, including inpatient rehabilitation services.
- The Rehabilitation Act of 1973 required the elimination of barriers and discrimination in the workplace for the disabled.
- In 1974 the Association of Rehabilitation Nurses (ARN) was established and soon after the *ARN Journal* was published. The Developmental Disability Assistance and Bill of Rights gave disabled individuals the right to treatment and services. The legislation included autism, cerebral palsy, epilepsy, and mental retardation. Each condition was assessed, and for the first time, individualized care plans were written, providing for accountability of outcomes.
- In 1975 the Education for All Handicapped Children Act moved rehabilitation nurses into the schools. The children not only were given the right to free education but also they were to be mainstreamed into regular classes. Mainstreaming required education of the teachers and adjustments appropriate to each child. A collaborative effort in the community resulted.
- In 1977 ARN defined rehabilitation nursing and its practice. Standards of practice were published.
- In 1978 the National Institute of Handicapped Research was created through amendments to the Rehabilitation Act. From this same legislation, independent living facilities were able to provide comprehensive services. Research was promoted strongly.
- In the late 1970s advances continued in traditional care and treatment for conditions requiring rehabilitation and in the introduction of innovative approaches, such as biofeedback interventions for paralysis and transcutaneous electrical nerve stimulation for pain control and mobility. The psychosocial impact of spinal cord injury was now a focus, drawing the psychiatrist, psychologist, and sex therapist into the rehabilitation team.

6. **What are the milestones of progress in rehabilitation in the United States from 1980 to 1990?**

- In 1981 ARN published a core curriculum in rehabilitation nursing. The same year was proclaimed the International Year of Disabled Persons. Between 1980 and 1983 legislation ensured more funding for vocational educational services for broader disabling conditions and for disadvantaged persons. Extreme stresses were occurring in all the realms of funding because of the

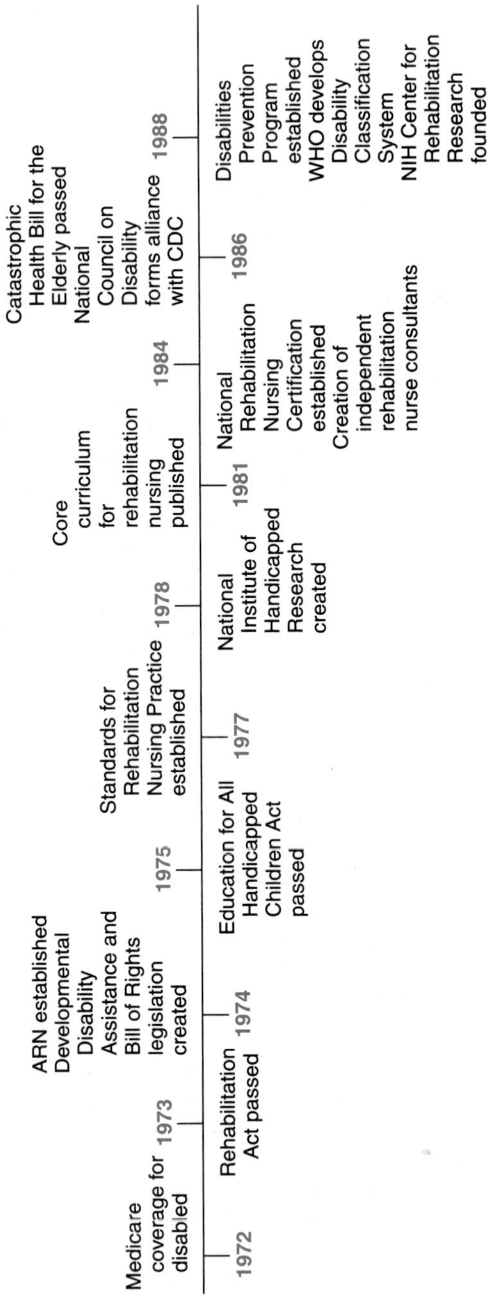

1972 — Medicare coverage for disabled

1973 — Rehabilitation Act passed

1974 — ARN established
Developmental Disability
Assistance and
Bill of Rights
legislation
created

1975 — Education for All Handicapped Children Act passed

1977 — Standards for Rehabilitation Nursing Practice established

1978 — National Institute of Handicapped Research created

1981 — Core curriculum for rehabilitation nursing published

1984 — National Rehabilitation Nursing Certification established
Creation of independent rehabilitation nurse consultants

1986 — Catastrophic Health Bill for the Elderly passed
National Council on Disability forms alliance with CDC

1988 — Disabilities Prevention Program established
WHO develops Disability Classification System
NIH Center for Rehabilitation Research founded

Figure 2-4. Rehabilitation milestones timeline: 1970s-1980s.

raised awareness of entitlements and the continuing increase in the number of individuals requiring rehabilitation measures.
- In 1984 ARN established the national certification examination in rehabilitation nursing.
- The mid-1980s birthed rehabilitation nurse consultants, who as entrepreneurs, established their own companies to provide contracted services such as case management, legal expertise, assessment, and monitoring.
- Prevention became a focus in 1986. The Catastrophic Health Bill for the Elderly focused on prevention of poverty as a result of catastrophic trauma or illness. Another bill addressed children at risk. The National Council on Disability also sought assistance from the Centers for Disease Control and Prevention to develop a program through the public health system.
- In 1988 the Disabilities Prevention Program came into existence. In 1988 the Disabilities Act provided for technologies for assistance to the disabled. The World Health Organization issued a supplement to the International Classification of Diseases, called International Classification of Impairments, Disabilities, and Handicaps. At this same time the National Center for Medical Rehabilitation Research at the National Institutes of Health was proposed. This center was the beginning of funded research specific to the realm of rehabilitation. Accountability for outcomes from services was becoming permanent.

7. **What are the milestones of progress in rehabilitation in the United States from 1990 to 2000?**

See Figure 2-5.

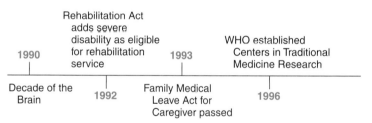

Figure 2-5. Rehabilitation milestones timeline: 1990s.

- In 1990 the Decade of the Brain was declared, leading to intense research and breakthroughs related to neurological diseases. Research centers were reporting recovery from paralysis through cellular biofeedback.
- By 1990 the attitude of society toward disabled persons had shifted and care had improved radically. Disabled persons not only were surviving but also were functioning in society, achieving educational goals, and competing for preferred employment.
- In 1992 the amendment to the Rehabilitation Act included the most severely disabled as eligible for rehabilitation. Patients gained the right to serve as members in their interdisciplinary teams and to be partners in the planning for their rehabilitation. Priority funding was given to minorities. Public interest in complementary modalities led to the establishment of the Office of Alternative Medicine.

- In 1993 the Family Leave Act supported the problems and needs of employed caregivers who at times may be required to place their family role first.
- In 1996 the World Health Organization Collaborative Centers in Traditional Medicine Research were established. These centers have assisted the international awareness that rehabilitation has a place in global health. Chronic, disabling conditions affect health care initiative in any country.

8. **What are the anticipated changes and initiatives from present to future?**

- The goals have remained consistent from the beginning in rehabilitation nursing. The methodology for accomplishing these goals has been effective: forming therapeutic relationships and partnerships with patients and communities and collaborative partnerships with other health professionals.
- The focus for the future is on increasing proactive interventions to prevent more disabling conditions and improve outcomes. The focus of rehabilitation nurses embraces Healthy People 2010. Some assistance from all stakeholders, including government, is needed for clarifying ethical issues related to rehabilitation, much of which is related to eligibility and funding. Rehabilitation nursing will be more involved in leading the community and patients to participate more actively to improve outcomes. The role of rehabilitation nursing will become more clear. As rehabilitation nurses improve their own understanding, they will be more willing to participate in international collaborative initiatives and research. This last opportunity has not yet been strongly embraced by the specialty.

9. **What paradigm shift has taken place in the health care industry since the 1930s?**

Acute care settings have had increased admissions of elders with chronic illnesses and increased evidence of chronic diseases such as acquired immunodeficiency syndrome. Diseases that were once fatal have become chronic. Patients have multiple medical problems and multisystem failure. Chronic care is the largest and fastest growing aspect of health care. Fee for service has shifted to capitation rates. The focus of care has moved from hospital inpatient care to ambulatory services, group practices, primary care, and promotion of health and wellness. Rehabilitation case management looks at reduced length of hospital stay with a shift to a lower-cost setting, effective management that produces patient satisfaction and is cost-effective, and responsiveness to treatment based on diagnosis.

10. **What is disease management?**

The model of disease management starts in the community and is driven by strategic management of costs, the most appropriate levels of care, and quality patient care outcomes. The rehabilitation nurse identifies the at-risk population and provides case management for the lifetime of the disease, from prevention to management of the disease and its comorbidities. Maximum wellness is maintained through preventive doctor office visits, home visits, phone triage to prevent emergency room visits and hospital admissions, linkings to required resources, and support groups. The model is an integrated approach that prepares and educates patients in their role in assuming responsibility for their own health.

11. What is the role of the rehabilitation nurse case manager?

The nurse's role is to coordinate care from entry into the system through the course of the disease/illness. The focus is on enhancing the quality of life through the appropriate selection and use of services in the most cost-effective approach. The nurse facilitates communication and collaboration while serving as a patient advocate. This nurse also may be a disease management coordinator.

12. What preparation should the case manager have?

Some disagreement still exists concerning preparation because many different caregivers have assumed this role in the past. The American Nurses' Association recommends a bachelor of science in nursing degree as the minimum education and 1 year of experience. The Case Management Society of America recommends 2 years of experience and certification. The American Association of Colleges of Nursing provides certification for nurses exclusively. The movement has become strong this century to fill the case manager role with a person who is a master's prepared advanced practice nurse, and the case manager is emerging as the newest advanced practice nurse role. Certification in the specialty area, such as rehabilitation, is highly recommended. This nurse must be assertive, creative, and flexible and must demonstrate skills in leadership, negotiation, collaboration, advocacy, and conflict resolution. The nurse must have effective verbal and written communication skills and must be able to see the whole picture. Knowledge of the health care system, discharge planning, estimation of costs, community resources, and appropriate use of health care services is also necessary.

13. What aspects of the rehabilitation nurse case manager's practice are influenced by ethics?

Case managers may be pulled between that which their employers see as the most cost-effective way to manage a patient and the most preferred, satisfying, effective, and ideal management. The nurse must treat all patients with respect and establish an authentic relationship based on truth. The inner conflict may be great, when the patient, who does not know, trusts the nurse to guide toward the best care. The nurse may know that the best, most appropriate care will not be approved, and the treatment that is covered must be "sold" to the patient. The case manager educates patients in their rights and assists as an advocate. The areas in which controversy arises include utilization review, precertification reimbursement, access to care, and denials.

14. Can care plans that have been designed specifically and standardized to medical diagnoses guide nurses in rehabilitation to achieve optimal outcomes?

Care plans specifically designed to meet medical diagnoses cannot effectively achieve optimal outcomes. Rehabilitation commonly must address multiple complex chronic and disabling conditions in one individual. A plan not based on individualized holistic family assessment and functional health system assessment will not provide the correct basis for interventions.

15. What is the status of disability?

Rehabilitation nurses have a variety of data collection systems in the United States, one of which is the National Health Interview Survey, which addresses impairments related to disability. Impairments are coded according to classifications of the Centers for Disease Control and Prevention. Diseases and injuries are coded according to the World Health Organization classification. About 40 million Americans report more than 40 million chronic diseases and more than 60 million disabling conditions. More than 13% of the disabling conditions are related to injuries. Heart disease leads the chronic diseases, with arthritis and other orthopedic conditions combined making up 25%. The figures are less than real-time estimates because of lag time in processing and publishing. The point is that the problem is extensive. Furthermore, this report was prepared from a self-report survey; therefore estimations are lower than actual prevalence. Estimations in 2001 from the Robert Wood Johnson Foundation of the extensiveness of chronic illness are 125 million, with 60 million having multiple conditions and 3 million of those persons having five chronic conditions. The Centers for Disease Control estimate that nearly 50 million Americans have a disability.

Key Points

- Rehabilitation began with the principles of Florence Nightingale.
- The first text for rehabilitation nursing was published in 1951.
- The importance of rehabilitation began to be accepted after World War II.
- The definition of and standards of practice for rehabilitation nursing were published in 1977 by the Association of Rehabilitation Nurses.
- The focus of nursing case management is on enhancing the quality of life through appropriate selection and use of services with the most cost-effective approach.
- Estimations indicate that Americans report more than 60 million disabling conditions.

Internet Resources

Association of Rehabilitation Nurses
http://www.rehabnurse.org/

The National Rehabilitation Information Center
http://www.naric.com

Bibliography

1. American Nurses' Association, Association of Rehabilitation Nurses: *Rehabilitation nursing: scope of practice—process and outcome criteria for selected diagnoses,* Kansas City, Mo, 1988, American Nurses' Association.

2. Hargrove SD, Derstine JB: Definition and philosophy of rehabilitation nursing: history and scope including chronicity and disability. In Dersine JB, Hargrove SD, editors: *Comprehensive rehabilitation nursing,* Philadelphia, 2001, WB Saunders.

3. Hoeman SP: History, issues and trends. In Hoeman SP, editor: *Rehabilitation nursing: process, application, & outcomes,* ed 3, St Louis, 2002, Mosby.

4. Partnership for Solutions. Retrieved May 31, 2002, from http://www.partnershipforsolutions.org/statistics/prevalence.htm (a partnership of Johns Hopkins University and the Robert Wood Johnson Foundation).

5. Remsburg R, Carson B: Rehabilitation. In Lubkin IM, Larsen PD, editors: *Chronic illness: impact and interventions,* ed 5, Boston, 2002, Jones and Bartlett.

6. Young M: A history of rehabilitation nursing. In *Association of Rehabilitation Nurses: fifteen years of making the difference,* Skokie, Ill, 1988, Sundance Press.

C h a p t e r 3

Ethical Issues

Jeanne Flannery

1. What is the emerging primary ethical dilemma in rehabilitation?

Scientific advances have permitted care providers to save lives, a feat that was once impossible. The value system in the United States drives care providers to continue improving the quality of care. As a result, this constant improvement has created a staggering cost to the health care industry to provide this level of care to the rapidly increasing number of persons who require it. The concern is whether dollars ultimately will need to be rationed for this level of care.

2. Is rehabilitation a right in America?

Rehabilitation is *not* a right; it is a privilege. For the most part, one must be able to pay for the services, either through third party reimbursement or out of one's own pocket. Few patients receive this care as a community service effort from a facility.

3. How do persons who require rehabilitation access the care?

The question opens the discussion that separates rehabilitation from other health care services in that individuals must go through a selection process, which may have many facets, before they are referred for services. Although inappropriate, persons go to emergency departments for minor problems, such as a cold, and are treated, even without any means to pay, accruing exorbitant charges because of the type of facility. No such open door exists for rehabilitation.

4. Do all providers consider a referral to rehabilitation?

Many times a referral to rehabilitation may not be made. Providers may lack the understanding or experience to perceive the benefits of rehabilitation for a particular patient or believe that they know how to manage the problem well enough without a referral.

5. Does the family desire rehabilitation when it is needed?

The patient/family may not have been educated in all options for care, or they may be unwilling to try these options. Family members may consider the patient too old, or they may not believe that rehabilitation can achieve positive outcomes; therefore they take the patient home or place the patient in a nursing home. Without exposure to experts who can demonstrate the possibilities for the patient, the family members just may not have adequate information on which to base their decision.

6. Can the patient/family afford rehabilitation?

Consideration of affordability is a selection mechanism itself. Criteria for coverage vary widely. Even well-established health insurance policies may provide coverage for only a certain number of days when weeks or months of rehabilitation may be needed. Some persons are covered marginally for limited services, some persons have no coverage, and some persons are not eligible ever to obtain any coverage.

7. Once determined eligible, can these patients all receive rehabilitation?

All eligible patients do not necessarily receive rehabilitation. Unless the patient participates actively in the designed program, the services will be discontinued. If the patient is in an acute rehabilitation facility and is unwilling or unable to participate in therapy a minimum of 3 hours daily, the patient will be discharged. Also, if the patient is not making progress for a period of time, even if the patient is participating, the patient is discharged.

8. Can the patient/family choose the facility if acute rehabilitation is required?

The patient/family does not necessarily have a choice of facility. Some facilities are not covered under specific insurance policies. Managed care invokes the initiative to divert patients away from acute rehabilitation facilities because of the expense and to direct them to subacute settings in which some therapy is provided, but not at the intense level as in the rehabilitation facility.

9. If the facility the patient/family prefers is covered under the patient's insurance, can the family make this decision?

Yes, the family can make this decision; however, if the rehabilitation nurse case manager is doing the appropriate level of teaching, the nurse may influence the family to reconsider in some cases. If the facility is expensive because it offers intense, specialized, cutting-edge care and the patient has severe problems that are going to require time to improve, the family might be wiser to save the days and dollars allowed by selecting a less intensive, less expensive type of care until the patient can gain the maximum benefit from the care that is offered at the preferred facility. The family needs to understand that if funds are depleted too quickly, the patient still will need rehabilitation, even when all the money is gone.

10. **Can American society accept an ethical distribution of health care services?**

A finite number of rehabilitation beds and services are available, and resources to provide more are scarce. Because not every patient requiring rehabilitation will be able to obtain all the desired, available, or needed services, how should the dilemma be resolved? If all resources were to be equally distributed, would minimally acceptable care be available for the masses? Currently, Americans have a value system focused on individuals more than on society as a whole. Americans desire the best care available, to the fullest extent, with the most current research applied, using all of the latest technology. Given anything less, Americans feel deprived. Americans would resist limiting care for those who can afford it to the same level as the masses so as to make more available in general.

11. **Who should determine the definitions of an acceptable minimum of care?**

No clear-cut answer to this question exists. Currently legislation has provided terms such as *basic services, universal access, basic packages,* and *fair access,* but these terms are described vaguely and tend to be ambiguous. Health care insurers, physicians, and other health care providers may misinterpret or misrepresent the intent, which leads to conflict. As a result, few persons are satisfied that the appropriate body is making the decision.

12. **How does the rehabilitation nurse handle the situation in which the patient has need for intensive rehabilitation, has been referred, has been accepted by the facility, and has reimbursement available to cover the needed services, yet the patient/family refuses to go?**

The patient ultimately has the right to decide. The rehabilitation nurse must weigh the patient's right to choose with the acceptable level of quality of life. The nurse must accept the patient's decisions whenever possible but at the same time must abide by the obligation to offer the best available care and cause no harm. After careful education about the disorder and the complications, the possibilities of improvement with the right care and support, opportunities to visit the facility and to talk with care providers, if the patient or family members still refuse, they have that right.

13. **What does the rehabilitation nurse do if a paraplegic patient expresses a goal to rehabilitate so as to return to a life of drug pushing by maintaining a presence on the street corner day and night?**

Although education related to the patients' own personal needs for maintaining well-being—such as weight shifts, skin checks, and limited hours in the wheelchair—is a part of their rehabilitation, how the patients intend to lead their lives is ultimately their decision to make. Functioning within the law and avoiding the responsibility of the negative effect of illegal drugs on others or themselves likewise would be discussed, and with positive opportunities for a vocation through training, patients might change their goals. Rehabilitation allows successful adaptation to a change in lifestyle, and in this case all aspects need consideration.

Key Points

Rehabilitation is not a right in America; it is a privilege that must be paid for.

Americans have a value system that would not readily embrace an equal distribution of rehabilitation services for the masses.

Internet Resources

The American Occupational Therapy Foundation
http://www.aotf.org/html/ethics.html

Codes of Ethics Online
http://www.iit.edu/departments/csep/PublicWWW/codes/health.html

Bibliography

1. Erlen JA: Ethics in chronic illness. In Lubkin IM, Larsen PD, editors: *Chronic illness: impact and interventions,* ed 5, Boston, 2002, Jones and Bartlett.
2. Hargrove SD, Woods JH: Ethics in rehabilitation nursing. In Derstine JB, Hargrove SD, editors: *Comprehensive rehabilitation nursing,* Philadelphia, 2001, WB Saunders.
3. Hoeman SP, Duchene PM: Ethical matters in rehabilitation. In Hoeman SP, editor: *Rehabilitation nursing: process, application, & outcomes,* ed 3, St Louis, 2002, Mosby.
4. Remsburg R, Carson B: Rehabilitation. In Lubkin IM, Larsen PD, editors: *Chronic illness: impact and interventions,* ed 5, Boston, 2002, Jones and Bartlett.

Chapter 4

Research in Rehabilitation Nursing

Jeanne Flannery

1. **What was the goal of research in rehabilitation before 1940?**

   Because rehabilitation was not a holistic focus yet, the majority of research focused on methods to provide a higher probability of surviving trauma and to find medications to combat infection. No evidence exists of published research in acute rehabilitation at that time.

2. **When in the 1950s rehabilitation research began to be published, what was the goal?**

   The goal of rehabilitation research included finding ways to enhance recovery, reduce complications, and maximize independence.

3. **When did the assessment and evaluation tools begin to be developed and tested?**

   Assessment and evaluation tools did not begin to be developed and tested until the 1970s. The Injury Severity Score and the Revised Trauma Score came into use at this time as some of the first.

4. **What societal focus prompted research in the 1970s?**

   A movement began in the 1970s toward independent living for those with disabilities. Many avenues of research were launched to determine appropriate ways to accomplish goals that were safe. Much information had to be evaluated in the realm of independence and what compensatory modalities could be created to support individuals with widely differing disabilities.

5. **What special rehabilitation procedures, equipment, and tests evolved from the technological explosion that began in the 1980s?**

   Tests such as ultrasonography, urodynamic tests, renal scanning, and new treatments such as lithotripsy were particularly helpful to patients with spinal cord injuries (SCIs). Additionally, the development of intrathecal catheters and pumps assisted in treating this same group for spasticity and pain through administration of neuroactive drugs directly into the spinal cord.

Equipment became more streamlined and esthetic to allow for more independence, such as the lightweight sports-focused wheelchairs used in the Special Olympics and one-handed, joystick-controlled motorized wheelchairs. Patients with little to no body movement were afforded empowerment over their environments with voice activated systems that raise/lower beds, operate wheelchairs, adjust the temperature of the room, turn lights and appliances on and off, and answer telephones. The sip/puff mechanism also was developed for similar operations when voice was not an option. Other devices exist, such as standing aids for patients in wheelchairs, but little use has been made of them because barriers still prevent the equipment from being used conveniently in society.

6. **What are the present goals of research in rehabilitation nursing?**

1. One goal focuses on the effect the present system of care has on
   - Delivery of care
   - Quality of care
   - Cost of care
   - Access to health care
   - Health outcomes
2. A second goal is to develop equipment that will enhance nursing practice to improve quality of life for patients with a variety of disabilities.
3. A third goal is to create new knowledge in the field that can lead to improvement in nursing diagnoses and patient problems in the following specific areas:
   - Prevention
   - Assessment
   - Intervention
4. A fourth goal is to improve quality of life through
   - Identification of needed improvements
   - Development of ways to improve
   - Evaluation of methods developed

7. **In what ways can rehabilitation nurses become involved in research?**

Rehabilitation nurses have three avenues by which to become involved in research:
- Being a consumer of research
- Conducting and disseminating research
- Applying research to practice

8. **What does being a consumer of research entail?**

- Education and experience have provided most rehabilitation nurses with basic knowledge of research design and methods and with basic understanding of analysis procedures. The nurse, through observation, can identify researchable problems and pose questions related to care.
- Nurses need to read the current research related to their particular practices to improve clinical knowledge and skills.

9. **What is the responsibility of rehabilitation nurses to conduct and disseminate research?**

   1. Professional nurses are obligated to contribute research-based knowledge to their discipline.
      - Advanced practice nurses, who have conducted research for a thesis or dissertation, or nurses with special training can be principal investigators who provide leadership in the design and execution of a study.
      - Nurses who are not comfortable yet with this degree of responsibility can participate as a co-investigator, a site coordinator in a multisite study, or a data collector for the research team.
   2. Any nurse, regardless of experience, can participate in the dissemination of the findings. This sharing of information, which must be done if research is to have any value, can take a variety of forms:
      a. Presentation within the organization
      b. Presentations on the local, regional, national, and international levels
      c. Publications in refereed journals
      d. Publications in books
      e. Lay publications to educate the consumer
      f. Development of policies, procedures, protocols, such as
         - Teaching guides
         - Guidelines for staff: standards of care, procedures for care
         - Clinical practice guidelines: protocols
         - Models of care delivery

10. **What does research use entail?**

    The process of using research does not imply that nurses should read a study and change their practice to incorporate the findings. Such an action could cause major problems. Using research is a process of analyzing research over time and synthesizing the conclusions from the studies for the purpose of determining whether change may be needed in practice, and if so, evaluating how to go about implementing such a change. The major components include
    - Evaluation of research outcomes
    - Implementation of research process
    - Planned change

11. **What specific steps should the rehabilitation nurse follow to use interdependent research appropriately?**

    - Identify the problem.
    - Review comprehensively the published research on the problem.
    - Evaluate the merit of each study, related to design, control, sample, methods, and scientific merit.
    - Analyze the conclusions from the set of studies.
    - Synthesize the conclusions into the prevailing recommendations.
    - Select one innovation to implement.
    - Gain administrative support to implement.

- Discuss the plan with all interested persons.
- Pilot the innovation.
- Evaluate the outcomes.
- Modify the plan; refine the procedure.
- Implement innovation fully.
- Publish the results.

12. **What research-based clinical guidelines specific to rehabilitation nursing have been developed to guide practice?**

1. The Agency for Health Care Policy and Research has developed many applicable guidelines (available on their Web site) such as those for
   - Urinary incontinence
   - Pressure ulcers
   - Depression
   - Sickle cell disease management
   - Management of cancer pain
   - Poststroke rehabilitation
   - Cardiac rehabilitation
2. The Paralyzed Veterans of America has developed guidelines for SCIs and disorders, such as neurogenic bowel.
3. The American Association of Spinal Cord Nurses published guidelines on dysreflexia.

The rehabilitation nurse should view these research-based guidelines as standards of best practice.

13. **How are priorities for research in rehabilitation for the future determined?**

Several professional organizations have contributed to the future research agenda. They include
- Association of Rehabilitation Nurses
- American Association of Spinal Cord Injury Nurses
- National Institutes of Disability Rehabilitation Research
- National Institute of Neurological Disorders and Stroke

In many cases, funding for research is based on how well the proposed research fits with the published agenda.

14. **What are some of the research priorities for rehabilitation for the future from the Association of Rehabilitation Nurses?**

- Health promotion and primary and secondary prevention to facilitate self-care and independence
- Interventions to maximize function of persons with disability
- Community-based care for at-risk populations
- Rehabilitation nurse–sensitive outcomes and costs
- Rehabilitation practice and roles in the changing health care system

15. **What are some of the research priorities determined by the American Association of Spinal Cord Nurses?**

   - Effectiveness of home care, outpatient, and other community-based programs
   - Aging with SCI and quality of life issues
   - Promoting community reentry
   - Attendant care or caregiver strain
   - Prediction of outcomes from SCI nurses' interventions
   - Fostering community independence
   - Effectiveness of teaching programs for SCI nurses

16. **What research initiatives have been published by the National Institute of Disability Rehabilitation Research?**

   Six areas of outcome research have been identified:
   1. Community reintegration
   2. Vocational rehabilitation
   3. Empowerment and independence
   4. Employment
   5. Human functioning
   6. Translation of knowledge into practice

   Additionally, six more issues common to these outcomes were identified:
   1. Promotion of positive attitudes toward persons with disabilities
   2. Promotion of environmental access
   3. Promotion of financial access
   4. Improvement of skills of persons with disabilities
   5. Improvement of support for and capacities of family members
   6. Improvement of the service system

17. **What are the research initiatives offered by the National Institute of Neurological Disorders and Stroke?**

   - Foster the new field of restorative neurology to devise new therapies for the long-term consequences of SCI.
   - Evaluate effectiveness of collaborative programs to educate health professionals and the general public about injury prevention and treatment.

🔑 Key Points

Rehabilitation research began to be published in the 1950s.

Independent living for those with disabilities was a societal movement in the 1970s, which prompted research to accomplish goals that were safe.

The Agency for Health Care Policy and Research has developed research-based clinical guidelines available for rehabilitation nursing.

Internet Resources

Kessler Rehabilitation Research and Education Corporation
http://www.kmrrec.org/

Rehabilitation Research
http://www.rehabinfo.net/training/lectures/

The Center for Neural Recovery and Rehabilitation Research
http://www.helenhayeshospital.org/CNRRRmain.htm

Bibliography

1. Germino BB: Research in chronic illness. In Lubkin IM, Larson PD, editors: *Chronic illness: impact and intervention,* ed 5, Boston, 2002, Jones and Bartlett.
2. Mumma CM: Research-based rehabilitation nursing practice. In Hoeman SP, editor: *Rehabilitation nursing: process, application, & outcomes,* ed 3, St Louis, 2002, Mosby.
3. Nelson A: Research in nursing. In Derstine JB, Hargrove SD, editors: *Comprehensive rehabilitation nursing,* Philadelphia, 2001, WB Saunders.

Chapter 5

Community-Based Rehabilitation Nursing

Jeanne Flannery

1. **What is community-based rehabilitation (CBR)?**

   This model of CBR is based on the components set forth in 1978 by the World Health Organization and aligned with Healthy People 2010 goals. These components include
   1. Focus: to prevent disabilities
   2. Goal: to reach a larger number of persons
   3. Target: entire community
   4. Control: create partnerships
   5. Expected outcomes:
      - Community members who take responsibility for their own health
      - Reduction in dependency on professionals
      - Enhancement of cultural sensitivity
      - Use of cost-effective approaches
      - Incorporation of volunteer consumer leaders

2. **What preparation do CBR nurses require?**

   Community-based rehabiliation nurses must have a comprehensive knowledge base and skill development based on public health core knowledge, including
   - Epidemiology
   - Communicable diseases
   - Disease prevention
   - Biological, physical, and behavioral sciences
   - Population-based care
   - Sanitation
   - Community value system
   - Spiritual beliefs

3. **How is the CBR nurse's practice described?**

   - The CBR nurse may provide direct care in the homes of patients with severe, complex illnesses who require a high level of care.

- The CBR nurse may provide consultation with some direct care in clinics, schools, or parishes.
- The CBR nurse may offer education in all sites.
- Advanced practice nurses may provide specialty care, such as wound management or cardiac rehabilitation.

4. What skills and knowledge does the CBR nurse use?

The CBR nurse requires the skills and knowledge special to the rehabilitation nurse, the public health nurse, the community nurse, and the nurse case manager. A few of these are
- Conflict resolution
- Cultural competence
- Legislative mandates
- Family systems theories
- Change theory
- Group dynamics
- Management of chronic illness
- Negotiation
- Communication skills
- Anatomy and physiology
- Counseling
- Disability management
- Health promotion
- Systems theory

5. The CBR nurse practices within the patient's own environment. How is *environment* defined?

Environment is not only the setting where the patient works and lives but also all of the contextual and residual processes that may affect the patient's functioning, such as
- Family dynamics
- Support systems
- Financial status
- Nutritional resource
- Medications resource
- Spiritual care
- Psychosocial state
- Culture

6. What purpose do lay community health workers serve?

Persons recruited from within the community may assist the CBR nurse to identify health needs and overcome barriers in providing care. Patients view community health workers as "one of their own" and are more likely to accept that which they ask or tell.

7. **What does community reintegration mean?**

The term *community reintegration* implies a synthesis of components applied to some degree:
- Living independently
- Enacting the normal roles as ascribed by a society to a person of similar demographics
- Participating in the mainstream of family and community
- Contributing to society

8. **What aspect of role theory prepares the CBR nurse to help the patient accept the disability?**

No aspect of role theory prepares the CBR nurse to help the patient accept the disability. This is a trick question. No person will ever accept the disability, so it should not be a goal of the nurse. Instead, the focus is on
- Reestablishing previous roles if the patient wishes
- Developing new roles
- Adapting to the effect of the disability on role functioning
- Providing education to the patient and family, with supportive written handouts
- Assisting the patient and family to develop necessary skills
- Providing support for caregivers

9. **What are primary barriers to community reintegration?**

The primary barriers to reintegration into the community are
- Inability to live independently
- Ineligibility for attendant programs
- Insufficient, inaccessible housing
- Delay in approval for home care
- Shortened length of hospital stay that does not permit thorough discharge planning
- Inadequate transportation
- Caregiver burden
- Inadequate coverage to provide needed home care visits and therapy

10. **What are some of the major interventions implemented to enhance CBR?**

Some of the major interventions are
1. Interdisciplinary collaborative teams between the hospital and community to meet holistic needs, adding to the acute rehabilitation team:
   - School nurse
   - Rescue squad
   - Department of human services
   - Providers of complementary therapy, such as acupuncturist
   - Neighbors

- Clergy
- Caregivers
2. Assistance to caregivers and patients to identify needs related to requirements for attendant care and to obtain resources for this service from a program for which eligibility can be met:
   - Medicare
   - Medicaid
   - Workers' compensation
   - Private health care insurance
   - Health maintenance organizations
   - Veterans Affairs
   - Preferred provider organizations
   - Auto liability policies
3. Referrals to centers for independent living that are based in the community and managed by persons with disabilities but supported with knowledgeable staff.
4. Assistance through return-to-work or return-to-school programs with assessments of needs, accommodations, and work site disability management programs.
5. Employee Assistance Programs to reduce the costs of worker absenteeism and inefficiency because of stress, family crisis, work problems, financial difficulties, or disability.
6. Supported employment programs to provide integrated work settings, services for persons with severe disabilities, ongoing job training and work-hardening, and extended support to keep the patient in employment.
7. Disability management programs provided at the work site in control of the employer, rather than the rehabilitation professionals, but a collaborative effort to
   - Reduce costs of workers' compensation
   - Provide safety
   - Enhance early return to work
   - Provide empathy
   - Make appropriate accommodations
   - Establish functional goals
8. Vocational rehabilitation programs that focus on assisting persons with disabilities to obtain gainful employment via
   - Making home or vehicle modifications or meeting other transportation requirements
   - Assessing the job market and providing job training and placement
   - Providing supportive employment
   - Recommending reasonable workplace accommodations
   - Educating employers and providing job coaches, work restructuring, and performance evaluations.
9. Early intervention programs to provide comprehensive family assessment, planning, and interventions to
   - Improve cognitive and developmental functioning of infants and children with disabilities while educating the parents and caregivers
   - Evaluate outcomes
   - Serve as advocates

Key Points

- The CBR nurse practices within the patient's own environment.
- The CBR nurse requires the skills and knowledge special to the rehabilitation nurse, the public health nurse, the community nurse, and the nurse case manager.

Internet Resources

Understanding Community-Based Rehabilitation
http://www.unescap.org/

Community-Based Rehabilitation
http://www.cbrresources.org/

Bibliography

1. Buchanan LC, Neal LJ: Community-based rehabilitation. In Hoeman SP, editor: *Rehabilitation nursing: process, application, & outcomes,* ed 3, St Louis, 2002, Mosby.
2. Nagy CL: Community-focused rehabilitation nursing. In Derstine JB, Hargrove SD, editors: *Comprehensive rehabilitation nursing,* Philadelphia, 2001, WB Saunders.
3. Travis SS, Piercy K: Family caregivers. In Lubkin IM, Larson PD, editors: *Chronic illness: impact and intervention,* ed 5, Boston, 2002, Jones and Bartlett.

Section 2

Approaches to Improvement of Outcomes

Roles, Competencies, and Standards of Accreditation

Jeanne Flannery

1. **What does a rehabilitation nurse do?**

   According to the Association of Rehabilitation Nurses (ARN), unique skills and knowledge base are required to achieve patient outcome realization and ensure quality of care. The rehabilitation nurse accomplishes these goals by performing within standards such as
   - Forming partnerships with patients/families and collaborating with other health care providers to achieve the best outcomes
   - Applying the nursing process with inclusion of understanding of the impact of the chronic disease or disability and available resources on all aspects of the process
   - Coordinating the interdisciplinary team with skill in team dynamics and integration
   - Providing holistic care with attention to the patient's physical, psychological, developmental, social, spiritual, economic, vocational, family, and recreational aspects
   - Attending to the patient's responses to health and illness with excellent knowledge and skill in assessment, considering the unique needs and problems of a rehabilitation patient
   - Maintaining communication with, and making referrals to, appropriate resources
   - Supporting outcomes through documented measurement of functional skills of patients
   - Providing patients/families with support in coping with lifelong issues through care that is ethical, humane, legal, informed, compassionate, and culturally sensitive
   - Educating patients/families and payers in the "enabling" philosophy and advocating for services that promote adaptation to the disability or chronic illness
   - Using research as a basis for practice
   - Viewing the patient through the continuum of illness to wellness

2. **In what settings is it appropriate for rehabilitation nurses to work?**

   The rehabilitation nurse may work in any setting. The ARN has proposed that unless, and until, rehabilitation nurses, particularly those nationally certified (certified rehabilitation registered nurse, [CRRN]), are used in all settings where principles and process of rehabilitation are included in the management of patients, the best outcomes will not be possible. Even acute care hospitals should have rehabilitation nurses who can serve as consultants and provide orientation to the new nurses, students, and technicians in the principles and expectations of rehabilitation nursing. Major complications could be avoided and readmissions reduced with this approach.

3. **What is the enabling-disabling process that rehabilitation nurses view as a standard?**

The enabling-disabling process is a model of rehabilitation developed by the Institute of Medicine in 1997 that has enhanced the World Health Organization's definition of disability (1980) and focuses on the uniqueness of each individual within each classification. The model conveys that each person will respond differently to an impairment; some will have no disability, and others all will have different levels of disability. The person's own personal characteristics in interaction with the environment, along with the degree of the pathological condition, can produce extreme differences in outcomes among patients with the same medical diagnosis. The model focuses on the contextual aspects of disability, which include biological, environmental, lifestyle, and behavioral factors. With understanding of how the disabling conditions occur, worsen, improve, and are affected by these factors, health care providers can strive to reverse the process. Thus rehabilitation can be called the enabling process, a positive process, leading to positive outcomes.

4. **What special competencies should a rehabilitation nurse manager have in addition to those required of a nurse manager in any aspect of nursing, such as adhering to a budget, upholding policies, and maintaining accountability?**

The rehabilitation nurse manager should have experience in routine management and rehabilitation clinical experience. The nurse should have a bachelor of science in nursing degree, and CRRN certification is preferred. This nurse should be able to

1. Promote professional rehabilitation nursing values and goals to nursing staff and rehabilitation team members. These goals include
   - Achievement of independence
   - Maintenance of optimum health and quality of life
   - Prevention of complications or worsening
   - Promotion of return to active participation in the community
2. Ensure continuity of care from admission to home.
3. Support nursing staff to perform rehabilitation clinical roles of caregiver, educator, counselor, consultant, and advocate.
4. Ensure research-based nursing practice.
5. Encourage staff to seek higher education and certification.
6. Provide support for nursing staff to participate in evaluating outcomes for patients with disabilities.

7. Articulate the value and contribution of the rehabilitation nurse to professionals.
8. Participate in interdisciplinary committees.
9. Support research initiatives in rehabilitation.
10. Advocate for persons with disabilities through participation in professional organizations and community activities.

5. What additional competencies are required for the leadership role?

The leader role may always include managerial competencies and skills, but managers are not always leaders.

1. A rehabilitation nurse leader must be a visionary. The nurse should construct a mental image of the desired future state for the organization. The process of implementing the vision into reality requires working backward from the outcome and identifying the steps. The nurse must articulate the vision and the steps to accomplish it with clarity and with passion. To move "out of the box" means being able to take risks. The leader must be able to motivate all who are involved to continue on the path until reaching the goal. The leader has raised the bar for everyone and ultimately will see everyone gaining. All team members will have set higher personal goals in the process.
2. The leader must embrace change theory, accepting that the role is never to maintain but to move the organization forward, changing to improve. Implementation of planned change is difficult and requires many skills to overcome the natural human resistance to change. An understanding of change theory assists one in making this process a positive experience.
3. The rehabilitation nurse leader must have a high level of emotional intelligence. This competency is the embodiment of interpersonal skills. The best leaders show their "heart." They anticipate how team members will react to change or difficult situations, and they help them deal with the emotional aspect of work. The responsibility of leaders to assist team members to improve their knowledge, skills, production, accomplishments, and relationships—a myriad of constant changes that are expected—can be accomplished only when the leaders can synchronize themselves with each member emotionally. The right words and actions, the encouragement at the right time, the praise at the bleakest moments, the motivational approach that matches the personality are only possible when assessment of each person has been holistic.
   Emotional intelligence is composed of components such as
   - Empathy: the ability to sense, understand, and consider carefully team members' feelings
   - Social skills: the ability to find common ground with a diverse population
   - Self-awareness: the honest assessment of one's own weaknesses, strengths, needs, and drives
   - Self-regulation: the ability to control one's feelings and impulses to create a positive environment, with trust and fairness evident
   - Motivation: an external drive to achieve or to improve with energy to persevere with passion
4. The nurse leader always serves as a mentor and a coach. Leaders must stimulate growth, improvement, development of new skills, and a desire to seek a higher

degree or to be certified in rehabilitation. Leaders must not only know the requirements each team member needs to accomplish these goals but also be able to provide the support, resources, reinforcement, or education to assist them. Leaders will need to provide different approaches for diverse persons. Just the difference in age among nurses will greatly affect the goals they set for themselves, how they measure satisfaction, and what motivates them to set higher goals.

For example, if a nurse is of the baby boomer generation (1946-1962), the nurse probably will be loyal to the organization, desiring to stay and work to improve outcomes, but will have struggled to keep up with technology.

If the nurse is a Generation X (1963-1977) nurse, the nurse is searching for meaning in work and wishes to incorporate fun into it. This nurse is accustomed to the information explosion through technology and sees everything as needing to be fast. The nurse requires frequent feedback, does not visualize long-term planning, and wants short-term rewards. Leaving may suit the needs of such nurses better than planning change.

If nurses are of the Generation Next (1978-1994) cohort, a much larger group than Generation X, they are certainly likely to be the most novice but also have a different view of the world. They will not have known a world without all the technology, conveniences, and economic promise. Money is the incentive, so they must see hope for pay increases to work harder. They will not be the "lone wolf" but will enjoy working on the team to accomplish goals. These nurses know no other life from "instant" everything; therefore, they may not appreciate how their perspective is different from older nurses. The nurse leader must stay abreast of technology to be in synchrony with these nurses.

6. **What standards does a rehabilitation nurse have to maintain?**
   - Standards of performance or practice are those that have been published by ARN and have been adopted as competencies required by the organization. The eight standards of professional performance are
     1. Quality of care: The nurse consistently evaluates effectiveness and quality.
     2. Performance appraisal: The nurse compares his or her own practice to professional practice standards, statutes, and rules.
     3. Education: The nurse maintains current knowledge in nursing.
     4. Collegiality: The nurse contributes to professional development of others.
     5. Ethics: The nurse's decisions are ethical.
     6. Collaboration: The nurse collaborates with the patient, family, and health care providers to provide care.
     7. Research: The nurse uses research as a basis for practice.
     8. Utilization: The nurse's plans of care include concern for cost, effectiveness, and safety.
   - Standards of care pertain to basic acceptable minimums for patients with particular problems published as general guidelines by the American Nurses

Association and specifically to rehabilitation nursing by ARN. The six standards of care are the nursing process:
1. Assessment: The nurse collects data regarding the patient's health status.
2. Diagnosis: The nurse analyzes the data to determine a diagnosis.
3. Outcome identification: The nurse lists expected outcomes, based on holistic assessment.
4. Planning: The nurse develops the plan of care, in collaboration, with prescribed interventions.
5. Implementation: The nurse implements the interventions.
6. Evaluation: The nurse evaluates the patient's progress toward the set outcomes.

- Additionally, the rehabilitation nurse also must abide by the standards of care expected by accrediting bodies of rehabilitation facilities. The Joint Commission on Accreditation of Healthcare Organizations and the Commission on Accreditation of Rehabilitation Facilities publish guidelines on which their routine site visits for evaluation are based. The Joint Commission on Accreditation of Healthcare Organizations now evaluates not only rehabilitation programs within hospitals but also free-standing rehabilitation facilities.

  A recent change in each of these is the refinement of the standard for patient and family education in 2000. The standards are specific and address detailed aspects of teaching/learning process, content that should be covered, discharge teaching, and individualized approach to promote healthy patient behaviors and improve outcomes.

  Currently, a new aspect of this evaluation process is the development of a standard set of performance measures against which the process and outcomes of the program are benchmarked.

- The rehabilitation nurse also must be cognizant of the standards to meet for eligibility to be reimbursed by government agencies, such as Medicare and Medicaid.

  Reimbursement from Medicare, a federal program serving patients over 65 or disabled, is based on a prospective payment system. The patient is classified into a case-mix group for monitoring the quality of care received. The patient's classification at discharge is based on impairment, age, functional abilities, and comorbidities. From this classification, a range of needed resources are determined; and those used to care for the patient are compared with those that are expected.

  Medicaid provides for medical assistance for patients without other means to pay for care. Although this is also a federal program, the standards one must follow are established in each state, and the program is administered by the state.

7. **What requirements must rehabilitation nurses meet to receive national certification?**

   - To be eligible to take the certification examination for CRRN, the currently licensed registered nurse must have at least 2 years of professional practice in rehabilitation nursing, or 1 year of professional practice in rehabilitation nursing and 1 year of advanced education toward a master's degree. These activities must have occurred within 5 years of the application date.

- The CRRN who has a master's degree or doctorate in nursing and has maintained the credential through current practice and continuing education may take the CRRN-A examination for advanced practice.
- Nurses may seek additional certifications to enhance the particular area of rehabilitation in which they specialize. For example, the nurse may add a gerontological clinical nurse specialist, a neuroscience, an oncology, a nurse case manager, or a pediatric certification. All certifications, whether through the American Nurses Credentialing Center or specialty organizations, require in the range of 2000 or more hours of professional practice in the area for eligibility and renewals every 2 to 5 years.

8. Why is the advanced practice nurse (APN) in rehabilitation needed?

The rehabilitation APN has a paramount role in enhancing growth of rehabilitation nursing as a specialty. The value of APNs is that all their activities are expected to lead to measurable outcomes, such as

- Improved cost-effectiveness of patient care
- Increased knowledge level and skill acquisition by staff nurses
- Reduced frequency of complications among patients
- Increased quality of care
- Increased patient/family satisfaction
- Increased staff satisfaction
- Reduction in costs of outside consultants

9. What are the competencies of the rehabilitation APN?

The rehabilitation APN is expected to function within the five APN roles of caregiver (although this may be indirect), consultant, educator, researcher, and leader. The APN must demonstrate competency in each role to function in the three spheres of influence: the patients, the nursing personnel, and the organization. Some of the expectations are

1. Caregiver
   - Manages independently the care of patients with complex needs.
   - Manages life-threatening, variant symptoms.
   - Ensures the appropriateness of admission of a patient.
   - Refers patients for appropriate care/services.
   - Provides discharge planning.
   - Develops a case management plan.
   - Manages the effect of interventions on restoring function.
   - Determines the effect of atypical variations of pathophysiology on the holistic patient functions.
   - Educates families in coping with catastrophic disabilities.

2. Educator
   - Provides education to improve staff knowledge and skills.
   - Presents in community conferences as an expert resource.
   - Mentors and teaches students.
   - Publishes in journals to increase nurses' knowledge level.
   - Presents at international and national conferences.
   - Teaches rehabilitation principles in university nursing classes as guest lecturer.
3. Consultant
   - Serves as a resource to staff in crisis situations.
   - Serves as a resource to staff for patients with unresolved problems, such as
     - Persistent infections
     - Irregular patterns of neurogenic bowel/bladder that remain uncontrolled
     - Patient's lack of motivation or inability to cope that delays activity goals
     - Abnormal sleep pattern that cannot be explained
     - Cognitive/behavioral changes that seem unrelated to the condition
     - Anxiety or depression that is worsening despite treatment
     - Family relationships that are interfering with therapy and progress
     - Sexual function expectations of the patient that are unrealistic, regardless of counseling
     - Ethical issues related to end-of-life that are unresolved
   - Serves in a marketing and public relations role.
   - Advocates for patient needs through negotiation.
   - Serves as expert witness in legal matters.
   - Creates programs to improve recruitment and retention of nurses.
   - Coordinates and evaluates the interdisciplinary care.
4. Researcher
   - Stays current with research in the literature and communicates relevant findings to staff regularly.
   - Identifies researchable problems in the organization.
   - Guides the establishment of research-based practice.
   - Conducts or assists in research projects.
   - Disseminates findings in publications and presentations.
   - Evaluates outcomes and directs needed practice changes.
5. Leader
   - Coordinates team in atypical situations.
   - Establishes new policies, procedures, and protocols based on research.
   - Is active politically to represent rehabilitation needs.
   - Markets for advanced practice nursing in the specialty.
   - Serves as liaison from staff nursing to all levels of administration and outside stakeholders.
   - Develops, implements, and evaluates new programs based on a needs assessment.
   - Participates in selection and rewarding of staff.

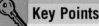

Key Points

- Rehabilitation nurses should be employed in acute care settings to prevent major complications and prevent readmissions.
- The rehabilitation APN serves as a role model to others in improving cost-effectiveness, increasing quality of care, improving patient/family and staff satisfaction, increasing knowledge and skill among staff, and reducing costs of outside consultants.

Internet Resources

Association of Rehabilitation Nurses Definition
http://www.rehabnurse.org/about/definition

Association of Rehabilitation Nurses Professional Resources
http://www.rehabnurse.org/profresources/index.html

Bibliography

1. Association of Rehabilitation Nurses: About ARN: rehabilitation nurses make a difference—what do rehabilitation nurses do? Retrieved June 1, 2003, from http://www.rehabnurse.org/about/definition
2. Association of Rehabilitation Nurses: Certification: CRRN. Retrieved June 1, 2003, from http://www.rehabnurse.org/profresources/certification/crrn.html
3. Association of Rehabilitation Nurses: Certification: CRRN-A. Retrieved June 1, 2003, from http://www.rehabnurse.org/profresources/crrna.html
4. Association of Rehabilitation Nurses: Professional resources: position statements—the appropriate inclusion of rehabilitation nurses wherever rehabilitation is provided, 1996. Retrieved May 28, 2003, from http://www.rehabnurse.org/profresources/papropr.html
5. Association of Rehabilitation Nurses: Professional resources: role descriptions—the advanced practice rehabilitation nurse. Retrieved May 28, 2003, from http://www.rehabnurse.org/profresources/advprac.html
6. Association of Rehabilitation Nurses: Professional resources: role descriptions—the rehabilitation nurse educator. Retrieved May 28, 2003, from http://www.rehabnurse.org/profresources/educator.html
7. Association of Rehabilitation Nurses: Professional resources: role descriptions—rehabilitation nurse manager. Retrieved May 28, 2003, from http://www.rehabnurse.org/profresources/nursemgr.html
8. Association of Rehabilitation Nurses: Professional resources: role descriptions—the rehabilitation staff nurse. Retrieved May 28, 2003, from http://www.rehabnurse.org/profresources/staffnurse.html
9. Gender AR, Benjamin JM: Administration and leadership. In Hoeman SP, editor: *Rehabilitation nursing: process, application, & outcomes,* ed 3, St Louis, 2002, Mosby.
10. O'Toole M: The rehabilitation team. In Destine JB, Hargrove SD, editor: *Comprehensive rehabilitation nursing,* Philadelphia, 2001, WB Saunders.
11. Remsburg R, Carson B: Rehabilitation. In Lubkin IM, Larsen PD, editors: *Chronic illness: impact and interventions,* ed 5, Boston, 2002, Jones and Bartlett.

Chapter 7

Quality Indicators and Outcome Measures

Jeanne Flannery

1. **How is quality defined?**

   Quality is a perception of the individual, based on the person's own philosophy, values system, experiential knowledge, education, and family. In the realm of care, even nurses with the same education define quality based on their different specialties. For example, a critical care nurse expects a comprehensive head-to-toe assessment to be done as a component of quality care, but a rehabilitation nurse would not expect to include this. The rehabilitation nurse would expect an assessment to include functional skills, independence, and adaptation to the impairments. The patient, however, may not consider either of these components of quality but rather the speed with which pain medication is delivered after a complaint of pain.

2. **How is quality health care measured by the Department of Health and Human Services?**

   Since 1998, when a policy council was formed for this task, four indicators have been published:
   - Underuse of services: failure to provide the recognized services that prevent complications, such as discharging a patient with an above-the-knee amputation without training in the use of the prosthesis.
   - Overuse of services: providing care that is unnecessary, such as antibiotics when they are not useful and may even be detrimental, or duplication of services that waste money and the time of the caregivers and the patient, such as every therapist on the team asking the same basic questions for each one's form.
   - Misuse of services: not providing timely diagnoses and not preventing medical errors that lead to complications, increased cost, and death. Things such as medication errors, pressure ulcer development, missed cancer diagnoses, and inappropriate pain management are examples of misuse.
   - Variation in services: not standardizing approach to care and services to be provided across America. For example, health care workers in the northeastern United States have been found to provide more preventive care and are more likely to provide rehabilitation to neurological and orthopedic patients than the rest of the country.

3. What are universal indicators of quality?

The universal indicators of quality vary considerably among groups, such as regulatory groups, professional organizations, advocacy groups, and consumer groups, just as the definition of quality does.

1. The Agency for Healthcare Research and Quality published indicators for consumers:
   - Outcome measures
   - Patient satisfaction reports
   - Accreditation reports
   - Clinical performance measures
2. The Centers for Medicare and Medicaid Services have developed indicators for programs seeking Medicare and Medicaid reimbursement on which such decisions are made. An example is patients' right to be free of restraints, which can bar participation unless the program is in compliance. This example provides the view of the difference in perceptions in quality, for the regulating agency sees no restraints as quality, whereas rehabilitation nurses see safety and prevention of harm to the patient or others as quality, and restraints often can provide that.
3. The Agency for Healthcare Research and Quality, the National Institute of Nursing Research, and the Division of Nursing of the Health Resources and Services Administration have focused on adequate staffing as a quality indicator. The influence of skill mix on nursing care is being researched.
4. Rehabilitation patients have particular expectations by which they judge nursing care. For nurses to be seen as credible, they must
   - Demonstrate caring.
   - Understand the patient's value system.
   - Use humor.
   - Demonstrate problem-solving skills.
   - Be creative and flexible.
   - Think in the future.
   - Demonstrate understanding of the effect of the disability or chronic condition on the patient's lifestyle.
   - Be tolerant of differences.
   - Accept the patient's interdependence on others.
   - Accept situations in which no resolution exists.

4. What are quality indicators for rehabilitation nursing practice?

The intent of quality indicators is to use a system approach to control the quality of care. The system must be intact with the relationships of the human, technological, and environmental elements functioning interdependently for the common outcomes of patient care. The system must be monitored for patterns of change. The American Nurses' Association combined elements with the Institute of Medicine to develop a system of quality assessment for rehabilitation nursing. The indicators include

1. Nursing skill mix
2. Nursing care hours provided per patient per day
3. Pressure ulcer incidence

4. Patient falls incidence
5. Medication errors incidence
6. Patient satisfaction with
   - Pain management
   - Education
   - Nursing care
7. Nosocomical infection rate (e.g., urinary tract infection)
8. Nursing staff satisfaction

5. What is the crucial next step once quality indicators have been selected?

The indicators selected must be measurable, and the measurements must have validity and reliability, or the whole effort will have no meaning to the rehabilitation team. The crucial next step, then, is to measure the indicators.

Though this sounds simplistic, measuring the indicators may be more difficult than anticipated, unless the method by which the indicators are measured is standardized. If nationwide disagreement exists about the tools to use, outcomes will be apples and oranges and cannot be analyzed or findings cannot be aggregated to establish national benchmarks.

6. What types of standardized tools are available to measure quality in rehabilitation?

1. Functional Independence Measurement (FIM)—a tool used worldwide with a database of about 2.5 million patient records. The FIM is probably the most well-known assessment tool. The FIM is a seven-level scale moving from 1 (total assistance) to 7 (complete independence), applied to six categories of activities of daily living:
   - Self-care
   - Sphincter control
   - Mobility
   - Locomotion
   - Communication
   - Social cognition

   The FIM can be used in the home and in the acute rehabilitation facility; however, it has not been reliable because of caregivers' inability to be consistent in their evaluations and the evaluations being biased. To access the FIM, visit **http://www.udsmr.com**

2. Computerized Needs Measures-Oriented Quality Measurement Evaluation System (CONQUEST)—created collaboratively and established by the Agency for Healthcare Research and Quality in 1999. This measure identifies quality as care being delivered to the right patient at the right time in the right way and is
   - Accessible.
   - Accountable.
   - Fair.
   - Effective.
   - Safe.

   To access CONQUEST, visit **http://www.ahcpr.gov/qual/conquest/htm**

3. Minimum Data Set (MDS)—a part of the Resident Assessment Instrument, which is used by staff in long-term care facilities to support the quality of care provided to the residents and is required by Medicare for reimbursement determination in the prospective payment system. This electronic tool allows monitoring of the quality indicators for all long-term residents nationwide by the Health Care Financing Administration. To access the tool, visit **http://www.hcfa.gov/medicaid/mds20**

4. MDS for Post Acute Care (MDS-PAC)—a modification of MDS for short-stay rehabilitation. The MDS-PAC is like MDS in that it determines Medicare reimbursement rates based on the functional level of the patient, the intensity of the illness, and the complexity of the nursing care required. To access the tool, visit **http://www.hcfa.gov/medicaid/rehabpac**

5. SF-36—a standardized instrument developed by the Medical Outcomes Trust that measures outcomes from the patient's perspective, including
   - Limitations in physical activities
   - Usual role activities
   - Body pain
   - Health perception
   - Vitality
   - Limitations in social or usual role activities
   - Mental health

   The SF-36 can be administered electronically, by telephone, or personal interview. To access the SF-36, visit **http://www.outcomes-trust.org/catalog/sf36.htm**

6. SF-12—a shorter version of SF-36 for repeated use with patients because it contains only 12 items. To access the SF-12, visit **http://www.outcomes-trust.org/catalog/sf12.htm**

7. What other methods can facilities use to measure quality?

Facilities, organizations, and individual teams have many approaches to measure their care within their units. Examples include

- **Brainstorming:** The group members contribute as many suggestions as they can think of, without critique. Everything is written and can be evaluated later in relation to resources, standards, and priorities.
- **Check sheets:** Unit-developed data collection tools allow a systematic method of recording patterns in areas that are difficult to maintain at top quality, such as pain management. The check sheet is a retrospective review of records to evaluate practice.
- **Audits:** Careful reviews of records when a problem surfaces allow one to see what might have been done to prevent the problem. The nurse can view issues holistically and objectively in this way. Perhaps the problem resulted from an undetected system delay that affected care at a later point. An APN rehabilitation nurse needs to be involved to coordinate this approach for the best systematic improvement.
- **Fishbone diagrams:** These diagrams are quality control instruments that identify a problem and issues that intensify the problem. The fishbone diagram serves to create a cause-and-effect picture that then can lead discussion directly to strategies in each (Figure 7-1).
- **Flowcharts:** Flowcharts outline a particular process in which a problem has been identified, such as patients from one unit being consistently late for 8 AM therapies.

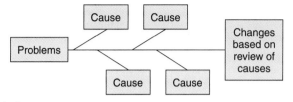

Figure 7-1. Example of a fishbone diagram.

Every step of the process is listed in a decision tree format, with all responsible positions identified, along with the time each step is allowed. The nursing team reviews all the steps to see what changes might be tried to improve the outcome. Flowcharts are more effective when the team considers them together to eliminate the "he didn't," "she did" finger-pointing, which serves no purpose. Many times team members who lodge the complaint are unaware of the process; and once they learn the intricacies, they are more positive. They may be able to contribute excellent help in resolving the issue (Figure 7-2).

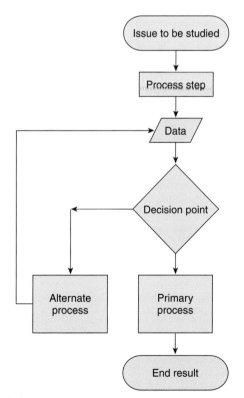

Figure 7-2. Example of a flowchart.

- **Pareto charts:** The nurse creates pareto charts by simply listing in descending order of frequency all problems identified in a process. The principle driving the approach is that 20% of the problems create 80% of the effects. Because no team can deal with all problems simultaneously and make progress measurably in a timely fashion, this technique allows the team to identify only the primary concerns with a focus on improving them. For example, if falls need to be reduced, and certainly a myriad of causes of falls exist, the team singles out factors that create 80% of the effect, such as incontinence, and addresses them actively, rather than focusing on all the causes that contribute only small percentages to the problem. The team might increase rounds to hourly and might establish a toileting schedule for each patient, as appropriate, as strategies to improve the outcome (Figure 7-3).

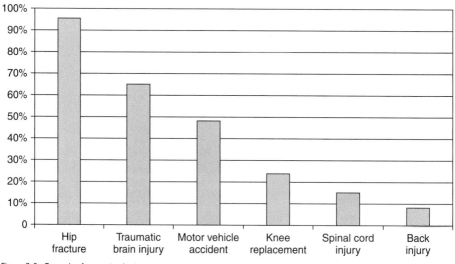

Figure 7-3. Example of a pareto chart.

- **Benchmarking:** Benchmarking is a national system within which the facility can compare specific care to the national norm of best practices, such as prevention and management of pressure sores. A chart is provided that shows how each quality indicator compared with the norm. This approach gives finite focus on those aspects needing attention and change and motivates the staff to try to move its results upward to match those systems that have better outcomes (Figure 7-4).

8. What is one major barrier to quality care?

Cost is one major barrier to quality care. Quality care always has a price, but it usually is an initial cost only, for in the long run the cost savings to the facility far outweigh the original cost. Yet this argument needs to be made with research-based support. Review of the literature can provide facts to assist in the argument. The APN rehabilitation nurse has the training to prepare this argument and project

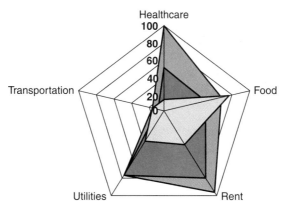

Figure 7-4. Example of a radar chart for benchmarking.

the cost savings accurately in terms of reduction in length of stay, improvement in patient/family satisfaction, and improvement in benchmarking.

9. **How should a team select an instrument that assesses outcomes?**

The team should consider the following characteristics:
- Validity: the ability of the tool to measure that which it is supposed to measure
- Reliability: the ability of the tool to measure consistently over time or among evaluators
- Sensitivity: the ability of the tool to measure small clinical changes
- Sensibility: the applicability of the tool to the situation and ease of use

10. **What should the team expect an instrument to provide?**

Each tool should
- Assess disability.
- Enhance communication.
- Measure effectiveness of treatment.
- Determine benefits of rehabilitation.

11. **What types of assessments may need to be done to measure outcomes?**

The following types of assessments measure outcomes:
1. Functional assessments, as with the FIM or the Barthel Index, are probably the most common outcome measures internationally. They measure degree of independence in these areas:
   - Feeding
   - Bathing
   - Grooming
   - Dressing
   - Bladder control

- Bowel control
- Toileting
- Chair/bed transfer
- Mobility
- Stair climbing

2. The multidimensional assessment of instrumental activities of daily living includes activities such as
   - Using a telephone
   - Shopping
   - Preparing meals
   - Managing money

   These skills are necessary for community reentry.

3. The rehabilitation nurse must monitor cognitive status consistently. Depending on the patient's impairment, one uses different approaches. The nurse can do a general assessment with the Mini-Mental State Examination. Specific tests may be required. For example, a patient with low responsivity will need an observational tool such as the LOCFAS (Levels of Cognitive Functioning Assessment Scale; 1993, 1995, 1997, 1998, 2003; see the appendix for the instrument, extension instrument, and management plan) that has strong psychometric support. This tool is derived from the Rancho Los Amigos scale and provides greater sensitivity to small changes and specificity to the degree that a nursing management plan has been published for each cognitive level. The assessment does not require patient participation to determine the status and design the specific nursing interventions required.
   As patients evidence higher cognitive function, the neuropsychologist who is a team member will administer specific tests to diagnose and prescribe specific therapies for each problem.

4. Depression may be a component of the disorder or may develop as a result of the patient's having to cope with the disorder. The CES-D Scale (the Centers for Epidemiological Studies—Depression Scale; Radloff, 1977) is one of the most widely used tools for screening depression.

5. Quality of life measures look at the patient's satisfaction and assess
   - Social roles and interactions
   - Functional performance
   - Intellectual functioning
   - Perceptions
   - Subjective health

Several measures exist, but few have reported validity. The Medical Outcomes Study (Ware and Sherbourne, 1992) and Sickness Impact Profile Scale (Bergner and others, 1981) assess these areas.

Key Points

- The intent of quality indicators is to use a system approach to control the quality of care.
- The indicators selected must be measurable; and the measurements must have validity and reliability, or the whole effort will have no meaning to the rehabilitation nurse.

Internet Resources

Agency for Healthcare Research and Quality
http://www.qualityindicators.ahrq.gov/

National Institute on Disability and Rehabilitation Research
http://www.ed.gov/about/offices/list/osers/nidrr/index.html

Bibliography

1. Duchene PM: Quality: indicators and management. In Hoeman SP, editor: *Rehabilitation nursing: process, application, & outcomes,* ed 3, St Louis, 2002, Mosby.

2. Joint Commission on Accreditation of Healthcare Organizations: Setting the standard: the Joint Commission & health care safety and quality, 2003. Retrieved July 1, 2003, from http://www.jcaho.org/accredited+organizations/patient&safety/setting&standard.htm

3. Kelly-Hayes M, Phipps H: Evaluation and outcomes measures. In Hoeman SP, editor: *Rehabilitation nursing: process, application, & outcomes,* ed 3, St Louis, 2002, Mosby.

4. Mahoney FI, Barthel D: Functional evaluation: the Barthel Index, *Md State Med J* 14:56-61, 1965.

Health Promotion: Maintenance of Health Patterns

Chapter 8

Skin Integrity

Susan R. Bulecza and Sharon A. Aronovitch

1. **Why do skin changes, such as reddened areas caused by pressure, become an open wound so quickly?**

   The epidermis is thin and avascular and regenerates every 4 to 6 weeks. The epidermis is up to 7 mm thick on palms of the hands and soles of the feet. The tissues located on the face, abdomen, and inner thighs are thinner and softer. Pressure ulcers usually occur over a bony prominence; the damage begins deep in the tissue near the bone, and the actual appearance of a pressure ulcer indicates that many layers of tissue damage have occurred already.

2. **Why does aging skin injure so easily?**

   The aging process results in a decrease in the thickness of the dermis and in a loss of subcutaneous tissue, which is the primary reason for increased skin injuries in the elderly. A loss of cohesion occurs between the epidermal and dermal layers of the skin. Aging also causes a decrease in the quantity of Langerhans' cells, resulting in a potential for increases in skin cancer and infection because of lowering of the immunocompetence of the skin. A decrease in vascular beds, sweat glands, sebaceous glands, and hair follicles also places the elderly at more risk for tissue injury.

3. **Is it appropriate to use talcum powder or cornstarch as a part of routine hygiene care, particularly in skin creases and skinfolds?**

   No, one should never use talcum powder or cornstarch as a part of a patient's routine hygiene care. The use of powders in skinfolds traps moisture that creates the perfect environment for fungal infections. A better choice of care would be to use an antiperspirant/deodorant in skinfolds. These products work just as well in skinfolds and creases as they do under the arm.

4. **How does inadequate oral intake affect the skin integrity?**

   Typically a patient with decreased oral intake is not receiving adequate hydration (at least 25 to 30 ml/kg in 24 hours) and less than the required calories in protein, carbohydrates, and fats. As the patient's oral intake decreases, the body begins to use muscle as its source of protein for energy. Decreased oral intake of protein is relative to decreased albumin and increases the risk for skin breakdown.

5. How are a patient's protein stores estimated?

Most health care providers use serum albumin as an indicator of the protein stores of the body. The normal range of serum albumin is 3.5 to 5.0 g/dl; however, this particular laboratory study has a half-life of 21 days, meaning the results are "old news" when one obtains them. A more reliable test for the current body state is serum prealbumin level (15 to 25 mg/dl and has a half-life of 2 days). A problem with serum prealbumin is that it is affected by the inflammatory response and decreases rapidly with a decrease in protein synthesis by the liver. The patient's level of hydration affects both of these tests such that dehydration produces falsely elevated values, and the opposite occurs with overhydration.

Another method of checking the patient's protein status is to evaluate the immune system because protein is a major component of this system. To do so, one calculates the total lymphocytic count by multiplying the percentage of lymphocytes by the white blood cell count. The resulting number should be in the range of 1500 to 3000 cells/mm^3. A value less than this normal range reflects malnutrition. The use of these blood tests is one important tool that the health care provider can use to determine whether the patient is more susceptible to skin injury.

6. What is the least caustic soap or cleanser to use when providing hygiene care?

The best cleanser to use is a low-alkali soap such as Neutrogena or Aveeno. The best cleansers are those that
• Are not soaps.
• Have a pH of 5.5.
• Clean the skin of bacteria and dirt.
• Are safe.
• Do not require a rinse.
Regular alkaline soaps eventually will reduce the thickness of the stratum corneum (upper most layer of the epidermis). Continued use of alkaline soaps increases the pH of the skin, which reverts back to its normal pH of 5 in about 45 minutes, though in prolonged exposure to alkaline soap this process can take as long as 19 hours. The change in the pH of the skin results in the body losing its protection from microorganisms and its ability to retain water.

7. Are moisturizers appropriate to use on patients?

Adequate hydration of the skin is important and is accomplished by a good intake of fluids and topical application of moisturizers. A good moisturizer should condition the skin and increase its moisture content, soothe irritation caused by dry or irritated skin, and have a clean base. Examples of ingredients that should be found in a moisturizer include allantoin, hydrolyzed protein, aloe vera extract, mineral oil, botanical oils, mucopolysaccharide, glycosamino-glycans, and petrolatum. The type of moisturizer selected for the patient depends on the condition of the patient's skin and how much moisture retention is required of the product.

8. **What is the difference between pressure relief surfaces and pressure reduction surfaces?**

   1. Pressure relief surfaces reduce the perpendicular force per area between the body and support surface below a level that closes capillaries (18 to 32 mm Hg); for example,
      - Alternating air mattress or overlay
      - Low-air-mass bed
   2. Pressure reduction surfaces reduce the perpendicular force per area between the body and support surface not usually below capillary closing level; for example,
      - Foam mattress overlay
      - Static air mattress
      - Gel cushions

9. **Why do some patients still develop changes in skin integrity while on a pressure relief surface?**

   Pressure relief surfaces are designed to reduce pressure consistently below capillary closing pressure, whereas a pressure reduction mattress system provides a lower pressure to the patient's body compared with a standard hospital mattress. The problem arises in that capillary closing pressure is a standard to which all patients are compared and is not necessarily appropriate for the young or extremely old. The gold standard for pressure relief is capillary closing pressure of 18 to 32 mm Hg, which is midpoint in the capillary. A patient's underlying biopathophysiological status also affects the ability to maintain an intact integumentary system. A patient with a history of arterial disease, diabetes, and hypertension with a poor nutritional status will have more likelihood of developing alterations in skin integrity than a healthy patient admitted for emergent repair of a fracture.

10. **Are moisture barriers really useful for patients with urinary or fecal incontinence?**

    Yes, moisture barriers are an important part of the patient's overall hygiene care. The nurse should use a moisture barrier after incontinence care. The moisture barrier of choice should not be removed easily with water because then it lacks the ability to provide an adequate barrier to urine or liquid stool. If an intact layer of ointment or paste is on the skin, the nurse has no need to remove all the ointment or paste each time the skin is cleansed. Mineral oil is a gentle and effective product for removal of ointments or pastes that are no longer providing an adequate barrier. Examples of product ingredients in a good moisture barrier include
    - Calamine
    - Petrolatum

- Dimethicone
- Glycerin
- Aluminum hydroxide gel
- Sodium bicarbonate
- Zinc oxide

11. Should all patients be assessed for risk of developing a pressure ulcer?

Yes, all patients need to be assessed for possible development of a pressure ulcer. The nurse can choose from many risk assessment tools, including Norton, Braden, Gosnell, Knoll, Waterlow, and Douglas, as well as instruments developed by manufacturers. An important note is that the Braden and Norton scales have been tested the most to determine reliability and validity. Whichever risk assessment tool the rehabilitation nurse chooses to use, the nurse must remember that as the patient's condition changes, so does the risk assessment score. For example, a patient can be considered as low risk for development of a pressure ulcer on admission to the facility but should be reassessed following any change in the medical condition, even following a minor surgical procedure. A recommendation is that the nurse assess a patient's risk for development of pressure ulcers at least once each week or when a change occurs in the patient's health status.

12. Are national guidelines available for use in assessing and treating pressure ulcers?

Yes, two guidelines are available from the Agency for Healthcare Research and Quality:
- Clinical Guideline Number 3: Pressure Ulcers in Adults—Prediction and Prevention
- Clinical Guideline Number 15: Treatment of Pressure Ulcers

13. What patients are most at risk for developing pressure ulcers?

- Patients who are bed- or chair-bound
- Patients who are unable to reposition themselves or have a mobility impairment
- Patients who have an altered level of consciousness
- Patients who have inadequate nutrition or incontinence or who are advanced in age

14. How can the nurse promote skin integrity?

The nurse can promote skin integrity in the following ways:
- Inspect the patient's skin daily and systematically.
- Establish a skin care routine that promotes cleanliness and minimizes skin dryness and irritation.
- Use moisturizers on dry skin.
- Do not massage skin over bony prominences, which can lead to tissue trauma.
- Reduce prolonged exposure of skin to wound drainage, urine, feces, or perspiration by using pads, barriers, and appropriate cleaning.

- Minimize shear and friction injuries by using proper turning, positioning, and moving techniques.
- Ensure adequate nutritional intake and calories.
- Maximize mobility and activity level.

15. What are the stages of pressure ulcers?

The National Pressure Ulcer Advisory Panel developed the following staging for pressure ulcers related to the deepest layer of tissue injury:
- Stage I: an observable change in an area of the skin related to pressure compared with surrounding skin. Change may occur in one or more of the following characteristics of the skin: temperature, consistency, color, or sensation. The skin does not blanch.
- Stage II: appearance of a superficial ulcer resembling an abrasion, blister, or shallow crater. Partial thickness skin loss has occurred.
- Stage III: appearance of a deep crater, with or without undermining of adjacent tissue, that may have intruded into surrounding tissue. Full-thickness skin loss to the fascia level has occurred and may include necrosis of subcutaneous tissue.
- Stage IV: appearance of a full-thickness deep crater with major destruction that may include damage to bone, muscle, or support structures. Tissue necrosis may be visible. Undermining and sinus tracts also may be present.

The nurse should not stage a wound covered by necrotic tissue until the necrotic tissue has been removed through débridement.

16. When a pressure ulcer is healing, should it be restaged?

No. The nurse always should refer to a pressure ulcer by the stage at which maximum depth of tissue injury was defined. As the ulcer heals, it is referred to as a healing ulcer. For example, Mrs. J. is being treated for a Stage IV ulcer on her left heel. The appearance of this ulcer is similar to a Stage II. The nurse's documentation would reflect this as a healing Stage IV ulcer.

17. Are any tools available to assess systematically pressure ulcer healing?

Tools available for systematic assessment of pressure ulcer healing are
- PUSH Scale: developed by the National Pressure Ulcer Advisory Panel
- Pressure Sore Status Tool: developed by Barbara Bates-Jensen

18. What are the basic components of a pressure ulcer care plan?

Although each patient's plan should be individualized to address the patient's specific needs, the plan should include the following four components:
- Necrotic tissue débridement
- Wound cleaning
- Infection prevention and control
- Dressing

19. **Are algorithms available to assist with pressure ulcer management?**

Yes. The Agency for Healthcare Research and Quality Guideline 15: Treatment of Pressure Ulcers has several algorithms that are helpful.

20. **What are some factors that affect skin integrity?**

The following are factors that affect skin integrity:
- Personal hygiene
- Nutrition and fluid status
- Exercise and activity
- Smoking
- Substance abuse
- Developmental stage
- Physiological issues
- Environmental influences
- Medications

21. **In addition to pressure ulcers, what other alterations in skin integrity may be present?**

Other alterations in skin integrity that may be present are
- Arterial ulcers on lower extremities
- Diabetic/neuropathic ulcers, primarily found on the feet
- Venous stasis ulcers, frequently found in the ankle area
- Mixed wounds (arterial, neuropathic, and venous)
- Skin abrasions, usually from rubbing or abrasive surface
- Skin tears, from friction or shearing
- Dryness
- Petechiae/ecchymoses, from bleeding into the tissue
- Surgical wounds
- Traumatic injury

 Key Points

- The best cleansers to use are low-alkali soaps such as Neutrogena or Aveeno to prevent change in the pH of the skin, which serves to protect the body from microorganisms and assists in its ability to retain water.
- The nurse should assess a patient's risk for developing pressure ulcers at least once a week or when a change occurs in the patient's condition.
- A healing pressure ulcer always should be referred to by the stage at which the maximum depth was defined.

Internet Resources

Skin Integrity
http://www.nih.gov/ninr/research/vol3/Skin.html

Center for Health Care Strategies: Developing a Skin Integrity Quality Program for Persons with Physical Disabilities
http://www.chcs.org/

Bibliography

1. Aronovitch SA: Intraoperatively acquired pressure ulcer prevalence: a national study, *J Wound Ostomy Continence Nurs* 26(3):130-136, 1999.

2. Scardillo J, Aronovitch SA: Successfully managing incontinence-related dermatitis across the lifespan, *Ostomy Wound Manage* 45(4):36-38, 1999.

3. Wysocli AB: Anatomy and physiology of skin and soft tissue. In Bryant R, editor: *Acute and chronic wounds: nursing management,* St Louis, 2000, Mosby.

Chapter 9

Nutrition Care

Louisa L. Dowling

1. **Why is nutrition assessment important?**

   A nutrition assessment is a comprehensive evaluation to determine nutrition status. The assessment identifies patients who are malnourished and those who are at risk of developing protein-energy malnutrition. A comprehensive nutrition assessment helps to identify nutrition-related complications, gives the nurse direction on how to provide the best therapy, and identifies the patient's response to the prescribed therapy.

2. **What are the essential components of a nutrition assessment?**

   A nutrition assessment, also referred to as metabolic assessment, includes a thorough review of the patient's medical history, physical examination, anthropometric measurements, and biochemical tests.

   Height and weight are used commonly to determine ideal or desirable body weight. These measurements help to determine estimated energy and protein requirements. Specifically, a comprehensive nutrition assessment should include the following components:
   1. History
      * Appetite
      * Elimination
      * Chewing/swallowing difficulties
      * Pain
      * Nutritional supplements
      * Percentage of meals consumed
      * Psychosocial status/rituals
      * Taste impairment
      * Type/consistency of foods
      * Weight loss/gain
   2. Diagnostics
      * Body mass index (BMI)
      * Complete blood count
      * Comprehensive metabolic panel
      * Lipid panel

- Medication profile
- Urinalysis
3. Examination
  - Fat distribution
  - Hair and scalp
  - Manual dexterity
  - Mental status
  - Respiratory status
  - Skin turgor
  - Teeth and gums
  - Wounds

3. How is height calculated?

Height is calculated from the following equations:

Men

Height (cm) = 64.19 − [0.04 × age (years)] + [2.02 × knee height (cm)]

Women

Height (cm) = 84.88 − [0.24 × age (years)] + [1.83 × knee height (cm)]²

4. How is ideal body weight calculated?

Weight is calculated to determine ideal body weight. A range of ±10 lb (4.5 kg) is used to interpret small, medium, or large frame size. The most common calculation used is the Hamwi "rule of thumb":

Men

106 lb (48 kg) for the first 5 ft (1.5 cm) and add 6 lb (2.7) kg for each inch (2.54 cm) over 5 ft

Women

100 lb (45 kg) for the first 5 ft and add 5 lb (2.3) kg for each inch (2.54 cm) over 5 ft

5. How is BMI calculated?

The BMI also can be used to approximate the severity of protein-energy malnutrition and obesity in adults. Body mass index is calculated using the following equations:

$$\text{BMI} = \frac{\text{Weight (kg)}}{\text{Height}^2 \ (\text{m}^2)} \quad or \quad \text{BMI} = [\text{weight (1b)} \div \text{Height}^2 \ (\text{in}^2)] \times 703$$

6. **How are children's weights compared with norms?**

   In children between the ages of 2 and 20 years, growth charts are used to determine body composition with measurements documented in percentiles.
   <5th percentile = underweight
   >85th percentile = at risk for overweight
   >95th percentile = overweight

7. **How are energy and protein requirements calculated?**

   The most commonly used equation to determine calorie and protein requirements is the Harris-Benedict equation. To provide an estimation of needed nutrients, a stress factor ranging from 1.2 for minor stress to 2.1 for severe stress is added. These measures provide estimations and may not be appropriate for critically ill patients but would be appropriate for rehabilitation patients.

   Men

   $$66.47 + [13.75 \times (\text{weight in kg})] + [5.0 \times (\text{height in cm})] - [6.75 \times (\text{age in years})]$$

   Women

   $$655.09 + [9.56 \times (\text{weight in kg})] + [1.85 \times (\text{height in cm})] - [4.68 \times (\text{age in years})]$$

8. **How are fluid requirements calculated?**

   The nurse can calculate daily water requirements using various methods. See Table 9-1.

Table 9-1. Calculation of daily water requirements

Method	Water requirements	
Method 1: body weight	First 10 kg	100 ml/kg
	Second 10 kg	50 ml/kg
	Each additional kilogram	20 ml/kg (≤50 years)
		15 ml/kg (>50 years)
Method 2: age	Young, athletic adult	40 ml/kg
	Most adults	35 ml/kg
	Elderly adults	30 ml/kg
Method 3: energy expenditure	1 ml/kcal energy expenditure	

9. **What is malnutrition?**

Malnutrition has been defined as a pathological state that results from a relative or an absolute deficiency, or from an excess, of one or more essential nutrients (Caldwell and others, 1990).

10. **What are the different types of malnutrition?**

- Marasmus is the result of long-term deprivation of nutrients and is recognized easily. Marasmus is manifested by weight loss, depleted fat stores, weakness, bradycardia, and hypothermia (Maloo and Forse, 2001).
- Kwashiorkor, or protein malnutrition, results from a deficit of protein in relation to calories and may develop over a shorter period. This type of malnutrition is more difficult to recognize because the patient appears healthy. However, marked protein depletion results in impaired immunocompetence. Patients generally develop edema as a result of hypoalbuminemia, muscle wasting, and delayed wound healing (Maloo and Forse, 2001; Shopbell and others, 2001).
- Protein-calorie malnutrition results when metabolic stress occurs in a patient with preexisting malnutrition.

11. **Which biochemical tests are helpful in identifying nutritional deficits?**

Various serum protein measurements help to detect and monitor protein and energy deficits. Though not one specific index is an ideal indicator of nutritional status, each marker provides useful baseline information. See Table 9-2.

Table 9-2. Protein markers for nutritional deficits

Protein	Half-life	Function
Albumin	14-20 days	Carrier protein, maintenance of plasma oncotic pressure; sensitive to hydration status
Transferrin	8-10 days	Carrier protein for iron; useful parameter in detection of liver disease
Prealbumin	2-3 days	Carrier protein for retinol-binding protein; transports thyroxine; sensitive to nonnutritional factors such as infection, bleeding, fever; sensitive indicator of protein-calorie malnutrition; not influenced by hydration or liver disease
Retinol-binding protein	12 hours	Bound to prealbumin; transports retinal; sensitive to nonnutritional variables; least commonly used in clinical settings because of short half-life

12. What is a nitrogen balance study?

A nitrogen balance study measures the difference between the amount of nitrogen ingested and the amount of nitrogen excreted. A nitrogen balance study helps to determine the adequacy of protein provision and rate of metabolism. Nitrogen balance is measured as a 24-hour total urinary nitrogen or urinary urea nitrogen (UUN). A factor of 4 is applied to the equation to account for insensible losses. The following formula is used:

Nitrogen balance = [(Protein intake in g) ÷ 6.25] − [(24-hour UUN in g) + 4]

13. What is nutritional support, and how does the rehabilitation nurse determine which type to use?

Nutritional support is the science of providing essential and nonessential nutrients when conventional consumption is inadequate, hindered, or deemed medically inappropriate. The nurse can provide support with enteral nutrition or parenteral nutrition.

The decision on how to choose which therapy is appropriate generally is guided by the basic principle "If the gut works, use it." Bowel sounds alone do not guarantee enteral nutrition delivery. Bowel function can be demonstrated by the presence of flatus, stool, or bowel sounds. Similarly, the absence of bowel sounds does not necessitate the use of parenteral nutrition. Postoperative ileus generally involves the colonic and stomach functions, sparing the small-bowel function. The presence of a soft, nontender, nondistended abdomen and hemodynamic stability are clinical indicators for the potential use of enteral nutrition. Enteral nutrition is safer, cost-effective, and more physiologically effective than parenteral nutrition. The patient with only minimal absorptive and digestive capabilities can be maintained on specialized enteral formulas via a gastric or a small-bowel feeding tube.

14. What type of questions should the nurse ask in a nutritional history?

General and specific areas of inquiry should include
• Appetite
• Unintentional weight loss or weight gain
• Elimination
• Functionality
• The presence of pain
• Quality and quantity of meals consumed
• Psychosocial status
• Existing chronic or acute illness

15. Which patients need nutritional intervention?

Every patient needs a nutritional status assessment to determine whether nutritional intervention is required. In general, patients in the following situations require nutritional intervention:
• Chronic or acute illnesses
• After trauma

- After surgery
- Pediatrics
- Pregnant or lactating women
- Geriatrics

16. When should nutritional therapy be initiated?

Nutritional therapy should be initiated as early as possible or within the first 24 hours after hospital admission. Because 50% to 70% of the total body immune function is in the gastrointestinal tract, early enteral feeding by mouth or through a feeding tube is needed to maintain luminal perfusion and gastrointestinal motility. Techniques to provide enteral nutrition have improved significantly over the years, making it possible to feed beyond the level of the pylorus. Small-bowel feedings, postpyloric or post–ligament of Treitz, are generally well tolerated.

17. What nutritional interventions are needed regarding specific health problems?

Table 9-3 provides guidelines for implementing nutritional interventions on an individual basis.

Table 9-3.   Guidelines for nutritional interventions

Disease/disorder	Nutritional interventions
Cardiovascular	Low saturated fats, cholesterol, and sodium High fiber (soluble and insoluble), low carbohydrates ω-3 fatty acids (fish oil) Lean beef, fish, poultry, low-fat dairy products, soy Enteral or parenteral therapy as indicated
Respiratory	Limit fluid intake High-fiber foods Discontinue use of tobacco, alcohol, and caffeine Provide calories to maintain energy level and weight Enteral or parenteral therapy as indicated
Gastrointestinal	Increase soluble and insoluble substances Increase fluid intake with increased fiber Assess if patient requires gluten-free, lactose-free diet Lean meats, low-fat dairy products Calcium, vitamin D Enteral or parenteral therapy as indicated

Table 9-3.   Guidelines for nutritional interventions *continued*

Renal	Limit fluid intake, sodium, protein
	Water-soluble vitamins
	Iron and vitamin D as indicated
	Enteral or parenteral therapy as indicated
Burns, trauma/ surgery, or infectious process	Increased calories and protein
	Vitamin C, zinc
	Selenium (begin 1 month after trauma/surgery)
	Monitor for lipid embolism with long-bone fractures
	Monitor blood urea nitrogen, serum creatinine, and hydration with high-protein intake
	Enteral or parenteral therapy as indicated
Cancer	Increase calories, proteins, fluid intake
	High-fiber foods
	Carotenoid; vitamins A, C, and E; and selenium
	Decrease caffeine intake
	Enteral or parenteral therapy as indicated
Diabetes, types 1 and 2	Assess for individual calorie, fats, and protein needs
	Increased soluble and insoluble fiber
	Avoid simple carbohydrates
	Enteral or parenteral therapy as indicated
Obesity	Decrease carbohydrates, high-fiber foods
	Cardiovascular guidelines
	Enteral or parenteral therapy as indicated
Eating disorder	Slow initiation of feeding
	Monitor fluid and electrolytes closely
	Multivitamin/mineral supplementation
	Interdisciplinary team approach
	Enteral or parenteral therapy as indicated
Neurological/ degenerative disease	Assess swallowing
	Flavored and textured foods
	Avoid thin liquids; use thickener
	Aspiration precautions
	Enteral or parenteral therapy as indicated

 Key Points

- Enteral nutrition should always be used, if possible.
- Nutrition assessment includes a thorough medical history, with a focus on nutrition, physical examination, anthropometric measurements, and biochemical tests.

Internet Resources

Food and Nutrition Information Center
http://www.nal.usda.gov/fnic

American Society for Nutritional Sciences
http://www.nutrition.org/

American Society for Parenteral and Enteral Nutrition
http://www.nutritioncare.org/

Bibliography

1. Caldwell MD, Kennedy-Caldwell C, Winkler ME: Micronutrients and enteral nutrition. In Rombeau JL, Caldwell MD, editors: *Clinical nutrition: enteral and tube feeding,* Washington, DC, 1990, Nutrition Screening Initiative.

2. Centers for Disease Control and Prevention: BMI for adults: what is BMI? Retrieved September 15, 2002, from http://www.cdc.gov/nccdphp/dnpa/bmi/bmi-adult.htm

3. Centers for Disease Control and Prevention: BMI for children and teens: BMI is used differently with children than it is with adults. Retrieved September 15, 2002, from http://www.cdc.gov/nccdphp/dnpa/bmi/bmi-for-age-htm

4. Coulstron AM, Rock CL, Monsen ER: *Nutrition in the prevention and treatment of disease,* San Diego, 2001, Academic Press.

5. Dowling LL: Advanced practice nurses' knowledge and assessment of nutrition. Unpublished master's thesis, Tallahassee, 2003, Florida State University.

6. Frankenfield DC, Muth ER, Rowe WA: The Harris-Benedict studies of human basal metabolism: history and limitations, *J Am Diet Assoc* 98:439-445, 1998.

7. Hamwi GJ: Changing dietary concepts. In Danowski TS, editor: *Diabetes mellitus: diagnosis and treatment,* New York, 1964, American Diabetes Association.

8. Mahan LK, Escott-Stump S: *Krause's food, nutrition, and diet therapy,* ed 9, Philadelphia, 1996, WB Saunders.

9. Maloo MK, Forse RA: Perioperative nutritional support. In Rombeau JL, Rolandelli RH, editors: *Clinical nutrition: parenteral nutrition,* ed 3, Philadelphia, 2001, WB Saunders.

10. Shopbell JM, Hopkins B, Shronts EP: Nutrition screening and assessment. In Gottschlich MM, editor: *The science and practice of nutrition support: a case-based core curriculum,* Dubuque, Iowa, 2001, Kendall Hunt.

11. Theriault L: Collaborating with nutritionists. In Goolsby MJ, editor: *Nurse practitioner secrets,* Philadelphia, 2002, Hanley & Belfus.

Chapter 10

Bowel Elimination

Sharon A. Aronovitch

1. What causes constipation?

Constipation is considered to be the passing of hard stool or an abnormally reduced frequency of eliminating stool, which for the majority of persons ranges from 3 times each day to every 3 or more days. Constipation can result from medication (e.g., opioids, anticholenergics, anticonvulsants, antidepressants, and calcium channel blockers), diabetes, hyperthyroidism, multiple sclerosis, and Parkinson's disease. For the hospitalized patient, constipation usually results from physical inactivity, stress, dietary changes, possible lack of fluids, and failure to respond to the urge to defecate.

Most often for the hospitalized patient, constipation results from decreased motility of the colon because of immobility. The longer stool remains in the colon, the more water is reabsorbed, and the stool becomes drier. Dry, hard stool is much more difficult to evacuate from the rectum than soft, formed stool.

2. Can chronic constipation be harmful to the patient?

Yes, chronic constipation can be unhealthy for the patient. When constipated, the patient has to increase the use of the Valsalva maneuver to bear down to try to remove the hard stool, which increases the likelihood of hemorrhoids developing. Chronic constipation also decreases the intestinal muscle tone. Untreated constipation can lead to fecal impaction in which the rectum overdistends. An overdistended rectum is unable to respond to the stimulus of stool in the rectal vault, which leads to rebound diarrhea and fecal incontinence.

3. What is rebound diarrhea?

Rebound diarrhea is the result of decreased motility of the intestinal tract that has resulted in severe constipation and fecal impaction. The obstructing fecal mass in the rectum causes a relaxation of the internal sphincter muscle, and bacterial action on the hard stool results in the production of liquid stool. The liquid stool that seeps out of the rectum is what many health care providers term *diarrhea.*

4. **How can constipation be prevented?**

The use of dietary fiber increases water content in the stool, making the stool easier to evacuate. Dietary fiber also promotes colonic motility by bacterial degradation. Other nursing interventions include dietary and fluid modifications, increasing the patient's activity within patient's limitations of movement, and establishing regular toileting patterns.

5. **What is the most common medication to prescribe for the patient with constipation?**

The most common medications given to patients with constipation are bulk formers, stool softeners, lubricants, hyperosmolar laxatives, saline laxatives, and stimulant/irritant laxatives.

- Bulk formers include psyllium and methylcellulose. The action of the bulk former is to combine with water and swell in the intestinal tract, causing peristalsis. The nurse must instruct the patient to drink plenty of fluid; otherwise, further constipation is possible or an obstruction may occur.
- Stool softeners (i.e., docusate sodium and docusate calcium) act as detergents in the intestinal tract, and by reducing the surface tension, they permit the incorporation of lipids and fat into stool to make it softer.
- Mineral oil is the lubricant of choice and acts by softening the fecal matter and lubricating the intestinal tract to facilitate evacuation of stool.
- Lactulose, polyethylene glycol (GoLYTELY), and sorbitol are hyperosmolar laxatives and work by degrading colonic bacteria and increasing stool osmolarity to increase intestinal peristalsis.
- Saline laxatives include magnesium citrate, magnesium sulfate (Epsom salts), and magnesium hydroxide (milk of magnesia). These laxatives cause the osmotic retention of fluid, which distends the intestine and increases peristalsis.
- Cascara sagrada, senna (Senokot), bisacodyl (Dulcolax), and castor oil are stimulant/irritant laxatives. This group of laxatives directly acts on the intestinal tract to cause irritation, thereby promoting peristalsis.

6. **Is there a dietary supplement the patient can take in place of a laxative?**

One of the most common dietary fibers is bran, though many patients do not like the taste. The recipes in Box 10-1 also can be used to increase the patient's fiber intake in a palatable form.

7. **What does the rehabilitation nurse do if the patient has an impaction?**

Removal of the mass is done manually by the insertion of a gloved finger into the rectum. Sometimes the nurse must give the patient an oil retention enema before digital removal of the stool to soften the mass.

Box 10-1. Palatable bran recipes

1. Take power pudding ¼ to 1 cup per day for desired results.
   - ½ cup prune juice
   - ½ cup applesauce
   - ½ cup wheat bran flakes
   - ½ cup canned or stewed prunes
2. Take bran formula 1 tablespoon/day and increase dose by 1 tablespoon each week until desired results are achieved.
   - 1 cup unprocessed miller's bran
   - 1 cup applesauce
   - ¼ cup prune juice

---

8. **Why do patients with diabetes seem always to develop constipation?**

   Diabetes mellitus eventually damages the efferent autonomic nerves, resulting in diminished intestinal motility and weaker contractions of the smooth muscle. Decreased motility (diabetic gastroparesis) results in slower colonic activity, leading to accumulation of stool in the colon. Patients developing diabetic neuropathy lose the gastrocolic reflex, which is the postprandial push that aids in the expulsion of stool from the rectum. Substance P, a sensory neuropeptide found in the rectal mucosa, is also decreased, resulting in a loss of sensory awareness that stool needs to be evacuated. Over time the patient has a decrease in the motility of the small intestine, allowing for bacterial proliferation and impaired absorption from ileocolonic denervation, which causes a cyclical pattern of diarrhea and constipation.

9. **What causes some patients to develop diarrhea with the use of antibiotics?**

   Many antibiotics given to treat an infection have a negative effect on the colon by decreasing the number of *Escherichia coli* bacteria. When *E. coli* are decreased in number, the bacterium *Clostridium difficile* overtakes the bowel, disturbing the normal flora. *Clostridium difficile* produces toxins that result in a secretory diarrhea and pseudomembranes that alter the absorptive capacity of the colon. Treatment for *C. difficile* includes orally administered metronidazole or orally administered vancomycin.

10. **What is an ileus?**

    Ileus is defined as impaired or absent peristalsis of the intestinal tract. Paralytic ileus is a temporary problem that usually follows abdominal surgery, particularly if the bowel has been handled for a long time. The nurse makes the diagnosis of ileus when no peristaltic activity has occurred for 72 hours. The patient will have symptoms of pain, nausea, and vomiting. Management of an ileus includes maintaining the patient by means other than the oral route and providing decompression of the bowel using a nasointestinal tube. Analgesics provide pain management, though they should be used sparingly so as not to continue the ileus, which is a nonmechanical intestinal obstruction. The patient may require medications to stimulate the parasympathetic nervous system, such as neostigmine (Prostigmine).

11. How do patients with paralysis of the lower extremities, such as with a spinal cord injury, maintain adequate elimination of stool?

Stool evacuation should be a planned program with spinal cord injury patients, for it is still a normal process. Spinal cord injury above the sixth thoracic vertebra has destroyed the patient's ability to bear down using the abdominal muscles to force stool out of the rectal vault. In planning for routine bowel elimination, the rehabilitation nurse needs to take into account what the patient's normal bowel habits were before injury and plan for evacuation of stool according to that preestablished time. Additionally, these patients will need special consideration in bowel management because of the risk for autonomic dysreflexia. Most patients typically have a bowel movement following breakfast, which is a natural stimulus of peristalsis for the intestinal tract. The nurse places the patient in a sitting position following digital stimulation of the anal sphincter by placing a gloved finger into the rectum. Some patients also may require a suppository to stimulate defecation and application of a topical anesthetic to avoid spastic reflex responses to digital stimulation. Once a pattern for fecal elimination has been established, digital stimulation may be adequate to initiate defecation.

Key Point

Although many factors cause constipation, immobility is most often the cause for hospitalized patients.

Internet Resources

International Foundation for Functional Gastrointestinal Disorders
http://www.aboutincontinence.org/BowelControl.html

Medline Plus: Bowel Retraining
http://www.nlm.nih.gov/medlineplus/ency/article/003971.htm

Bibliography

1. Heitkemper MM: Physiology of defecation. In Doughty DB, editor: *Urinary and fecal incontinence: nursing management,* St Louis, 2000, Mosby.
2. Sands JK: Intestinal problems. In Phipps WJ, Monahan FD, Sands JK, and others, editors: *Medical-surgical nursing: health and illness perspectives,* ed 7, St Louis, 2003, Mosby.
3. Waldrop J, Doughty DB: Pathophysiology of bowel dysfunction and fecal incontinence. In Doughty DB, editor: *Urinary and fecal incontinence: nursing management,* St Louis, 2000, Mosby.

Chapter 11

Bladder Elimination

Jeanne Flannery and Susan R. Bulecza

1. What is the definition of urinary incontinence?

As defined by the American Urological Association and the Agency for Healthcare Research and Quality, *urinary incontinence* is the involuntary loss of urine to the degree it becomes problematic to the individual. The ramifications of this problem are far-reaching and have significant impact on the individual's psychological, social, and physical well-being.

2. Who is most at risk for urinary incontinence?

A number of populations are considered at risk, the elderly being one of the largest. However, incontinence is not a normal part of aging. Other groups include individuals with neurological diseases and disorders, individuals who participate in high-impact sports or training, and individuals who are obese.

3. What is the prevalence of incontinence?

About 10% to 35% of adult Americans have been reported to suffer from urinary incontinence. Furthermore, more than one half of nursing home residents are incontinent, and incontinence is often the primary reason for placement in a facility. In the over 60-year-old populations, women are twice as likely as men to suffer from incontinence. The prevalence for women in this age group is 12% to 49% compared with 7% to 22% of men. Although most persons associate incontinence primarily with the elderly, incontinence does occur in the younger population. As with the elders, women are affected more frequently than men. For women less than 30 years old the prevalence is 5% to 16% compared with 6% to 10% for men of the same age. Research with female elite athletes has shown an increased prevalence, especially in high-impact sports such as gymnastics. Incontinence also can be a problem for women who have had multiple pregnancies or traumatic deliveries.

4. What is the cost associated with incontinence?

The cost of urinary incontinence is greater than $26 billion annually, which is approximately $3,500 per person with the disorder. Although these costs may seem excessive, the real cost is much more because of the underreporting of

the condition. Several factors have contributed to the increasing costs of urinary incontinence:
- Increased availability and development of incontinence management products
- Increase in the older population
- Change in prevalence of the disorder

5. How does culture affect individuals with urinary incontinence?

In the Western culture, certain mores exist that place value and worth on cleanliness and continence. Therefore individuals who are unable to achieve these expectations are viewed negatively. Subsequently, individuals who suffer from incontinence tend to isolate themselves, limit activity, and suffer tremendous loss of self-esteem. Additionally, culture can influence an individual's response to management. African American or Mexican American males may not seek treatment because of cultural influences that consider bowel and bladder issues private and because any alteration from the expected norm is significantly damaging to their self-esteem. Another cultural myth that affects an individual to seek care is the belief that incontinence is a normal part of the aging process.

6. How is urinary incontinence classified?

The Clinical Practice Guidelines for Urinary Incontinence in Adults gives four classifications of incontinence. Box 11-1 presents these classifications.

Box 11-1.   Classifications of incontinence

- **Stress incontinence** occurs when pelvic floor muscles have become weak. Reasons for this are varied and include injury during childbirth, decreased function, straining, estrogen deficiency, and genetics.
- **Urge incontinence** occurs with detrusser instability creating a sudden urge to urinate, with or without loss of urine. Reasons for this include infection, vaginal prolapse, or cystocele.
- **Retention/overlow incontinence** occurs with inadequate bladder emptying and subsequent overdistention, resulting in constant urine dribbling. Pain and pressure in the lower abdomen are frequent symptoms.
- **Functional incontinence** is involuntary loss of urine because of medications or physical or mental disorders outside the urinary tract

---

7. What are neurological causes of urinary incontinence?

- Suprapontine and higher cervical lesions: Possible symptoms include retention or uncontrollable micturition reflex.
- Upper motor neuron lesions: Possible symptoms include lack of detrusor sphincter coordination and urethrovesical reflux.
- Peripheral and autonomic nervous system and lower motor neuron lesions: Symptoms include detrusor muscle areflexia, incontinence, or diffuse pain.

8. **What types of bladder dysfunction occur, based on disruption of the central nervous system?**

   - An upper motor neuron injury that causes disruption in the brainstem pontine level will disrupt the coordination of bladder contraction and sphincter relaxation, which results in a hyperreflexic bladder.
   - Disruptions in the medial frontal lobes of the cortex or the hypothalamus will interrupt the pathways that control initiation and cessation of micturition. This disruption results in involuntary micturition, or an uninhibited bladder.

9. **What type of bladder function occurs, based on disruption of the peripheral nervous system?**

   Disruption of the sacral reflex control center, which is located in the spinal segments S2 to S4, or the peripheral nervous system is a lower motor neuron injury and results in an areflexic bladder.

10. **What is a neurogenic bladder?**

    A neurogenic bladder results from any disruption of any of the motor or sensory pathways that supply the bladder, both central nervous system and peripheral nervous system (upper and lower motor neuron injuries). The nurse must understand five different variations of neurogenic bladder to assist the patient appropriately. See Table 11-1.

Table 11-1. Types of neurogenic bladder

Type	Level	Characteristics	Related problems
Uninhibited	Frontal brain or pontine	Cortical control diminished Urgency, frequency Urge incontinence, nocturia Reduced bladder capacity	Stroke, traumatic brain injury, multiple sclerosis (MS), brain tumor
Reflex	Spinal cord above T12 to L1	Upper motor neuron (above S2 to S4) problem Involuntary emptying, controlled by reflex arc Inadequate emptying; large residual amounts	Lower spinal cord injury or inadequate circulation from vascular lesion, MS
Areflexic (autonomic)	Spinal cord at or below T12 to L1	Lower motor neuron (S2 to S4) problem Increased bladder capacity Decreased sensation of bladder fullness Loss of voluntary voiding Overflow incontinence	Herniated disk with nerve injury, spina bifida, spinal shock

Table 11-1.   Types of neurogenic bladder *continued*

Type	Level	Characteristics	Related problems
Motor paralytic	Anterior horn cells of S2 to S4 ventral roots	Intact sensation Partial or total loss of voluntary voiding Overflow incontinence	Herniated disc, poliomyelitis, spinal tumor
Sensory paralytic	Dorsal roots of S2 to S4 (sacral reflex arc) or sensory pathways	Partial or total loss of sensation Increased bladder capacity Infrequent voiding Overflow incontinence	Diabetic neuropathy, MS, tabes dorsalis, syringomyelia

11. **Are there other causes for urinary incontinence?**

Yes. These causes can be psychogenic (e.g., schizophrenia), endocrine (e.g., diabetes), hormonal deficiencies (e.g., estrogen deficiency), inflammatory (e.g., cystitis), obstructive (e.g., tumor), or pharmacological (e.g., hypertension medication). Symptoms related to these causes manifest like stress, urge, and retention/overflow incontinence.

12. **What is functional incontinence?**

Functional incontinence is incontinence not related to abnormalities in the genitourinary tract. Generally, the cause is related to physical or cognitive impairments such as inability to access a bathroom or decreased awareness of the urge to urinate.

13. **What are common causes of transient incontinence?**

A rehabilitation nurse needs to consider all the possible reasons for a patient's incontinence to design the approach to care. Box 11-2 lists general causes of transient incontinence.

14. **What method helps the rehabilitation nurse to remember the extensive range of possible factors contributing to transient incontinence?**

The nurse can remember the mnemonic DIAPPERS. See Box 11-3.

15. **In assessing the patient for bladder function, on which specific areas in the history must the rehabilitation nurse focus?**

1. Characteristics of voiding pattern, such as
   • Frequency during day and night
   • Amount

Box 11-2. Causes for transient incontinence

- Excessive fluid intake
- Diuretics
- Restricted mobility
- Bed rest
- Fecal impaction
- Depression
- Dementia
- Confusion
- Altered level of consciousness
- Parkinson's disease
- Diabetes mellitus
- Orthostatic hypotension
- Generalized weakness
- Fatigue
- Sedation
- Medications that act on bladder muscles and sphincters
- Calcium channel blockers, antidepressants, narcotics, over-the-counter cold preparations (retention with overflow)
- Urinary tract infections
- Vaginitis
- Postprostatectomy
- Hypercalcemia
- Volume overload (venous insufficiency, edema, congestive heart failure)
- Alcohol
- Renal disease
- Cancer

Box 11-3. Mnemonic (DIAPPERS): contributing factors to transient incontinence

Delirium
Infection or **I**nflammation
Atrophic vaginitis or uretheritis
Pharmaceuticals
Psychological conditions
Excess urine production
Restricted mobility
Stool impaction

- Urgency
- Ability to delay
- Amount of leakage
- Precipitating circumstances for incontinence
- Difficulty initiating
- Dysuria
- Awareness of full bladder
- Sensation of incomplete emptying
- Use of pads or briefs
- Bladder distention
- Foul-smelling urine

2. Relevant medical history, related to problems such as those discussed in question 12.
3. Medications
4. Environmental factors (distance to travel to bathroom, barriers in bathroom, manual dexterity, toileting aids)

16. The physical examination conducted by the rehabilitation nurse should include which focal points?

The specific areas on which to focus include

1. Functional assessment
   - Mobility
   - Manual dexterity
   - Ability to disrobe
   - Ability to perceive the need to void
   - Understanding of how to get to toilet or substitute
   - Gait and balance
   - Mood
2. Abdominal examination
   - Scars indicative of previous surgery
   - Masses
   - Suprapubic tenderness
   - Distended bladder
3. Genital examination
   - Abnormalities of the foreskin, penis, or perineum
   - Pelvic examination with gloved fingers to detect mass, prolapse, tenderness, discharge, ability to contract pelvic floor, and paravaginal muscles
   - Signs of infection
4. Rectal examination
   - Perineal sensation
   - Sphincter tone
   - Mass
   - Fecal impaction
   - Size and consistency of prostate
   - Bulbocavernosus reflex (status of sacral reflex arc)
5. General and neurological examination

6. Stress test with full bladder
   - Lithotomy position: Have patient cough vigorously; observe urethra for leakage.
   - Standing position: Have patient cough vigorously; observe urethra for leakage.

17. What are the major treatment options for urinary incontinence?

The treatment options include
1. Behavioral techniques
   - Bladder training
   - Habit training (timed voiding)
   - Prompted voiding
   - Pelvic muscle exercises (Kegel)
2. Bladder-triggering techniques
   - Suprapubic stimulation: pulling pubic hairs, stroking medial thighs, tapping suprabubic area
   - Valsalva's maneuver: straining against a closed epiglottis
   - Credé's maneuver: pressing firmly down and inward on abdomen below umbilicus
3. Catheters and catheterizations
4. Padding

18. What does a bladder training program entail?

Bladder training is of primary importance to those who have cerebral damage, spinal cord damage, or regional dysfunction resulting in areflexia, hyperflexia, urinary frequency, and incontinence. The purpose of the program is to
- Prevent bladder overfilling
- Prevent infection in the bladder and kidneys
A bladder training program includes three primary components. See Box 11-4.

Box 11-4. Bladder training components

- Education: physiology, pathophysiology, technique, and outcome
- Scheduled voiding: resist or inhibit urgency; postpone voiding; maintain timetable
- Positive reinforcement

---

19. What strategies does the rehabilitation nurse use to improve the outcome in bladder training?

The rehabilitation nurse can use the following strategies to improve bladder training outcome:
- Adjust fluid intake to match timetables.
- Progressively postpone voiding so that large volumes of urine distend the bladder (initial goal may be to achieve a 2- to 3-hour interval, except during sleep).
- Prompt to void on a timetable.

- Praise the patient and reinforce education.
- Provide a written discharge bladder training manual.

20. How should the rehabilitation nurse explain Kegel exercises to a patient who has no familiarity with them?

The nurse should start by having the patient go into the bathroom and sit on the commode. The nurse should ask the patient to initiate voiding and then attempt to stop the stream. The nurse can ask the patient to notice the muscles used in the pelvic floor to accomplish this. The patient should try the maneuver several more times during this emptying of the bladder to become familiar with the sensation of the muscle contraction.

Then the nurse should discuss the exercise. The patient should squeeze these muscles, without tensing the buttocks or abdomen for a slow count of 3 and then relax for a slow count of 3. This is one repetition. The patient should plan to do 45 repetitions a day in the following pattern:
- Lying: 15 repetitions
- Sitting: 15 repetitions
- Standing: 15 repetitions

The nurse directs the patient to establish a regular time of day so that the patient does not forget. If the patient is unable to do 15 repetitions at a time, the patient can do fewer more frequently.

21. What are issues specific to the elder population regarding urinary incontinence?

Because many of the problems causing urinary incontinence are treatable, resulting in a cure or significant improvement in the problem, an important aspect of treatment is for an elder to understand that urinary incontinence is not a normal part of aging. The following factors can contribute to incontinence in elders:
- Immobility
- Urinary tract infection
- Medication
- Depression
- Dementia
- Isolation
- Cognitive deficits
- Physical barriers
- Chronic diseases
- Disability

22. What are the main complications from urinary incontinence?

- Skin breakdown: Prolonged exposure to urine can result in skin breakdown and ulcer formation.
- Rashes: Irritation from urine can result in the development or rashes.
- Infections: Disruption in the skin surface can result in wound infection.

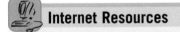

Key Points

- Urinary incontinence is the involuntary loss of urine to the degree it becomes problematic to the individual.
- Individuals who suffer from incontinence tend to isolate themselves, limit activity, and suffer tremendous loss of self-esteem.
- Bladder dysfunction can be caused from central nervous system or peripheral nervous system disruption; psychogenic, endocrine, inflammatory, obstructive, or pharmacological causes; or hormonal deficiencies.
- DIAPPERS is a mnemonic to help the nurse remember the extensive range of possible factors contributing to transient incontinence.
- Assessment of bladder function should include voiding pattern history, medical history, medications, environmental factors, and a physical examination.
- An important aspect of treatment is for an elderly patient to understand that incontinence is not a normal process of aging.

Internet Resources

Bladder Disorders
http://www.bladder-disorders.com

Incontinence Information
http://www.types-of-incontinence.com/

Bibliography

1. Carrière B: The pelvic floor treatment of incontinence and other urinary dysfunctions in men and women. In Umphred DA, editor: *Neurological rehabilitation,* ed 4, St Louis, 2001, Mosby.

2. Easton KL: Establishing bowel and bladder patterns. In *Gerontological rehabilitation nursing,* Philadelphia, 1999, WB Saunders.

3. Fried KM, Fried GW, Farnan C: Elimination. In Derstine JB, Hargrove SD, editors: *Comprehensive rehabilitation nursing,* Philadelphia, 2001, WB Saunders.

4. Hickey JV: Rehabilitation of neuroscience patients. In Hickey JV, editor: *The clinical practice of neurological and neurosurgical nursing,* ed 5, Philadelphia, 2003, Lippincott.

5. Pires M: Bladder elimination. In Hoeman SP, editor: *Rehabilitation nursing: process, application, & outcomes,* ed 3, St Louis, 2002, Mosby.

Chapter 12

Sleep and Relaxation

Jeanne Flannery

1. **How much of one's life is spent in sleep?**

   About one third of an adult's life is spent sleeping.

2. **What is the definition of sleep?**

   Sleep is a specific state of consciousness with relative unconsciousness to the environment. Sleep occurs in a circadian pattern (24-hour cycle) during the point of low energy and alertness. A person has reduced, selective vigilance and minimal physical activity. Sleep is a biological rhythm, occurs in cyclical stages, and is terminated by stimuli appropriate to produce arousal. Sleep is differentiated from those states of unconsciousness produced by deep anesthesia, coma, or grand mal seizures in which the reticular activating system is inactive or excessively active and in which brain activity is channeled in proper directions. However, these conditions do have characteristics similar to deep sleep.

3. **The reticular activating system (RAS) is involved in sleep production. What is the function of the RAS?**

   The RAS begins in the lower brainstem, and pathways extend to the medulla, pons, and midbrain through the hypothalamus. The RAS transmits impulses to the cortex by pathways through the hypothalamus and, more importantly, through the thalamus.

   The brainstem portion of the RAS causes generalized activation of the entire brain (cortex, thalamic, nuclei, basal ganglions, hypothalamus, other sections of the brainstem, and also the spinal cord). The RAS is considered responsible for wakefulness. The thalamic pathway has the ability to activate selected areas of the cortex and has an important role in the function of attention. A severe lesion (i.e., a brain tumor, hemorrhage, or tissue damage from an infectious organism) in the brainstem portion of the RAS below the pons produces coma, and the person is nonresponsive to normal awakening stimuli. Severe damage from the midpons upward in the RAS, including the nuclei of the raphe and locus caeruleus, may produce lethal exhaustion because of absolute inability to sleep.

4. What causes sleep?

Box 12-1 presents three explanations of what causes sleep.

Box 12-1.   Reasons for sleep

- A passive process: neurons controlling wakefulness become fatigued
- An active process: sleep centers produce sleep
- Biochemical process: neurotransmitters produce sleep

---

5. What is the physiology of the passive theory of sleep?

The RAS is established on a positive feedback theory, in which two systems work to keep the RAS active once it becomes excited. One system of positive feedback includes the stimulation of the cortex by the RAS and the return stimulation of the RAS from the excited cortex. This aspect of the theory explains why active concentration on vital data is used to try to maintain wakefulness. The second system of positive feedback includes the circular stimulation of the RAS to the cortex but stimulation also to the peripheral musculature. Only peripheral movement sends signals back to the RAS, many of which serve to stimulate it. This aspect of the theory explains why movement is used to try to maintain wakefulness.

Once an arousal signal activates the system, return signals from both areas continue to increase the level of response until the level of activity reaches neuronal saturation and stabilizes at a wakefulness plateau. This theory could explain the rapid onset of wakefulness. The theory is built on the premise that the neurons controlling wakefulness become fatigued. In this passive theory, for reasons yet to be explained, neurons become fatigued after 16 hours of wakefulness and decrease the cortical and peripheral stimulation. The decrease in activity of one neuron reduces the excitability of all the others so that at some point the feedback activity is not strong enough to maintain excitability in the RAS. Thus gradual drowsiness leads finally to an abrupt change from wakefulness to sleep. The cause of the change in the neuronal excitability may be due to some environmental change created by a chemical, such as secretion of a neurotransmitter substance. If this theory proved true, then it would support one of the other theories to explain the onset of sleep. See Figure 12-1.

6. What is the physiology of the active theory of sleep?

The theory that presents sleep as an active process postulates that areas of the brain that are considered to be sleep centers, when activated, produce inhibition of the RAS. These sleep centers include three identified areas:
- Rostral tracts in the brainstem, located bilaterally in the pons
- Diffuse nuclei of the thalamus
- A region between the hypothalamus and the supraorbital areas of the frontal lobes

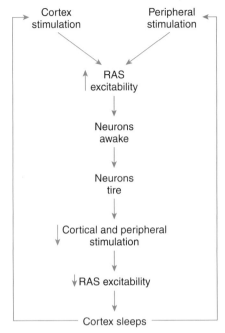

Figure 12-1. Passive theory of sleep. *RAS,* Reticular activating system.

This active theory of sleep is supported by the fact that stimulation in these areas in the same frequency as alpha brain waves produces sleep. See Figure 12-2.

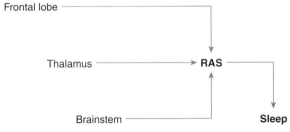
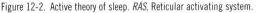

Figure 12-2. Active theory of sleep. *RAS,* Reticular activating system.

7. **What is the physiology of the biochemical theory of sleep?**

The biochemical theory of sleep production has evolved from the discovery of a small polypeptide present in the cerebrospinal fluid from animals kept awake for days. When this polypeptide is injected into the cerebral ventricular system of another animal, sleep results. In addition, the nuclei of raphe in the midline of the brainstem contain a neuronal system that secretes serotonin into the RAS, producing slow wave sleep (discussion to follow). What stimulates the secretion has not been explained.

Lastly, the locus caeruleus, located bilaterally in the upper middle pons contains a neuronal system that secretes norepinephrine, which causes the RAS to produce paradoxical sleep, also called rapid eye movement (REM) sleep. Once again, the mechanisms triggering the locus caeruleus to secrete are unknown. Studies in human beings have begun to suggest more recently the existence of an unexplained role reversal of these substances. Evidence indicates that the higher the serotonin level and the lower the noradrenaline level, the greater the amount of REM sleep.

8. What are the types of sleep?

The two types of sleep are (1) paradoxical or REM sleep and (2) sleep resulting from decreased activity of the RAS; that is, slow wave, quiescent (quiet), or non–rapid eye movement (NREM) sleep.

9. How is paradoxical, or REM, sleep described?

Paradoxical sleep, or REM sleep, occurs during peaks of periodic excitability cycles, occurring about every 90 minutes in the RAS. Rapid eye movement sleep time is about 25% of total sleep time. First decreased activity and then increased activity occur, cycling throughout the 24-hour period. This greater and lesser excitability has been demonstrated during wakefulness and during sleep. This period of RAS activity is superimposed over a sleep state, causing vivid, full-color, emotionally charged dreaming that may be bizarre. This period of sleep also has an auditory component but is not enough to wake the person. Nightmares occur during this stage.

Another proposal is that this RAS activity also stimulates the bulboreticular inhibitory area in the lower brainstem, which explains the depressed motor function of the cord during REM. The electromyogram displays almost flat muscle tone. The neurons in the brainstem and spinal cord have been described as hyperpolarized at this time, meaning they are overexcited and subsequently unable to transmit impulses. Although immobility, much like paralysis, exists in the skeletal muscles, cerebral activity generally increases. Cerebral metabolism and blood flow increase, and the electrooculogram shows rapid, darting eye movements. The sympathetic branch of the autonomic system is stimulated, thereby increasing cardiac output, blood pressure, and heart rate to a point that may surpass waking values. The heart rhythm may become erratic.

Respiratory rates are erratic and highly variable, with oxygen consumption and body temperature higher than during quiescent or NREM sleep. The physiological basis for the increased oxygen consumption during a period when skeletal muscle is paralyzed is the excessive cerebral activity. Respiratory drive is reduced, responsiveness to hypoxia and hypercarbia are reduced, and arousal response to these conditions and laryngeal stimulation are blunted.

Central and obstructive apnea can occur during this type sleep. The electroencephalogram shows beta waves that are similar to waves typical of wakefulness. Gastric secretions increase. In a sense the patient is experiencing brain activity of wakefulness but is asleep. Rapid eye movement sleep is believed to be important in the maintenance of mental-emotional equilibrium and that input from the previous day is sorted, stored in memory or cleared, and psychological concerns are dealt with adequately to clear the phenomena from the conscious level.

10. How is slow wave, or NREM, sleep described?

Most sleep (75%) during a night is slow wave, or deep restful, quiescent, dreamless sleep. During this type of sleep, vascular tone, blood pressure, pulse rate, respiratory rate, metabolic rate, and muscular tone are decreased. Sympathetic activity decreases, and parasympathetic activity increases to some extent with gastrointestinal tract activity increased and skin vessels dilated.

Non–rapid eye movement sleep is subdivided into four stages according to depth, as presented in Box 12-2.

Box 12-2. Stages of non–rapid eye movement sleep

- The individual progresses from wakefulness to **stage I** in which muscle relaxation occurs. Alpha rhythm gives way to low-voltage theta waves in this transitional stage. Tests indicate that responses are slower and intellectual acuity is decreased. This stage lasts between 30 seconds and 7 minutes. If asked, the individual will deny being asleep. About 5% of total sleep time is spent in this transition stage.
- The individual enters **stage II** or light sleep, where the background of theta waves is interspersed with alpha sleep spindles and high-voltage K complexes. The patient still is aroused easily, although the patient is more relaxed. Slow, rolling eye movement of stage I disappears. Stage II occurs before and after rapid eye movement sleep; 50% of sleep occurs in this stage.
- In **stage III,** relaxation continues with slowing of functions that are innervated by the sympathetic system (i.e., decreased cardiac and respiratory rates, metabolic rate, blood pressure, body temperature). Large, slow, low-frequency delta waves occupy 20% to 40% of the sleep activity. The individual is more difficult to awaken. About 10% of sleep time occurs in this stage.
- **Stage IV** is deep sleep with delta waves predominating (50% or more) on the electroencephalogram. The individual is profoundly relaxed, rarely moves, and is difficult to arouse. During this stage parasomnias (i.e., somnambulism [sleepwalking], enuresis [bed-wetting], and night terrors) occur. Dreams may occur that are realistic but unemotional and difficult to recall. About 10% of sleep time occurs in this stage. Growth hormone is secreted consistently by the anterior pituitary during the reduced availability of fuel and therefore serves as an anabolic state for tissue formation. Cerebral blood flow is reduced.

The process of progressing from wakefulness to stage IV takes about 20 to 30 minutes. The stages then are reversed slowly, taking 60 to 90 minutes to ascend back to Stage II. The usual pattern during an uninterrupted night will be several cycles of I, II, III, IV, III, II, REM, II, III, IV, III, II, REM, II, III, IV. The cycle progresses to I periodically, depending on age of the patient, varying from 4 times in children to 14 times in elders during a 7-hour sleep period. Children actually may awaken twice, whereas elders may awaken 11 times.

11. How does REM sleep relate to the stages of NREM sleep?

At the point in the cycle of ascension toward light sleep from slow wave sleep when stage II has been reached, the other type of sleep—paradoxical or REM sleep—occurs. This type of sleep never occurs alone but is superimposed on NREM sleep. The paradoxical episodes occur about every 90 minutes and last from 5 to 20 minutes, depending on the fatigue of the individual. The saw-tooth waves on the electroencephalogram are unique to REM sleep. Muscle tone is nearly absent or absent, yet phasic rapid eye movement occurs. Penile tumescence or clitoral engorgement, increased brain temperature, increased blood pressure, tachycardia, vasoconstriction, and increased oxygen consumption occur during this stage as phasic events. However, hypotension, brachycardia, loss of deep tendon reflexes, decreased tones in smooth muscles, and vasodilation also occur during tonic events in REM. With extreme fatigue, the episodes are extremely short or absent. As the person becomes more rested, the duration of these episodes increases.

12. What is rebound sleep?

If the patient has been deprived of stage IV NREM or REM sleep, a compensatory mechanism, or rebound, occurs. In rebound sleep, during the next subsequent sleep period, the percentage of total sleep time is greatly increased in the stage of sleep that was deprived.

13. What is included in a polysomnogram?

Research done with a polysomnogram to monitor sleep has provided accurate data related to the four stages of NREM sleep and REM sleep. A polysomnogram includes the electroencephalogram, electrooculogram, and electromyelogram (through electrodes on the chin). Other devices to measure respiratory effort and airflow, leg movements, oxygen saturation, heart activity, and penile tumescence (erection) may be used. The electroencephalogram displays alpha waves, which are slow and shallow during presleep and in "sleep spindles" in stage II. Stage I slows to theta rhythm; delta waves, the wide and slow waves, are characteristic of deeper sleep in stages III and IV.

14. What are the objective signs and subjective account for each of the stages of sleep?

Table 12-1 presents the signs and patient descriptions for each stage of sleep.

15. What is the purpose of sleep?

Sleep is postulated to be the time allowed to the central nervous system to evaluate its status and to rebalance its various activities, storing input into memory. Without this time to "regroup," as in prolonged wakefulness, difficulty in cerebration occurs,

Table 12-1. **Comparison of stages of sleep**

Type of sleep	Behaviors and findings	Report of client
Non–rapid eye movement sleep stages		
I	Slow, rolling, eye movements; easily awakened (transition state); involuntary jerking may occur; alpha waves to theta waves	Somewhat aware of surroundings, fleeting thoughts, floating sensation; would deny being asleep if awakened
II	Relaxed; light sleep; fairly easily aroused; respirations more even and regular; pulse slowing; theta waves with alpha "sleep spindles" and K complexes	Unaware of surroundings; able to recall fragmented thoughts if awakened
III	Deeper, quiet sleep; harder to awaken; vital signs decreased; beginning of anabolic state for protein synthesis; delta waves (20%-40%)	Unaware of surroundings; rarely able to recall thoughts of dreams if awakened
IV	Profound sleep providing essential rest for physical health; awakened only with difficulty; if parasomnias occur, occur in this stage (enuresis, somnambulism, night terrors); normally, little movement; metabolism approaches basal level, but with anabolism of protein, though growth hormone secretions occur; delta waves (50%)	Would report having slept well if awakened; dreams may be recalled, but are realistic and factual in nature, with no exciting effect
Rapid eye movement sleep		
	Body muscles atonic (like paralysis), but some muscle twitching may occur; rapid, darting eye movements; total atony of jaw; penile erection in male of any age; oxygen consumption increased but breathing is decreased; autonomic activity is increased; vital signs fluctuate; respiratory drive reduced (lack of response to P_{CO_2}) pulse may be irregular; temperature varies; gastric secretions increased; awakened with extreme difficulty	Dreaming occurs during 80%-85% of the time spent asleep in this stage; dreams may or may not be remembered, but if so, they are vivid and exciting to all senses and may be bizarre

accompanied by irritability and finally psychosis. Box 12-3 presents processes occurring during sleep.

Box 12-3.   Processes occurring during sleep

- Reduction of stress on pulmonary, cardiovascular, nervous, endocrine, and excretory systems and reduction of anxiety and tension
- Formation of new neuronal connections and repair and reorganization of cells and functions in the nervous system
- Nourishment, growth, and repair of body cells, release of hormones, and biochemical changes in the body

---

16. How do the requirements for sleep vary among age groups?

Table 12-2 presents the comparison of sleep requirements through the life span.

Table 12-2.   Hours of sleep needed daily according to age groups and percentage of REM sleep for each age group

Age	Hours of sleep needed daily	REM sleep (%)
Newborn	16	50
1 year	14-15	35
Toddler	12, plus naps during the day	25
Preschool	11-12	20
6-11 years	10-11	18.5 (more stages III and IV than adult)
Adolescent	8.5	20 (stages III and IV begin to decrease)
Adult	6-7.75	19-22
Elderly	5.75 (napping returns) Longer sleep latency, more awakenings during night; sleeping only 70%-80% of the time while in bed; earlier rising	15 (stages III and IV are greatly decreased; may be totally absent)

REM, rapid eye movement.

17. What factors, besides age, influence sleep?

Factors that influence sleep include
- Environment
- Interference with circadian rhythm

- Emotional and physical stimulation
- Bedtime rituals
- The patient's expectations
- Fatigue
- Illness
- Medications

18. How does environment influence sleep?

An environment that is familiar and to which the person is accustomed enhances sleep. A strange bed or pillow; different lighting through windows; uncontrolled temperature of a new room, which differs from the usual; different sounds; and sleeping alone when used to sleeping with another or sleeping with a different person can cause sleep disturbances.

19. What factors are most likely to interfere with circadian rhythm?

A change or interruption in accustomed sleep times can make sleep difficult. Traveling across time zones or working during usual sleep times can produce this desynchronization. Most persons sleep at night. Patients having to resynchronize their sleep pattern to work at night require 3 to 5 days to stabilize. These patients can experience chronic fatigue because they must change sleep patterns constantly on nights off.

20. What types of emotional and physical stimulation should one avoid?

Emotional and physical stimulation before sleep time can prevent sleep. A calm time with the patient in a relaxed state needs to occur to create a transition from wakefulness to sleep. Leaving a shift in the emergency department or hours of vigorous dancing or a terrible argument requires a calming time before sleep can occur.

21. What are some bedtime rituals that enhance sleep?

Bedtime rituals assist the individual to prepare mentally for sleep. If hair brushing, reading, a bath, or a light snack is usual and is prevented, sleep latency (the time spent going to sleep) may be increased. What the ritual entails is not important, but rather that the activity is important to the patient to become relaxed enough to go to sleep.

22. How does fatigue influence sleep?

Fatigue promotes sleep when the degree is within a usual range. Complete exhaustion is detrimental and discourages sleep, severely decreasing REM sleep. Lack of sleep produces a tiredness that prevents normal activities; too much sleep can prevent sleep from occurring at the usual time and can leave the individual with a feeling of tiredness throughout wakefulness.

23. How do the client's expectations related to sleep influence sleep?

The client's expectations of either staying awake or hurrying to fall asleep impact sleep. If it is important to remain awake for some event or responsibility, such as caring for another or working, sleep onset is delayed until this expectation is relaxed.

24. What effect does illness, particularly hospitalized illness, have on sleep?

Illness and stress increase sleep needs. Patients hospitalized for these problems, and particularly those who require surgery or intensive care, have environmental factors that prevent and disturb this needed sleep. Comfort is a necessity for sleep and yet pain, unusual or uncomfortable positions, and discomfort from devices (i.e., intravenous catheter or ventilator) are frequently present in illness.

Patients having an exacerbation that requires care in an intensive care unit are prime candidates for sleep deprivation, sometimes to the point of having behavioral manifestations similar to psychosis, with hallucinations, delusions, alterations in cognition, mood, and affect. The constant monitoring, noise from alarms and machines, frequent invasive procedures, continual medications, and constant 24-hour care with lights required creates high stress and exhaustion. Pain is frequently present that prevents sleep. Disorders that affect the central nervous system may disturb the sleep-wake cycle as well.

25. What effect do medications that affect sleep have on the quality of sleep?

Medications influence sleep, and for that reason patients are given tranquilizers and sedatives for the specific purpose of enhancing sleep. Hypnotics and barbiturates increase slow wave sleep but decrease REM sleep. Stimulants, such as amphetamines, methylphenidate (Ritalin), and caffeine discourage sleep. Tricyclic antidepressants decrease stage IV sleep. Alcohol, a depressant, decreases REM sleep and produces REM rebound. Withdrawal of drugs that have decreased REM sleep for a prolonged period frequently may cause nightmares during REM rebound.

26. How does sleep influence the status of a patient's medical disorder?

Although sleep itself does not cause disease and disorders, the changes that occur during sleep may allow manifestations of disorders to present more readily than during wakefulness. During the longer REM sleep periods that occur toward the end of the night, dangerous problems such as cardiac arrhythmias, angina, myocardial infarctions, and strokes may occur during sleep. Attacks of asthma frequently occur at night, especially in early morning during stage II sleep. The pain experienced by patients with duodenal ulcers is more intense at night, especially during the peak of REM sleep from 1 to 3 AM because of increased gastric secretions that may be 3 to 20 times that in a normal person. Patients with hypothyroidism remain drowsy all the time because they mainly have stage I and II sleep only. Patients with chronic lung disorders may have the condition worsened during REM sleep and generally suffer from sleep deprivation that in turn worsens the condition because of decreased respiratory drive. Studies indicate that increased serum endorphin concentration from sleep loss produces this blunted ventilatory drive.

Depression, as well as other mental illnesses, change the sleeping pattern. Assessment of these changes may indicate the type of progression of the disease to expect such as in schizophrenia or organic brain syndrome. Organic brain disturbances such as encephalitis may produce reversal of the sleep pattern, with wakefulness at night and sleep during the day. Seizures frequently occur at night in some types of epilepsy; the activity is correlated with a decrease in inhibiting impulses that normally prevent pyramidal discharges. Vascular headaches normally begin in early morning just before waking.

27. Why are sleep disorders important to rehabilitation nurses?

Sleep disorders are important to rehabilitation nurses because about 60 million Americans have chronic insomnia, with women and older adults more frequently affected. Estimated direct costs are reported to be more than $15.4 billion in the United States. These patients also have been reported to have 2.5 as many traffic accidents as those without insomnia. Additionally, about 135,000 Americans have narcolepsy, who are diagnosed between 15 and 30 years of age, which frequently leads to disability.

28. What are the types of sleep disorders?

Table 12-3 presents the type of sleep disorders and their characteristics.

Table 12-3. Sleep disorders

Category	Specific disorder	Characteristic
Disorders of initiating and maintaining sleep	Insomnias	Difficulty falling asleep, frequent wakefulness for long periods or awakening too early
Disorders of excessive somnolence	Hypersomnias • Sleep apnea syndrome (18 million Americans)	*Central:* respiratory effort lacking; respiration ceases *Obstructive:* oropharyngeal airway collapses and occludes airway *Mixed:* combination of central and obstructive
	• Narcolepsy	Rapid eye movement (REM) sleep stage intruding into wakefulness, producing sleep attacks, cataplexy (muscle atony), sleep paralysis, and hypnagogic hallucinations; disturbed nocturnal sleep; sleep attack; daytime sleepiness
	• Nocturnal myoclonus	Twitching of legs; frequency: every 20 to 40 seconds; duration: 5 minutes to 2 hours
Disorders related to sleep stages or partial arousals	Parasomnias	Enuresis, night terror, and somnambulism (sleepwalking) occur during delta wage sleep (stages III and IV). Violent sleep (REM sleep behavior disorder) Sleep paralysis, nightmares (REM)

29. The major sleep disorder patients complain of is insomnia. How is insomnia described?

Insomnia is the most common problem related to sleep, with about 30% of the population complaining of the condition. The problem intensifies with age, but the lifestyle, background, and personality factors profoundly influence the development of insomnia. Patients with insomnia are characteristically more tense, anxious, and worried than those without insomnia. The problem is totally subjective, being described as the inability to fall asleep or to stay asleep according to the person's expectations. Regardless of the amount of time spent sleeping, the condition is not a problem unless the person perceives it as such. Some persons are delighted to have much more time available for activities by sleeping only a fraction of the time that others sleep and do not perceive themselves as having any problems.

Insomnia generally is precipitated by psychological disturbances such as bereavement, work concerns, or marital or financial stresses. Physical illness also may cause insomnia. The quality of sleep of insomniacs is poor in that they spend more time in stages I and II and have less REM. Their body functions do not decrease to the same level as a normal sleeper.

In addition, a similar category of pseudoinsomnia occurs in which the patients actually sleep an adequate amount of time but spend a large percent of sleep time in REM, dreaming they are awake. These persons then believe that they are in need of medical assistance to sleep normally.

30. How should the health care provider treat insomnia?

The treatment for insomnia must be directed toward the cause. Drug therapy with short-acting hypnotics may not be effective over a long period and is not the treatment of choice. In fact, some sedatives such as barbiturates disturb sleep even further with REM sleep deprivation. The patient must be assisted to evaluate any emotional problems and set realistic goals to alleviate the stress. If an emotional problem exists, relaxation training, biofeedback, or hypnosis may be useful to improve sleep. The patient must not depend on drugs alone. The patient may use benzodiazepines intermittently over a period of time to assist with the problem, but most drugs lose their effectiveness if used more than 2 weeks.

A common approach to management of insomnia is to increase physical activity during waking hours with a planned exercise pattern several hours before bedtime to promote muscle relaxation. In addition, the ingestion of L-tryptophan before retiring, an amino acid found in many high-protein foods such as milk, tends to reduce sleep latency (shorten the period of time required to fall asleep). This supports the approach of drinking warm milk to promote sleep. Reducing excitement during the evening and performing a satisfying bedtime ritual may be helpful in promoting sleep.

31. **What measures can the nurse recommend for improving sleep?**

The nurse may refer the patient to a sleep clinic for evaluation if the problem is severe. Depending on the patient's complaints, general recommendations might include the activities described in Box 12-4.

Box 12-4.   Measures for improving sleep

- Avoid afternoon naps (increases non–rapid eye movement sleep and may interfere with nighttime sleep).
- Take 20- to 40-minute morning naps (replenishes rapid eye movement sleep).
- Control pain before bedtime.
- Encourage the patient to join a self-help group.
- Remind the patient to limit the bed to sleeping (and sex) only.
- Set a regular bedtime.
- Do relaxing activities in the evening: a relaxing walk, warm bath, soothing music, warm milk.
- Do not go to bed hungry but eat only a light snack.
- Get up out of bed if not asleep in 15 minutes and read.
- Keep the temperature of the room cool.
- Eliminate use of caffeine, tobacco, alcohol, and psychoactive drugs.
- Move clock so that one cannot see the time.
- Avoid hypnotics.
- Increase exercise during the day.
- Consider aromatherapy.
- Use stress-reduction tapes.
- Use relaxation tapes.
- Reduce fluid intake after dinner.
- Avoid spicy foods.
- Avoid sleeping excessively on weekends.
- Do not go to bed until sleepy.

---

32. **What is the effect of sleep deprivation?**

Because sleep generally is considered to be an integrative and restorative process, the lack of sleep may cause physical symptoms and changes in behaviors. Sleep deprivation results when periods of sleep are interrupted frequently, causing deprivation of the REM stage. A cycle of sleep measured from REM stage to REM stage requires from 90 to 100 minutes. Rapid eye movement sleep is necessary for mental restoration and occurs later in the sleep cycle. During REM sleep, the patient not only dreams but also is able to review the events of the day, clear out nonessential data, and integrate other information into the storage system of the brain. This sleep is critical for memory and psychological adaptation. Processes may be reviewed and refined for up to 3 years before being filed finally into memory.

When REM sleep is lost, the person may experience anxiety, irritability, lack of alertness, poor judgment, apathy, depression, and decreased tolerance to pain or discomfort. Prolonged REM deprivation may lead to confusion, disorientation, and hallucinations. Non-REM sleep deprivation may produce neurofibrositis, a neuromuscular arthritic syndrome, and the person is very sleepy during waking hours.

An overall sleep loss creates the symptoms described in Box 12-5.

Box 12-5.   Symptoms produced by sleep loss

- Physical exhaustion
- General fatigue
- Labile emotional states
- Disruption of metabolic function
- Increased sensitivity to pain and discomfort
- Impaired ventilatory responsiveness to hypercapnia and hypoxia
- Lapses in attention and inability to concentrate
- Loss of memory
- Decreased intellectual function
- Blurred vision
- Itching eyes
- Nausea
- Headache
- Paresthesias and unsteadiness
- Loss of ability to perform tasks normally

---

33. **When a patient complains of chronic sleep disruption, what should the rehabilitation nurse include in the assessment?**

A detailed interview is required, during which the nurse takes a general health history, including medication history, and performs a complete physical examination. Evaluation of upper airway patency is important. The nurse may order specific blood work, pulmonary studies, and psychological inventories. Box 12-6 lists specific information needed for a sleep assessment.

34. **What is hypersomnia?**

Hypersomnia is the tendency to sleep excessively. The patient has difficulty becoming alert and is confused on awakening. The patient may accept the behavior as a normal pattern. The behavior may be periodic or chronic and may be a mechanism of escape from psychological stressors. Depression may be an underlying mechanism and may be improved with tricyclic antidepressants such as imipramine (Tofranil).

Box 12-6. **Information needed for a sleep assessment**

1. Relaxation methods
2. Times favored for relaxation
3. Sleep pattern
   - Time of sleep; number of hours
   - Awakenings during sleep: number and reason
   - Time and number of naps taken during day
4. Sleep environment
   - Type of bed
   - Amount of cover
   - Number of pillows
   - Amount of light
   - Noise
   - Persons in the room
   - Temperature of the room
5. Bedtime routine
6. Sedatives used
7. Beliefs about sleep
8. Characteristics of the patient's lifestyle (work, home, school, leisure)
9. Caffeine intake
10. Alcohol use
11. Tobacco use
12. Living conditions
13. Severity of the complaint
14. Duration of the problem
15. Symptoms that occur during sleep
16. Symptoms that occur during nocturnal awakenings
17. Patient's perception of the cause
18. Degree of daytime impairment
19. Corroboration from sleep partner

Hypersomnia frequently occurs with eating disorders and morbid obesity, as is seen in the pickwickian syndrome (named for the fat boy in Charles Dickens' *The Pickwick Papers*). This relationship has led to the thought that an altered hypothalamic function, the hunger-satiety center, also may produce hypersomnias. Evidence exists of abuse of alcohol and tobacco in many of these same patients, which may intensify the problem. The patient remains sleepy all the time and will fall asleep when at rest, sleeping several hours if not awakened. The patient is difficult to arouse and may be confused on awakening.

35. What is sleep apnea?

Sleep apnea is the most frequent cause of hypersomnia. Sleep apnea is a transient cessation of breathing during sleep. In a normal individual a 5- to 10-second episode may occur as often as 3 times a night. In a patient with sleep apnea episodes from 15 seconds to 2 minutes occur hundreds of times per night.

The two types of sleep apnea are central and obstructive. Central apnea may result from a REM-related failure in the brainstem respiratory drive center because of hyperpolarization of the brainstem neurons. No innervation is sent to the diaphragm; therefore it becomes immobile and causes a peaceful cessation of breathing. These apneic periods occur during REM sleep.

Obstructive apnea occurs during NREM and REM sleep when the muscles that normally maintain a patent airway become hypotonic (most pronounced in REM sleep), causing the negative pressure needed to permit air to flow in and out to increase steadily as this pressure increases, and the airway further lengthens and narrows, causing greater resistance to airflow. Most patients are obese males whose added weight further increases airflow resistance. The intense negative pressure results in collapse of the upper airway, but the patient ceases to breathe only after heavy labored snoring, gasping, and grunting.

The physiological changes occurring as a result of sleep apnea are greater in obstructive apnea and depend on the number and duration of apneic events. With cessation of airflow, arterial blood becomes desaturated, resulting in hypoxemia. The severely decreased oxygen content in the blood reaching the respiratory center in the brainstem stimulates arousal, removing the sleep-related hypotonia and allowing stimulation of the diaphragm to move air once again. Patients suffering from sleep apnea generally have chronic systemic and pulmonary hypertension. Cardiac arrhythmias frequently occur during apneic events. The high negative pressure may stimulate the vagus nerve and result in second-degree heart block or cardiac arrest.

36. How does the health care provider treat sleep apnea?

The treatment of choice to manage this problem is the use of continuous positive alveolar pressure ventilation during sleep to prevent airway collapse. Other approaches include use of tricyclic antidepressants, such as protriptyline, to reduce REM sleep, cessation of excessive alcohol and tobacco use, and weight loss. The approaches are not greatly effective. Patients may need to consider surgery if they have large tonsils or narrow airway inlets. The treatment of choice some years ago was a tracheostomy and still may be used in some individuals.

37. What is narcolepsy?

Narcolepsy has a prevalence of approximately 1:1000 population with the onset in 75% of the cases occurring before age 30. Evidence indicates a much greater risk for the disease if it is present in other members of a family. Narcolepsy is a syndrome of four symptoms:
- *Sleep attacks* are the most important. These attacks are brief (5 to 10 minutes), irresistible episodes of sleep that may occur many times a day when sensory stimulation is decreased, regardless of the situation. The individual feels refreshed on awakening.

- *Hypnagogic hallucinations* are vivid auditory or visual hallucinations occurring on awakening. Although the person is aware of the surroundings, the person feels as if experiencing a "waking dream."
- *Cataplexy* is a sudden relaxation of muscle tone that causes the person to slump or fall. The response usually is precipitated by an emotion such as laughing. The person remains conscious during the response.
- *Sleep paralysis* is a brief (1 minute or less) period on awakening in which the person is unable to move. Even though the episodes may be frequent, the person is frightened each time. The attack is terminated instantly if the person is stimulated gently as by a touch.

This syndrome of symptoms related to narcolepsy would be considered a normal part of REM sleep, but it occurs during wakefulness. When the person experiences all the symptoms described, the sleep attacks are typical of REM sleep in that the person dreams vividly (hypnagogic hallucinations) and motor inhibition is apparent (cataplexy and sleep paralysis).

38. How does the health care provider treat narcolepsy?

The management of narcolepsy requires constant support by the patient's family, friends, and employer until a satisfactory therapy can be found. During this period, the patient should not drive. Amphetamines such as dextroamphetamine were used previously, but the addictive response outweighed the effective control of the disorder. Methylphenidate (Ritalin) is often effective as a stimulant to abort the sleep attacks. Imipramine (Tofranil) or monoamine oxidase inhibitors may help the cataplexy, sleep paralysis, and hypnagogic hallucinations. Propranolol (Inderal) or protriptyline (Vivactil) may be used if imipramine is not effective, for all these drugs reduce REM sleep. Experimentation continues with other medications such as γ-hydroxybutyrate, which may be effective in treating narcolepsy.

39. What is nocturnal myoclonus?

Normal individuals experience myoclonic jerks rarely as the gradual progression of drowsiness changes abruptly to sleep. The jerk actually may arouse the person to wakefulness. Nocturnal myoclonus, characterized by repetitive contractions of the leg muscles, may cause excessive daytime drowsiness resulting from insomnia. The stereotypical twitches may occur every 20 to 40 seconds for periods lasting from 5 minutes to 2 hours. The cause has not been determined clearly; therefore treatment is not well established. Some patients have responded to clonazepam (Klonopin) or carbamazepine (Tegretol), even though the condition is not a seizure disorder.

40. How is enuresis, an important parasomnia, described?

Enuresis (bed-wetting) is frequent in childhood, but some incidence still occurs in adulthood. Enuresis may be due to an organic cause relative to the urinary tract, such as a hypertonic bladder, or may be psychogenic. Patients with psychogenic enuresis (enuresis from psychological causes) may have long, dry periods, with the problem occurring during bouts of insomnia (with an organic cause), whereas primary enuresis continues from infancy. Enuresis usually occurs in the first third of the night and begins with stage IV of NREM sleep. When the sleep pattern reverts to stage I or II, micturition occurs.

41. How can the rehabilitation nurse manage enuresis?

The treatment depends on the underlying cause. If an organic cause is found and treated, the problem will subside. If the problem has no organic basis, family education is the highest priority, along with support for the patient. The nurse must take care to maintain a positive self-image for the patient during the problem period. Lack of empathy from loved ones may cause psychological trauma that worsens the condition.

Physical measures include a rigid pattern of fluid intake with restriction in the evening. Measuring the time the patient can extend the period between voidings during the day is another method that helps expand the bladder capacity and reduce irritability. Setting an alarm to get up during the night to empty the bladder sometimes helps. The use of antidepressants, such as imipramine or amitriptyline, may prevent stage IV sleep and abort the incident, generally with no ill effects. Another measure may be the use of a device that provides a mild shock when a drop of urine touches a pad under the patient. This method has proved effective in a high percentage of cases within a few months. The nurse must provide much support, explanation, and encouragement during the use of this equipment.

42. What is a night terror?

A night terror ("pavor nocturnus") is a parasomnia in which the patient suddenly awakens from stage IV NREM sleep, usually about an hour after falling asleep, with no memory of the event, but with intense anxiety. The patient is difficult to arouse completely, but the electroencephalogram pattern has alpha waves of a normal waking pattern. The patient is mobile, has terrified screams, has autonomic stimulation that accompanies intense fear, and respiratory restriction from the sense of a tight band around the chest and a sense of impending doom.

43. How can the rehabilitation nurse manage night terrors?

Treatment includes support and explanation because no recall of a dream exists, and the patient feels threatened for his or her life and a sense of lasting dread remains. In some instances, medications, such as strong hypnotics, may be impairing the arousal mechanism and should be evaluated. The nurse should consider a psychopathological cause if no organic cause is apparent.

44. How is nightmare described?

The parasomnia nightmare ("incubus") is a frightening dream in REM stage sleep that produces arousal. The patient recalls the dream vividly and understands the cause for the fright.

45. **What management plan should the nurse suggest?**

Treatment includes offering support and understanding to the patient who experiences nightmares frequently. Nightmares are not unusual in a patient who has REM sleep suppressed by medication or other factors and is in a withdrawal state with rebound REM sleep. If the nightmares are persistent, a psychological evaluation may be needed. If medications that must be continued for concurrent medical problems are increasing the dreaming, such as propranolol or L-dopa, then diazepam or flurazepam may be used to counteract their effect. One should not use barbiturates, which may intensify the problem.

46. **How can somnambulism be explained?**

Somnambulism (sleepwalking) may be a familial parasomnia and may be accompanied by enuresis and night terrors. Generally the problem is more frequent in children from ages 4 to 12. This behavior occurs entirely in stage IV NREM sleep and lasts about 10 minutes. Adults may have an underlying psychological problem. When awakened, the patient will have no recall of the event.

47. **How does the rehabilitation nurse manage sleepwalking?**

Although the patient perceives enough of the environment to avoid persons and objects, management still focuses on providing safety from falls or areas of danger. Latches on doors and windows that are not easily accessible often are used. A dose of amitriptyline nightly may be of some value to some patients. In general, benzodiazepines are the best treatment because they suppress stage IV sleep.

48. **What is violent sleep?**

One of the less common but extremely important parasomnias, violent sleep is an REM behavior disorder. This disorder causes violent dream reenactment in the form of aggressive behavior that can lead to serious injury to the patient or the bed partner. The bed partner is in grave danger of being battered or suffocated. The disorder generally affects middle-aged men. The violence emerges in the middle and final third of the night, often during nightmares in which the patient is being attacked. Patients awaken believing they have slept well, and they feel rested.

The disorder is defined by intermittent loss of electromyographic atonia with shouting, flailing, grabbing, reaching, body jerking during REM, and limb twitching during NREM. Stages III and IV of NREM are increased. An underlying neurological disorder may be the cause (up to 40%); therefore a neurological evaluation is necessary. Some patients do not have the aggressive behavior but instead wake up frequently during dreams and have trouble falling back asleep. A third group just complains of having frightening nightmares and twitching of their arms and legs.

49. What is the treatment for violent sleep?

The nurse should refer the patient to a sleep-disorder center for evaluation. Once diagnosed, clonazepam (Klonopin) 0.5 to 1.5 mg/day, given at bedtime, is effective. The drug often works the very first night. Because REM behavior disorder is a life-long progressive disorder, the patient will have to continue to use the medication. The patient should control stress because it may precipitate breakthrough episodes. The bedroom also should be made safe by moving breakables and sharp objects away from the bed and placing cushions around the bed, in case of a breakthrough.

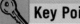 Key Points

- Sleep is thought to allow the central nervous system time to evaluate its status and rebalance, thus preventing disruption in cognition and psychosis.
- Sleep requirements vary throughout the life span.
- Illness and stress increase sleep needs. The hospital environment and discomfort can be barriers to sleep.
- Insomnia is the major sleep disorder complained of by patients.
- For the rehabilitation nurse to assess the quality and adequacy of the patient's sleep thoroughly is important.

Internet Resources

American Academy of Sleep Medicine
http://www.aasmnet.org

Mayo Clinic Sleep Disorders Center
http://www.mayohealth.org

Narcolepsy Network, Inc.
http://www.narcolepsynetwork.org

National Center for Sleep Disorders Research
http://www.nhlbi.nih.gov/about/ncsdr/index.htm

National Sleep Foundation
http://www.sleepfoundation.org

Bibliography

1. Barker E: Sleep disorders. In Barker E, editor: *Neuroscience nursing: a spectrum of care,* ed 2, St Louis, 2002, Mosby.
2. Kirkwood CK: *Treatment of insomnia,* Littleton, Colo, 2001, Medical Education Resources.
3. Rogers AE: Rhythmic alterations in consciousness: sleep. In Stewart-Amidei C, editor: *AANN's neuroscience nursing: human responses to neurologic dysfunction,* ed 2, Philadelphia, 2001, WB Saunders.
4. Zaidat OO, Lerner AJ: *The little black book of neurology,* ed 4, St Louis, 2002, Mosby.

Chapter 13

Functional Mobility: Activities of Daily Living

Susan R. Bulecza

1. What is the definition of functional assessment?

Functional assessment means the measurement of the patient's ability to interact purposefully with the environment within a given context. This definition guides the rehabilitation professional in evaluating the patient to determine ability to function in a dynamic environment by producing goal-directed behaviors to achieve optimal outcomes as independently as possible. Functional assessments also assist the rehabilitation professional in identifying patient limitations. Rehabilitation nurses have been instrumental in the development of functional assessment tools and in conducting functional assessments.

2. How are the terms *impairment, disability,* and *handicap* differentiated?

In 1980 the World Health Organization adopted the Disablement Model, which provided international definition for these terms. *Impairment* is defined as a loss of normal function or structure from psychological, physiological, or anatomical conditions that result in a temporary or permanent change in structure or function. *Disability* is the result of the impairment causing deficits that require assistance to perform essential activities of daily living. The type of assistance may be another person, adaptive equipment, or longer time frame for completion. *Handicap* refers to the inability of the patient with disability to integrate personally and socially into the community because of problems with coping, adaptation, and transition. The interrelatedness of these three outcomes can affect the patient's ability to function positively or negatively. For example, a patient with a significant impairment such as a spinal cord injury that results in major disability may have a small handicap because the patient is able to adapt and participate fully in community and social areas. Whereas, a patient with minimal impairment such as low back pain that creates minimal disability may have significant handicap because of disruption in relationships or employment.

3. What are two conceptual distinctions made in functional assessment models?

An important point for rehabilitation nurses to understand is the difference between the rehabilitation model of functional assessment, which focuses on capability or the capacity to do a task, and the psychosocial model, which focuses on the patient's behavior or what the patient actually does. Therefore if one has the capability to perform a task but does not do so, the assessment would be of behavior not capability. An important note is the role environment plays in behavior, resulting in positive or negative outcomes. So the rehabiliation nurse must control the environment as much as possible when assessing functional performance.

4. What are categorical assessment instruments?

Categorical assessment instruments assess a specific functional parameter for patients with a particular condition or disease. The Glasgow Coma Scale and muscle strength scale are examples of categorical assessment instruments.

5. What are some activities of daily living assessment scales?

The following are activities of daily living assessment scales:
1. Barthel Index: Assesses 10 areas of functional ability and uses a 3-point scale for each area with a total assessment score determined and ranked on a scale of 0 to 100. Areas assessed are
   • Feeding
   • Grooming
   • Bathing
   • Stairs
   • Bladder control
   • Wheelchair transfer
   • Toilet transfer
   • Level walking
   • Dressing
   • Bowel control
2. Katz Index: Assesses six areas of function; each area is rated as dependent or independent. Overall functional status is ranked as A to G based on the number of areas independent or dependent, with A as fully independent. Areas assessed are
   • Bathing
   • Toileting
   • Continence
   • Dressing
   • Transfers
   • Feeding
3. Kenny Self-Care Evaluation: Assesses six areas of function, with each area scored using a 5-point scale. Total score is determined and ranked on scale of 0 to 24, with 24 being independent. Areas assessed are
   • Bed mobility
   • Transfers
   • Locomotion
   • Dressing
   • Personal hygiene
   • Feeding activities

6. What are other tools used in functional assessment?

The following are other functional assessment tools:
1. PULSES Profile
   - Measures ability to use all four extremities in performing activities independently.
   - Takes into consideration the presence of disease and patient's ability to perceive correctly and respond appropriately in situations.
   - Evaluates six areas:
     1. **Physical** conditioning
     2. **Upper** limb functions
     3. **Lower** limb functions
     4. **Sensory** components
     5. **Excretory** function
     6. **Situation** factors
   - Uses negative scoring; a lower score equals more independence.
   - Uses a 4-point scale, with 1 as independent.
2. Level of Rehabilitation Scale
   - Adapted from Functional Life Scale.
   - Assesses five functional categories:
     1. Cognition
     2. Activities of daily living
     3. Activities in the home
     4. Outside activities
     5. Social interactions
   - Uses a 5-point scale (0 to 4); 4 equals normal performance.
3. Uniform Data System for Medical Rehabilitation Functional Independence Measures (UDSMRFIM)
   - Measures effect of physical and psychosocial disabilities on function.
   - Assesses 18 functional items using a 7-point scale; 1 equals dependent, unsafe to perform, or not performed.
   - Covers six categories:
     1. Self-care
     2. Sphincter control
     3. Transfers
     4. Locomotion
     5. Communication
     6. Social cognition
   - Requires passing of a credentialing test to be able to administer.
   - Can be administered by credentialed person from any discipline.
   - Considered a global assessment tool.
   - Endorsed by Association of Rehabilitation Nurses because it provides a uniform framework for evaluation across disciplines.
4. Functional Assessment Measure
   - Measures high-level cognitive function following brain injury.
   - Assesses 12 areas:
     1. Swallowing
     2. Community access

3. Writing
4. Intelligibility
5. Adjustment to limitations
6. Attention
7. Car transfers
8. Reading
9. Speech
10. Emotional status
11. Employability
12. Safety judgment

5. Levels of Cognitive Functioning Assessment Scale (LOCFAS; see Appendix 1). Box 13-1 provides an overview.

Box 13-1.   Levels of Cognitive Functioning Assessment Scale (LOCFAS) overview

1. This cognitive assessment tool, derived from the first five levels of the Rancho Los Amigos Levels of Cognitive Functioning instrument, assesses patient's behavior through observation when the patient is unable or unwilling to participate in testing.
2. The tool is designed for ongoing assessment to measure improvement and identify appropriate interventions for patients with low level of responsivity.
3. Ten subcategories are assessed with each level:
   - Attention to environment
   - Behavior status
   - Ability to follow commands
   - Awareness of time
   - Ability to converse
   - Response to stimuli
   - Ability to process information
   - Awareness of person
   - Ability to perform self-care
   - Ability to learn new information
4. Scoring
   - Behaviors are marked if present.
   - Level of functioning is determined by the greatest number of behaviors present in a given level.
   - Accompanying management plan is implemented according to the current level (see Appendix 3).

---

6. Patient Evaluation and Conference System (PECS)
   - Comprehensive global functional assessment tool measures 15 major categories.
   - Uses a scale of 1 to 7 (1 equals dependent) throughout rehabilitation.
   - Each discipline assesses appropriate categories.
     - Rehabilitation medicine
     - Activities of daily living
     - Nutrition
     - Neuropsychology

- Recreation
- Rehabilitation nursing
- Communication
- Assistive devices
- Social issues
- Pain
- Physical mobility
- Medications
- Psychology
- Vocational educational activity
- Pulmonary rehabilitation

7. **What is a key point to remember about functional assessment?**

Functional assessment is ongoing and dynamic. Functional assessment provides quantitative and qualitative data about the patient so that interventions are appropriate and provided at the optimal time, ensuring successful achievement of rehabilitation goals.

8. **Why is it important for rehabilitation nurses to understand how comorbidity affects functional mobility and activity?**

With increasing frequency, rehabilitation nurses are involved with patients who have more than one disabling condition, resulting in increased disability and more complex problems. This situation is especially prevalent in older individuals. Research has shown that different combinations of conditions resulted in functional outcomes different from each condition independently. Additionally, individuals over the age of 70 without a diagnosed disability had more difficulty with activities of daily living and independent activities of daily living (such as housekeeping and budgeting) than with physical activity. Therefore comprehensive assessment is necessary to ascertain true functional ability for all complex patients and elders who may have only one diagnosed disorder.

9. **What is the Bobath neurodevelopmental therapy approach?**

Neurodevelopmental therapy is an approach that helps the patient relearn movement sensation after brain damage. Through nurse-led interventions, patients attempt to regain control of motor output mitigating the abnormal posture and movement patterns that developed through sensation shunting following injury. The approach does not attempt to modify sensory input; rather the approach is to inhibit abnormal patterns. Interventions start at a basic level, with the nurse providing stimuli for learning basic position and movement patterns and progress to the patient performing functional skills.

10. **What is the Feldenkrais method?**

The Feldenkrais method is a neuropsychomotor approach that combines patient perceptions and lifestyle with sensory, emotional, cognitive, and movement components. The method is based on the premise that an individual's personal movement habits occur without thought and can be regained when lost by active stimulus of sensory and motor systems to learn and adapt. This method is patient-centered, with the therapist providing cues that are specific and that can be verbal, visual, and/or kinesthetic.

11. **What is the recovery pattern following cerebral cortical damage?**

First, one must understand what effect damage has on the cerebral cortical area. The ability of the patient to plan, sequence, coordinate, and time movements is disrupted. The patient also may be unable to predict movement based on received sensory data. Additionally, the patient may have coordination problems if the cerebellum has been injured. Although disruption in motor function may be the obvious outcome from cortical injury, one must remember the inherent relationship that motor function has with sensory. For that reason, recovery is going to follow a developmental sequence such as reflex to voluntary control. However, one must realize that recovery may stop at any point or level and recovery speed may be indicative of attainable function.

12. **Is exercise important for maintaining or regaining function?**

Yes. Exercise in various forms can help prevent contractures or atrophy, minimize joint damage, reduce pain, and maintain or increase muscle tone, strength, and function. However, a comprehensive assessment is necessary before initiating any type of exercise to prevent injury or complications.

13. **List some appropriate exercises for maintaining mobility.**

- Range of motion
- Isometric exercise
- Yoga
- Tai chi
- Stretching

14. **What are systems or factors that influence functional mobility?**

Systems or factors that influence functional mobility are
- Central nervous system impairment such as paralysis, muscle atrophy, or cognitive disruption
- Musculoskeletal system impairment such as contractures or joint instability
- Sensory impairment such as blindness or pain
- Cognitive-perceptual factors such as dementia or impaired judgment
- Psychosocial and emotional factors such as coping ability or depression
- Environment and technical barriers such as lack of assistive devices or physical barriers
- Social, cultural, and economic factors such as lack of financial resources to acquire equipment or cultural stigma about disability

15. What are the goals related to functional mobility?

The goals related to functional mobility are
- Optimize independence and function.
- Prevent further disability and complications.
- Enhance coping and reduce stress.
- Ensure community and environmental access.
- Foster positive social and personal interaction.
- Ensure safe environment and injury prevention.

Key Points

- The interrelatedness of impairment, disability, and handicap can affect the patient's ability to function positively or negatively.
- Functional assessment is ongoing and dynamic and provides quantitative and qualitative data for development of appropriate interventions.
- A number of standardized assessment tools are available that provide uniformity to patient evaluation.

Internet Resources

The Patricia Neal Rehabilitation Center—Physical Therapy
http://www.patneal.org/pnrc-pt.cfm

American Kinesiotherapy Association
http://www.akta.org/

NeuroCom International Inc.
http://www.onbalance.com/

Bibliography

1. Hoeman SP: Movement, functional mobility, and activities of daily living. In Hoeman SP, editor: *Rehabilitation nursing process, application, & outcomes,* ed 3, St Louis, 2002, Mosby.
2. Quigley P: Functional assessment. In Derstine JB, Hargrove SD, editors: *Comprehensive rehabilitation nursing,* Philadelphia, 2001, WB Saunders.

Chapter 14

Complementary Modalities

Jeanne Flannery

1. How does rehabilitation relate to alternative or complementary medicine?

Rehabilitation, when first addressed from the view of Western medicine or the allopathic model, was seen as an alternative modality. American culture, being based on Cartesian thinking, requires that medical practices follow systematic supportive research, including research that is published in scientific, peer-reviewed journals. Early on, research was lacking in the area of rehabilitation, and some conventional practitioners discounted approaches that they viewed as being strange or different from accepted practices. The outcome of being discounted meant that these "alternative practices" were excluded from "legitimate" status, which in turn prevented reimbursement. Only the expensive procedures, cutting-edge surgery, latest technology, and most highly trained physicians were seen as the way to a cure. Modalities that focused on preventive care and self-care were viewed as illogical. Thus not until after World War II was rehabilitation allowed into the "accepted" circle as a specialty.

2. Does the government provide any oversight for complementary medicine in the United States?

Yes. The National Center for Complementary and Alternative Medicine (NCCAM) is located in the National Institutes of Health, U.S. Public Health Service. The NCCAM is part of the U.S. Department of Health and Human Services. This center was mandated by Congress in 1998.

3. What is the mission of NCCAM?

The mission of NCCAM includes the following major activities:
- Identifying complementary therapies
- Examining patterns of use
- Investigating efficacy and safety
- Disseminating information
- Validating outcomes
- Training practitioners to integrate tested therapies into traditional Western medicine and to gain reimbursement

4. What is the highest priority of NCCAM?

The highest priority of NCCAM is clinical research. The intent is to run clinical trials to evaluate complementary therapies for safety, efficacy, and potential problems. Funded studies across the United States have addressed topics such as
- Acupuncture for treating knee osteoarthritis, fibromyalgia, and back pain
- Melatonin for sleep disorders related to Parkinson's disease
- Saw palmetto for benign prostate hypertrophy
- Triple antioxidant therapy for improvement in multiple sclerosis symptoms
- Self-hypnosis, acupuncture, and osteopathic manipulation for spasticity in cerebal palsy
- *Ginkgo biloba* for decreasing dementia in Alzheimer's disease

5. What is the explanation for the large difference between the belief systems of Western medicine and alternative modalities?

The difference comes from the historical origins of each. One way to place them in historical perspective is to relate them to four worldviews:
- *Premodern, or first, worldview:* Human beings from prehistoric times to sixteenth century held the view of all things being cyclical (moon, sun, tide, seasons, stars, life, death) and that human beings were connected mysteriously and mystically. Practices such as acupuncture, yoga, meditation, herbal remedies, and prayer emerged from this worldview.
- *Modern worldview:* This view began with Copernicus and Descartes and extended to the twentieth century (1500s to 1900s). This view strongly influenced Western medicine and is built on the premise that human beings are discrete entities, separate from the environment and universe, and that the world is rational and predictable. The whole is precisely equal to the sum of its parts. Time is linear, with progress from beginning to end. The scientist is an objective observer, discovering perfectly logical outcomes. Furthermore, the scientist changes no factor because of observation. All things can be reduced to numbers, and if the numbers do not fit, the thing is not accepted as real. Followers of this view were comforted by their own inflexibility.
- *Fracturing or splintering worldview:* The view began in the early 1900s when so many discoveries were being made in the realm of physics, including quantum mechanics. The world, as it had been accepted, was no longer true. The components human beings had believed to be the basis for the environment were found to be far from accurate. The world was so much more. Individuals were beginning to question the logical, predictable, linear, clockwork-like world that had been described.
- *Postmodern worldview:* This view emerged as the fourth view, in the present, with a systems organization, holding beliefs that the whole is greater than the sum of its parts. Organization is integrated and nonlinear, and the search for patterns is a focus. Self-organizing and self-regulating systems are addressed. The relationship of time and space is variable. New technology that has opened up pure sciences research leads to vastly different interpretations of outcomes. No longer is the science based on purely objective data, but scientists

consider the epistemological aspect as well. The first worldview is a strong influence.

6. How has Western medicine evolved?

Western medicine began in 400 BC with Hippocrates, who wrote about the relation of the body, mind, and environment in creating holistic health (first worldview), but changed direction with Descartes to viewing the body as a machine, with body completely separate from mind and human beings completely separate from nature. Human beings believed that one could observe others or nature without affecting what was being observed, affording complete objectivity (modern worldview). The medical model resulted, called biomedicine, and was established strongly by the middle of the nineteenth century. The principles on which Western medicine was established included

- Disease is a measurable deviation from the norm.
- Treatments are used to cure or improve the deviations.
- Objective findings are more important than subjective findings.
- Biomedicine can address basically all medical problems at least satisfactorily, if not completely, with adequate knowledge and research.

7. Why has there not been the same amount of research to support complementary medicine as has been done in Western medicine, and why does the research that has been done not make a strong statement to the Western world?

Complementary medicine focuses on the patient as a whole, including all body systems and mind-body interactions together, inseparably. Complementary medicine recognizes no reductionistic, linear aspect in existence. Therefore the type of research accepted by Western medicine cannot be done. Scientists do not have the instruments to measure multiple systems and multiple levels of consciousness simultaneously. Scientists have not developed the research skill to measure the efficacy of these modalities. In many instances, scientists cannot even explain anatomically or physiologically what is at work.

8. What realms of approach might be used in alternative or complementary modalities?

Approaches that are outside traditional allopathic medicine include
1. Movement therapy such as
   - Feldenkrais
   - Tai chi
   - Tae kwon do
2. Energetic therapy such as
   - Therapeutic touch
   - Medical intuitive diagnostic

- Myofascial release
- Reiki

3. Health care belief systems such as
   - Acupuncture
   - Native American healing
   - Asian medicine
   - Indian medicine (ayurveda)
   - Homeopathy
   - Curanderismo (Puerto Rican, Mexican, Latin American)
   - Naturopathic

4. Mind-body interventions such as
   - Hypnotherapy
   - Meditation
   - Guided imagery
   - Pet therapy
   - Prayer
   - Humor
   - Music therapy
   - Biofeedback

5. Biological-based therapies such as
   - Nutritional programs
   - Herbal preparations
   - Aromatherapy
   - Hydrotherapy

6. Manipulative or body-based therapies such as
   - Reflexology
   - Rolfing
   - Acupressure
   - Massage

9. Why are complementary therapies so appropriate for the rehabilitation nurse?

Nurses were some of the first professionals to promote complementary therapies because these modalities fit well with the holistic approach, which is part of the foundation of nursing. Nursing is about caring, not curing, and engaging the patient in planning and implementing the care is an expected behavior. The ultimate expected outcome is self-care. Nurses are also trusted advisors and can warn patients about the risks of complementary and alternative medicine, such as the increased bleeding risk when taking supplements such as vitamin E, gingko, and St. John's wort, or the increased cancer risk in smokers who take vitamin A supplements. Many supplements interfere with the serum levels or the effects of other common medications, such as digoxin.

Furthermore, nurses see the family and environment as integral to the patient's health and to the systems with which patient interacts. A practical approach is to promote health within the parameters of the spiritual, emotional, social, and psychological components, as well as the biophysiological aspect.

Within the realm of health promotion are
- Primary prevention: interventions to maintain health
- Secondary prevention: interventions to regain or maintain health in the face of illness or disease
- Tertiary prevention: rehabilitation interventions to restore function, adapt to chronic illness or disability, and maintain health

10. Which of the complementary modalities are an integral part of nursing practice?

Many nurses not only routinely use imagery, stress management, relaxation techniques, meditation, therapeutic exercise, life management, herbals, massage, therapeutic humor, pain management, acupressure, support and self-help groups, art and music therapy, diet and nutrition, sports, pet therapy, smoking cessation and weight reduction techniques, and counseling, but also some have been trained to do therapeutic touch, Reiki, Feldenkrais, acupuncture, reflexology, and hypnotherapy.

11. What is the rehabilitation nurse's responsibility to the patient regarding complementary or alternative interventions?

- First, the nurse needs to be aware of the patient's philosophy regarding complementary modalities. The nurse must know whether the patient intends to use these modalities, and if so, which ones.
- Next, the nurse must assess the selected modality for safety, feasibility, and ethical application and determine whether it is reasonable to do.
- Next, the nurse must research the efficacy of the modality in relation to the problem it will be used to treat. The nurse must evaluate side effects, the effect of this modality on medications the patient requires, and traditional treatments.
- The nurse must assess the overall rehabilitation plan to determine whether the desired modality is compatible.
- The nurse must learn whether the use of this modality is driven by religion or culture. The nurse may need to make adjustments to the traditional approach if the patient feels required to use the modality.
- Finally, the nurse must share knowledge with the patient/family of the potential outcomes or consequences of the use of the modality. Education is always the nurse's responsibility, and the nurse is expected to share any research relative to the chosen modality on the effects on the patient's problem.

12. Does the nurse have any responsibility in suggesting complementary or alternative therapies?

Yes. The nurse should offer as suggestions those modalities that do have research supporting their use in improving the patient's condition when traditional methods have brought little satisfaction. The nurse must take care not to suggest anything harmful. Likewise, the nurse should suggest nothing that would impede the effects of current therapy. The nurse should provide resources for information that is impartial (not a marketing article). To provide an estimation of cost to the patient is also wise because many of these modalities are not yet covered under health insurance.

13. **How does biofeedback work on such a wide variety of conditions, ranging from pain, spasms, migraine and tension headaches, and functional disorders of any system to paralysis?**

Because the therapy integrates the mind-body concepts, the patient can learn to isolate and control functions that are basically involuntary responses. With the use of immediate external signals through electronic instrumentation, the patient can detect changes in the system being pinpointed and, with concentration, can control the response. Such control may involve immune function, blood pressure, heart rate and rhythm, sensation, brain wave activity, balance, or other realms. The patient can learn how the body is supposed to work and bring change toward that outcome through raised awareness of the process. The therapy acts as a sixth sense, establishing a new association between a stimulus and a response. Reinforcement for the voluntary effort the patient is making comes from the improvement in function or the elimination of a negative stimulus. The patient accepts the whole responsibility for making the change. The instrumentation simply helps the patient measure progress toward the goal.

14. **Has there been research on the effects of biofeedback?**

Current research is ongoing to reestablish function of neurons in the central nervous system after a traumatic brain injury or a spinal cord injury. Although biofeedback does not work on all patients, a small number who have been paralyzed for a number of years ultimately regained some function in clinical trials. In these situations the biofeedback is focused on one cell at a time. The wide application, the long history, the general acceptance, and the extensive supportive research on biofeedback serves well in rehabilitation to empower the patient to help himself or herself.

15. **Why would a selected modality work well with one patient and not at all with another who has the identical problem?**

First and foremost, each patient is a unique individual. No surgery, medication, or treatment works the same for all patients. However, another aspect needs to be considered. The nurse must assess the patient's belief system carefully to learn whether it is compatible with the complementary approach. For example, if the patient thinks hypnosis is all a sham, the patient will unconsciously resist the process and outcomes. However, therapeutic touch does not require the patient to believe it will work, for it does not require mental cooperation to gain the outcome. Such a technique can be used with positive outcomes with patients who do not have the capacity to understand because the patient is a passive recipient. A nurse can provide therapeutic touch while sitting with a patient, providing hygienic care, or during a back rub.

Key Points

* Complementary therapies fit tightly with the holistic approach, the foundation of nursing.
* Complementary therapies support the nursing philosophy of self-care being an expected outcome.
* Complementary therapy is a practical approach to promote health within the biophysiological, spiritual, emotional, social, and psychological parameters.

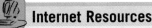

Internet Resources

Complementary Wellness Professional Association
http://www.compwellness.com

Complementary/Alternative Medical Association
http://www.camaweb.org/links/index.php

Bibliography

1. Bottomley JM, Galantine ML, Umphred DA, and others: Alternative and complementary therapies: beyond traditional approaches to intervention in neurological diseases, syndromes, and disorders. In Umphred DA, editor: *Neurological rehabilitation,* ed 4, St Louis, 2001, Mosby.

2. Fontanarosa PB, Lundberg GD: Alternative medicine meets science, *JAMA* 280(18):1618-1619, 1998.

3. Geddes N, Henry JK: Nursing and alternative medicine, *J Holist Nurs* 15(3):271-282, 1997.

4. Hoeman SP, Cappello TP: Culture and medical systems: conventional alternative, and complementary health patterns. In Hoeman SP, editor: *Rehabilitation nursing: process, application, & outcomes,* ed 3, St Louis, 2002, Mosby.

5. Laszlo E: *The systems view of the world,* Cresskill, NJ, 1996, Hampton Press.

Chapter 15

Culture

Jeanne Flannery

1. Why is the knowledge of culture important to a rehabilitation nurse specifically?

Knowledge of culture is important to rehabilitation nurses specifically because a position statement by the Association of Rehabilitation Nurses indicated in 1996 that rehabilitation nurses "provide holistic care and attend to the full range of human experiences and responses to health and illness" (Association of Rehabilitation Nurses, 1996).

2. What effect does culture have on an American rehabilitation nurse?

The population of the world continues to increase rapidly from 5.6 billion in 1994 to an expected 7.9 billion by 2020, with 90% of this increase in developing countries; a 1 billion increase is predicted in Asia alone. The majority of immigrants to the United States come from the 20 most populous countries, the top six being Mexico, Philippines, Vietnam, China, India, and Iran. Currently, one in every four persons in America is a member of a minority group. By 2050 Asians are expected to have increased to 11%, African American to 16%, and Hispanics to 21% of the U.S. population.

3. What American ideal has created a barrier for providing culturally competent care?

Americans value individualism and personal freedom. The ability to make one's decisions based on that which one believes is best is the ideal. Americans do not wish to be confined or manipulated by others' decisions of what should be. The value of individualism is integral to the American's character and nourishes the mind against all obstacles. Nursing is based on individuality, supporting the patient to enhance self-reliance and increase the patient's self-empowerment.

Many other cultures never have, nor will, embrace the concept of individualism. Their whole society is based on groups. Better transportation for all, better lifestyles, better environment is the focus, not individual health. Encounters with patients bring family decision making—what is best for all, not for just the patient. This is difficult for American nurses to understand when the decision does not seem to be the best for the patient, such as the denial of a rehabilitation facility best suited to provide for the patient's needs.

4. What is the definition of culture?

Culture can be defined comprehensively as the composite of all the social behavioral patterns, customs, values, beliefs, and lifestyles, including their products, such as art, music, clothing, and literary writings and speech, which guide the members' thoughts or worldview and decision making.

5. What is included in cultural competence?

Cultural competence is a complex process that is conscious and nonlinear and includes
- Becoming aware of one's own self and all that goes into creating one's existence, such as values, beliefs, thoughts, sensations, motivations, and controlling them so that they do not influence those from different backgrounds
- Demonstrating knowledge of others' cultures
- Accepting cultural difference
- Adapting one's behaviors to be congruent with others' cultures

6. How is cultural competence applied to nursing care?

Because cultural competence is not a linear process, it is probably never truly achieved. Nurses are striving continually to *become* culturally competent, rather than seeing themselves as *being* culturally competent in providing nursing care.

7. What are the essential components of cultural competence?

Nurses must focus and work on each of five components in the process of becoming culturally competent, which are presented in Box 15-1.

Box 15-1.   Components of cultural competence

- Cultural awareness
- Cultural knowledge
- Cultural encounters
- Cultural skill
- Cultural desire

---

8. How is cultural awareness described?

Cultural awareness is a process in which nurses commit to a lifelong self-evaluation and critique about their own biases and become respectful, appreciative, and sensitive to the patient's values, beliefs, practices, and decision-making strategies.

9. **What does cultural knowledge encompass?**

Cultural knowledge is a process of obtaining an educational foundation about the worldviews of different cultures. Without understanding the worldview of the patient's culture, the rehabilitation nurse cannot appreciate the meaning the patient attaches to health, illness, or disability. Without this knowledge, the rehabilitation nurse cannot understand the patient's decision to have or refuse surgery, to go through rehabilitation or not, to accept the disability or not, or to give up or to start a new life. The nurse may not be able to understand even the way the patient's family and friends act in the presence of the disability.

10. **What are the stages of acquiring cultural knowledge?**

Box 15-2 presents the four stages in acquiring an educational foundation of culture.

Box 15-2.   Stages of acquisition of cultural competence

- Unconscious incompetence: the lack of awareness that one does not have cultural knowledge, such as knowing that drug metabolism or risk factors for diseases are different among races
- Conscious incompetence: awareness that one does not have adequate knowledge of a given culture, which may have been acquired through reading, workshops, or exposure to patients with different backgrounds
- Conscious competence: the intentional act of learning about a patient's culture and responding with interventions that are culturally sensitive; but the nurse may be uncomfortable for fear of offending by using the incorrect term, such as whether to address a Spanish-speaking patient as Latino, Chicano, or Hispanic
- Unconscious competence: the ability to provide culturally congruent care to patients from different cultures naturally, without thinking about it. This level is unlikely to be achieved.

---

11. **What does having cultural encounters entail?**

Having an encounter with a patient from a different culture does not qualify for the extent of cultural knowledge that is intended here; in fact, not even encounters with three or four patients from the same culture qualify. The intent is to be able to generate a wide variety of verbal responses and to send and receive verbal and nonverbal messages accurately and appropriately (within each culture).

12. **How is *cultural skill* defined?**

Cultural skill requires the combination of cultural awareness and cultural knowledge to assess the patient's relative cultural data, health history, and health concern/disorder and to perform a physical examination in a culturally sensitive manner. Such skill would include appropriate eye contact or not, acceptable physical distance, touch or not, awareness of gender restrictions, and needs for certain clothing or other persons' participation during the physical examination. Furthermore, cultural skill requires the appropriate description of the findings and strategies to include necessary family in setting acceptable mutual goals to address the problem.

13. How is cultural desire described?

Nurses reflect cultural desire when they convey authentic caring in their actions that match their words. The nurses' motivation to care for patients from different cultures demonstrates a congruency between their inner feelings and cultural skill. Patients have been found to say in cultural research that they do not seek knowledge first, but the degree to which the nurse demonstrates caring from the heart. Often caring is something as simple as sitting down and asking how each of the family members is and listening to stories the patient may choose to tell. Time spent with interest in the patient's family, as individuals, is important in many cultures.

14. What are some standard questions the rehabilitation nurse should ask for a cultural assessment?

The nurse should listen attentively in a nonjudgmental fashion to the answers to the questions in Box 15-3.

Box 15-3.   Standard questions in a cultural assessment of a patient

- What is your understanding of this disability?
- What do you think caused this problem?
- What kind of treatment do you think you should receive?
- What do you fear?
- How will your family need to participate in the treatment of your disability?
- How will your family react to your disability when you go home with them?
- What do you expect of your family as far as their duties and obligations?

---

15. What is ethnocentrism?

Ethnocentrism is the assumption that a person's values, beliefs, and practices are the correct worldview. "Noncompliance" is frequently the result of a nurse's nonresponsiveness to the patient's worldview.

16. What is a culture broker?

A culture broker links the cultural concerns of a group of patients to the health care system. The broker is skilled in advocating, negotiating, mediating, and intervening for the patient. The broker is not restrained by the health care institution but is knowledgeable of its culture and has an ongoing relationship so as to seek a balance between the recommended treatment and the patient's desired treatment.

17. What concepts are important to the nurse in understanding a patient's culture?

Box 15-4 presents concepts that a nurse needs to understand regarding a patient's culture.

Box 15-4.   Cultural concepts nurses need to understand

- **Family definition:** who's involved; rituals, holidays, festivities, rites of passage; family duties; childbearing, child-rearing practices
- **Communication:** language, use of space, nonverbal patterns; expectations for visitors, rules for polite behavior, and norms for verbal and nonverbal communication
- **Health practices:** type of providers used; methods used to prevent sickness, promote health, and prevent death
- **Health beliefs:** what is considered health or illness; what is believed to cause illness; what kind of state is considered a problem; and how problem solving is done
- **Religious/death beliefs:** what the meaning of pain/suffering is; how the dying process is viewed; what religious beliefs may need to be followed during illness that the nurse should know about, such as rituals; how death may need to be handled
- **Dietary practices:** special food requirements, unacceptable foods, special preparations required; how to handle modifications necessary for treatment
- **Geography:** where has the family emigrated from, reasons for coming to America, what their country/society is like; what problems they are having in America

---

18. What are some cultural differences the nurse may need to know about African Americans?

Some cultural differences the nurse may need to know about African Americans are
- Have a high prevalence of hypertension, diabetes, and cancer.
- Grandmother may have central role and is a matriarch.
- Health may be threatened by their preference for fried foods and dried beans and greens cooked with salt pork.
- May use folk medicine and root doctors.
- Are tolerant of obesity.

19. What are some cultural differences the nurse may need to know about Jewish individuals?

Some cultural differences the nurse may need to know about Jewish individuals are
- May use Hebrew language for prayers.
- Observe Sabbath from Friday sunset to Saturday sunset.

- Do not eat pork or shellfish (Orthodox).
- Eat only kosher foods (Orthodox).
- Do not mix milk and meat (Orthodox).
- Perform circumcision on eighth day after delivery.
- Do not believe in use of condoms/diaphragms (Orthodox).

20. **What are some cultural differences the nurse may need to know about South Asians?**

Some cultural differences the nurse may need to know about South Asians are
- Oldest woman is the authority on health matters.
- May deny psychiatric symptoms.
- May not view rehabilitation positively; view the disabled negatively and hide them.
- Extended families may be under one roof.
- May speak in soft tones; females may not make eye contact with males; may not express anger or pain.
- May feel compelled to greet oldest male first, then other males, then females by age.
- May not accept right to die.
- May mourn death through loud chanting.
- May forbid telling a dying patient of prognosis.
- No one may touch a body but family and a priest (Muslim).
- Do not eat meat (Hindu).

21. **What are some cultural differences the nurse may need to know about Asian Americans?**

Some cultural differences the nurse may need to know about Asian Americans are
- May prefer stir-fried foods over typically prepared institutional meals; may avoid milk; may fast 1 day for purification.
- May be uncomfortable with face-to-face communication; may avoid eye contact.
- Should address the patient by whole name (family name first, then given name); maintain formal distance.
- The patient/family may consistently agree with the nurse's suggestions, but then not follow them (do not wish to show overt conflict).
- Usually follow the belief that health is a balance between yin and yang, and practice acupuncture to create the balance.

22. **What are some cultural differences the nurse may need to know about Latinos?**

Some cultural differences the nurse may need to know about Latinos are
- May consult folk healers and use folk medicine.
- Usually believe in treating hot diseases with cold remedies and cold diseases with hot remedies; may resist prescribed treatment if not viewed in correct category.

- May believe disease is caused by evil eye or hex.
- May be expressive and emotional in communication.
- May classify foods as hot or cold for use with hot or cold diseases.
- Older male is usually the central figure with the most respect.

23. **What are some cultural differences the nurse may need to know about Native Americans?**

Some cultural differences the nurse may need to know about Native Americans are
- May use medicine man and hand tremblers; may need a series of ceremonies to cure illness or drive away evil; wear turquoise to ward off evil.
- Often use herbal remedies.
- Are highly vulnerable to type 2 diabetes, with poor control and likely complications.
- Have high incidence of gall bladder disease.
- View mental illness as a curse.
- Typically refuse organ transplants and autopsy.
- Usually perceive silence as supportive.
- May be suspicious when health care workers ask questions.
- May not relate to time concept.
- May not drink milk; may prefer mutton and brains over typical meats served in institutions.

Key Points

- Currently one in four persons in the United States is a member of a minority group.
- Cultural competence involves becoming aware of one's own holistic self and not allowing it to influence those from different backgrounds, being knowledgeable of and accepting cultural differences, and adapting one's behaviors to be congruent with others' cultures.

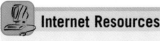

Internet Resources

Cultural Competence Standards
http://www.omhrc.gov/clas/

Culturally Competent Care
http://et12.library.musc.edu/cultural/competent_care/index.php

Toward Culturally Competent Care
http://www.oandp.com/news/jmcorner/2002-07/2.asp

Bibliography

1. Association of Rehabilitation Nurses: *The appropriate inclusion of rehabilitation nurses wherever rehabilitation is provided.* Position statement. Glenview, Ill, 1996, The Association.

2. Compinha-Bacote J: A model of practice to address cultural competence in rehabilitation nursing, *Rehabil Nurs* 26(1):8-11, 2001.

3. Hoeman SP, Cappello TP: Culture and medical systems: conventional, alternative, and complementary health patterns. In Hoeman SP, editor: *Rehabilitation nursing,* ed 3, St Louis, 2002, Mosby.

4. Petrinos D, White N: Culturally competent rehabilitation care. In Derstine JB, Hargrove SD, editors: *Comprehensive rehabilitation nursing,* Philadelphia, 2001, WB Saunders.

5. Purnell LD, Paulouka BJ: Purnell's model for cultural competence. In Purnell LD, editor: *Transcultural health care: a culturally competent approach,* Philadelphia, 1998, FA Davis.

6. Purnell LD, Paulouka BJ: Transcultural diversity and health care. In Purnell LD, editor: *Transcultural health care: a culturally competent approach,* Philadelphia, 1998, FA Davis.

Section 4

Rehabilitation Nursing with a Special Focus

Chapter 16

End-Stage Renal Disease Rehabilitation

Denise A. Tucker

1. **The patient is diagnosed with end-stage renal disease (ESRD), or chronic renal failure. How does this disease alter the patient's lifestyle?**

   Because the diseased kidneys can no longer function, patients need other methods to cleanse the blood of waste products. They may need dialysis treatments, using a dialyzer and dialysate solution, to cleanse their blood and pull off excess fluid regularly. Hemodialysis, peritoneal dialysis, and continuous ambulatory peritoneal dialysis (CAPD) are several methods commonly used for patients with ESRD. Although hemodialysis typically is performed every other day, or about 3 times a week, peritoneal dialysis may be performed daily (perhaps at night, while the patient is sleeping). The nurse must tell patients what to expect before, during, and after the treatments.

   Before hemodialysis is possible, a surgeon must create an arteriovenous fistula or graft in a suitable site (usually the arm) to arterialize the blood flow in the vein. When the site has matured (8 to 12 weeks later), it will be used as the venipuncture site during dialysis treatments. One set of lines draws out the patient's blood to be taken through the dialyzer, where the blood is cleansed of waste products and toxins; and one set of lines returns the cleansed blood back to the body.

   Before peritoneal dialysis or CAPD, a surgeon places a dialysis catheter in the abdomen. This catheter is not used for 10 days to 2 weeks after insertion to give the site time to heal before it is stressed by the dialysis procedure. The CAPD exchanges usually are done by the patient or family member in the home environment. The CAPD exchanges usually are timed at 4- to 6-hour intervals during waking hours and the last exchange is left to dwell overnight.

   These treatments are physically exhausting. Hemodialysis treatments last several hours, during which time patients are connected physically to the dialyzer. Fluid and electrolyte shifts may cause distressing symptoms such as fainting or lightheadedness, cramping, nausea, or malaise as excess fluid and waste products are drawn off and the balance in the body is restored. The nurse should encourage patients to rest after treatments and avoid stressful stimulation for the rest of the day. Although patients may be thirsty, the nurse should remind them that they must maintain appropriate fluid restrictions at all times.

Patients requiring hemodialysis must protect the arteriovenous fistula or graft site. They must keep the arteriovenous fistula free from contamination and safe from disruption that may cause hemorrhage. Swimming and contact sports are not recommended, which could further limit the patient's lifestyle.

Based on the number of times per week the patient needs dialysis, treatment becomes an extreme barrier to continuing a prior lifestyle. The patient cannot work during the time hemodialysis or peritoneal dialysis is provided; the number of days it occupies per week probably will preclude the patient's being able to retain a previous position. The problem involves not only the number of hours per treatment, which may vary from 3 to 7, but also the fact that the patient should rest following the treatment. Additionally, the confinement to the routine of an every-other-day dialysis prevents travel with family or planned vacations unless dialysis can be arranged in the area to which the family is traveling. Such adjustments certainly affect the patient's quality of life. If the patient is married and has children, all the members' quality of life is affected to an extent because of their inability to be free to participate spontaneously, as a family, in many activities they might desire.

If peritoneal dialysis is provided at a facility, the same restrictions would exist. If peritoneal dialysis is provided at home, then it usually is done overnight so that days are free; but the home routine is disturbed and responsibility for the proper procedure falls on at least one family member. If the patient uses ambulatory peritoneal dialysis, the patient may experience a distorted body image because of the padded appearance and loose clothing one must wear.

If the patient has an abdominal catheter, the patient must keep it clean and dry. The nurse teaches the patient and family to access the catheter using aseptic technique. Usually a single room in the home is designated for CAPD, and the supplies are stored there. The nurse teaches the patient and family to avoid strain on the catheter and abdominal trauma and to observe for signs of infection and report them immediately to prevent peritonitis.

Finally, the whole family is likely to be affected by the patient's strict diet and fluid restriction. Not only does the patient feel deprived of not having a choice, but the restrictions prevent family dinners out and probably cause some concern to family members who may feel guilty or inhibited when eating "forbidden" food in front of the patient. Mealtime may become less than the positive family time it otherwise might be. Fluid restriction is an enormous problem to the patient because the American culture expects to have refreshments as a routine at most any gathering; therefore the patient is challenged to refrain.

2. **What type of teaching is necessary for these patients and why?**

Teaching is a nurse's top priority for patients newly diagnosed with ESRD. Lifestyle changes are necessary for patients to maintain their health status while undergoing dialysis treatments. The nurse must instruct patients on dietary and fluid intake restrictions, medications, and symptom recognition. Additionally, the nurse must give information about the arteriovenous fistula or graft or abdominal catheter.

3. **What are dietary and fluid intake restrictions for patients with ESRD?**

Dietary and fluid intake restrictions must be instituted to prevent fluid overload and toxin buildup in the body during the time the patient is not undergoing the dialysis treatments. Patients must maintain their nutritional status while avoiding the buildup of toxins in the blood.
- Because the kidney cannot concentrate urine to excrete electrolytes properly, foods and medications with potassium and magnesium must be restricted. Hyperkalemic and hypermagnesemic states are toxic to the cardiac muscle. Although specific restrictions must be individualized for each patient, patients may be allowed to consume about 50 mEq, or 2 g, of potassium daily (or approximately 0.5 mEq/kg of body mass daily).
- Because of fluid buildup in the body, patients must also restrict sodium and water. Once again, the amount must be individualized for each patient. Patients must be warned against using salt substitutes; many contain potassium iodide. Fluid is restricted as well. Because many patients with ESRD void small amounts of urine daily, the daily fluid allowance typically includes the amount voided the day before, plus an allowance for insensible water losses, such as sweating. The additional allowance, individualized for the patient, may be from 500 to 1000 ml of fluid. The nurse should caution patients to count as liquid foods that are liquid when melted, such as ice cream and popsicles.
- Protein also must be limited, often from 40 to 60 g a day; the end product wastes of protein breakdown increase the blood urea nitrogen in the blood, increasing the possibility of toxic uremia. Carbohydrates and fats are useful in maintaining energy, and patients should maintain a caloric intake of about 35 calories/kg of body mass daily. Patients should not fast or eat less than their body requirements because they will begin breaking down their own body proteins and fats, increasing the load of waste products in their blood. Increased levels of toxins may make the person more uremic, or symptomatic. The rehabilitation nurse may request a consultation from the nutritionist on the team to assist the patient and family to plan appealing, nourishing meals.

4. **What kind of teaching will patients with ESRD need about medications?**

The rehabilitation nurse will need to explain the importance of the many medications required.
- Typical medications needed by the patient with ESRD include phosphate binders (such as antacids), with calcium and vitamin D supplements to maintain serum calcium levels.
- Folic acid and multivitamin supplements also may be given to maintain hemoglobin levels.
- Epoetin injections also may be given to stimulate the bone marrow to produce red blood cells.

These medications must be timed to coincide with other medications the patient is receiving. Many patients with ESRD also have cardiovascular disease and receive antihypertensive and antiarrhythmic medications. The nurse should consult a pharmacist to ensure that medications are given correctly. Additionally, patients may be asked to take certain medications (such as antihypertensive agents) after dialysis treatments are completed; the treatments will remove the medication from the bloodstream if taken immediately before the treatment.

The nurse must warn patients that they most likely will need lower doses of medications to achieve therapeutic effects. Therefore serum levels of some medications may need to be checked regularly. The nurse must give instructions informing patients how often they need to have blood drawn for testing.

5. What must patients with ESRD know about anticoagulation?

During hemodialysis treatments, patients are given anticoagulation medications to prevent the artificial kidney from clotting. The nurse will check the clotting times throughout the treatment to ensure they are at the appropriate level. Although anticoagulation effects are reversed at the end of the treatment, some effects may linger after the treatments. Thus patients should observe for signs and symptoms of bleeding, such as easy bruising, bleeding, tea colored urine, and blood in the stools. Additionally, the nurse should encourage patients to avoid contact sports or physical activities in which they may be injured.

The rehabilitation nurse also should stress that patients must not take over-the-counter medications or herbal supplements/remedies without consulting their health care provider. Common herbal supplements such as St. John's wort, *Gingko biloba,* and vitamin E may increase clotting time and promote bleeding.

6. Why should patients with ESRD be careful about their immune function?

End-stage renal disease affects every body system and depresses the immune functioning of the body. The nurse must teach patients to watch for signs and symptoms of infection, such as a low-grade fever, feeling of malaise, or redness, swelling, or warmth of an infected site. Because their immune systems function poorly, these patients may not be able to mount an effective systemic defense to infection. Thus they should notify their health care provider when their temperature is 100.0° F or higher.

Patients should avoid crowds, especially in the winter when upper respiratory infections are prevalent. They should limit exposure to persons who are ill to avoid catching contagious diseases themselves.

7. What should patients know about the arteriovenous fistula or graft?

Patients should monitor the arteriovenous fistula or graft daily to ensure its patency. See Box 16-1.

Patients should treat the site gently, keep it clean and dry, and avoid wearing constricting clothing or objects on the arm in which the graft is located.

Box 16-1.   Monitoring information for patients

- One should feel a palpable pulse distal to the fistula.
- When one places a hand on the fistula, the person should feel a "thrill" where the arterialized blood rushes through the graft (this may feel like a cat purring).
- The fistula should be clean and dry, free from the swelling, redness, and warmth of an infection.
- If one places a stethoscope over the graft, the person should hear the blood rush through the graft; it will sound similar to a murmur, or bruit.

Health care personnel must never take blood pressures or draw blood from the affected arm to avoid compromising the blood flow. The patient must protect the site when outside gardening; the patient should wear gloves or long sleeves to avoid irritating or injuring the site.

8. **Why do so many patients with ESRD have mental status changes?**

   End-stage renal disease affects every system of the body, and the brain is not spared. Circulating toxins in the body affect the mental status and the physical status. Thus patients may have differing levels of consciousness, may become confused or anxious, or may become depressed. A risk also exists of mental status changes resulting from elevated levels of medications that usually are cleared from the body by the kidneys or are taken inadvertently by a confused patient.

   The rehabilitation nurse should monitor patients with ESRD for mental status changes and teach the patients and their family members to be alert for changes in mental functioning and to monitor carefully the patient's medication schedule. The patient may need a psychiatric consultation for further follow-up and treatment with antidepressant medications. Patients and family members may benefit from counseling. Additionally, support groups may be useful for all involved.

9. **What is the uremic state?**

   Patients suffering from ESRD develop the toxic state of uremia if and when enough toxins, waste products, and other end products of metabolism build up in the blood to cause symptoms. The blood urea nitrogen and creatinine levels also will be elevated. Although uremic toxemia may occur in every body system, gastrointestinal symptoms such as nausea, vomiting, anorexia, diarrhea, and weight loss typically occur. Additionally, these patients also may suffer from integumentary problems such as pruritis and may develop dependent edema. Patients also may experience neurological changes and dysfunction, including mental status changes and peripheral neuropathies.

   Dialysis can control the symptoms of uremia and maintain the patient's comfort level. However, uremia has no cure, unless the patient receives a kidney transplant.

10. **Do patients requiring dialysis sometimes decide to stop their treatments and die?**

No clear figure is available for the percentage of deaths from discontinuation of dialysis at the end of life. Patients may elect to stop coming to dialysis treatments because they wish to die. Less overt actions for the same purpose may include deliberate noncompliance with fluid and food restrictions and refusal of required medications.

Although the choice to withdraw from treatment should rest with the patients themselves, they should be given the opportunity to ventilate and explore their feelings about their situation and should be offered adequate counseling. The rehabilitation nurse should offer opportunities for discussion or provide information for counseling and referral if needed.

Key Points

- Because of toxicity to the cardiac muscle, foods and medications with potassium and magnesium are restricted; for example, salt substitutes are not allowed.
- Fluid restriction is individualized and allows an amount each day to match the urinary output from the previous day plus 500 to 1000 ml to cover insensible losses such as sweating.
- Protein intake is restricted to 40 to 60 g/day to prevent the possibility of toxic uremia.
- Serum levels of medications may need to be checked routinely to be sure overdosage does not occur because lower doses usually are needed.

Internet Resources

The Renal Network
http://www.therenalnetwork.org

Centers for Medicare & Medicaid Services: ESRD Information Resource
http://www.cms.hhs.gov/providers/esrd.asp

National Institute of Diabetes and Digestive and Kidney Disorders
http://www.niddk.nih.gov

Bibliography

1. Holechek M J: Nursing management: acute renal failure and chronic kidney disease. In Lewis SM, Heitkemper MM, Dirksen SR, editors: *Medical-surgical nursing: assessment and management of clinical problems,* ed 6, St Louis, 2004, Mosby.
2. Huether S: Alterations of renal and urinary tract function. In McCance KL, Huether SE, editors: *Pathophysiology: the biologic basis for disease in adults and children,* ed 4, St Louis, 2002, Mosby.

Chapter 17

Kidney Transplant Rehabilitation

Denise A. Tucker

1. **The patient has been approved for a kidney transplant. What is important for the patient to know before and after the transplant?**

   Patients should have teaching on what to expect before and after surgery. The nurse also must provide additional information about nutrition, hydration, medications, and monitoring instructions. The rehabilitation nurse has had the opportunity to discuss the lifelong impact of transplant during the time the patient has been on dialysis.

2. **What should the patient know about the surgery?**
   - Unless patients are to receive a living related donor kidney and the surgery is set for a specified date and time, they will not know when the surgery will take place. They must be notified immediately on the receipt of a potential cadaver donor kidney so that they can go to the hospital and be prepared for surgery as soon as possible. Many transplant centers use a beeper system for notification.
   - Waiting for a kidney to become available may be stressful for patients and families. The fact that another person must die for the organ to become available also may cause feelings of guilt or depression. The rehabilitation nurse may recommend attending a support group to provide help during this difficult time.
   - Once patients are notified, they are rushed through to surgery to receive the organ. The surgery itself is rather simple and requires few incisions; the new kidney is nestled in the abdomen near the bladder, and the new and existing ureters are anastomosed together. The new kidney should turn pink immediately after perfusion. Patients typically feel well right away because the kidney now is functioning normally, and the patient no longer has toxic wastes circulating in the blood. However, patients also should be aware that complications such as rejection are possible and may require additional treatment and monitoring; sometimes severe reactions occur, and patients may be seriously ill postoperatively.
   - The rehabilitation nurse should teach typical postoperative measures such as turning, coughing, deep breathing, and ankle exercises preoperatively and reinforce them postoperatively. Patients will be encouraged to get out of bed and ambulate as soon as possible to avoid postoperative complications of surgery. Vital signs, intake and output, and daily weights also will be recorded to monitor the patient's progress. Recovery is routinely relatively quick with early discharge.

• After discharge, patients should continue to observe the surgical site daily for signs and symptoms of infection such as redness, warmth, swelling, foul-smelling discharge from the wound, increased temperature, or sharp pain from the surgical site. They should notify the physician if any of these signs or symptoms appear so that they can be treated immediately.

3. **What should posttransplant patients know about nutrition and activities of daily living?**

After a kidney transplant, patients feel better than they may have felt for years. After the previous spartan restrictions in proteins and other nutrients, a risk is that patients may make poor food choices. Therefore, the rehabilitation nurse should caution patients to eat a healthful, nutritious diet and avoid overindulging in foods high in fats, cholesterol, and sugars. The nurse should encourage patients to drink water to maintain hydration and the health of the new kidney.

The nurse also should encourage patients to exercise regularly to maintain overall health. Walking is an excellent activity that can be increased gradually as the patient's endurance increases. Patients should remember to remain hydrated during exercise and to avoid exercising to exhaustion.

4. **When should the posttransplant patient contact the health care provider? Does keeping a diary help?**

Posttransplant patients are encouraged to monitor their health after the transplant. By monitoring daily trends in intake and output, weight, vital signs with temperature, and symptoms such as edema, shortness of breath, and difficulty in breathing, these patients can feel a change in their health and may detect problems early. Early detection ensures early treatment and may prevent rejection of the organ. Box 17-1 provides points to teach the patient.

Box 17-1.   When posttransplant patients should notify the health care provider

Patients should notify their health care provider if
• Their blood pressure rises.
• They gain several pounds in less than a week.
• They have symptoms such as edema (observe for shoes feeling too tight as a sign of pedal edema).
• They have problems with breathing.

The foregoing may be signs and symptoms of fluid retention from a failing or rejected kidney. Organ rejection may be reversed if treated aggressively and quickly with increased doses of immunosuppressive medications.

Rehabilitation nurses also should encourage patients to keep all follow-up appointments with their health care providers. Follow-up appointments ensure that patients are monitored closely to maintain their health.

5. Why should the posttransplant patient be hypervigilant against infection?

Posttransplant patients receive massive amounts of immunosuppressive medications, especially in the beginning, immediately after receiving the transplant. Immunosuppressive medications maintain depression of the immune system to avoid rejection of the new organ.

Because the patient's immune function is decreased from the immunosuppressive medications, posttransplant patients are not able to mount an effective systemic defense to infection. In this way they are similar to the patient with end-stage renal disease, although the reason for the response is different. Therefore posttransplant patients need to watch for subtle signs and symptoms of infection, such as a low-grade fever, feeling of malaise, or redness, swelling, or warmth of an infected site. Thus they should notify their health care provider when their temperature is 99.0°F or higher.

As in end-stage renal disease, posttransplant patients should avoid crowds, especially in the winter when upper respiratory infections are prevalent. They also should avoid exposure to persons who are ill to avoid catching contagious diseases themselves.

6. What should posttransplant patients know about immunosuppressive medications?

Posttransplant patients are given immunosuppressive medication therapy to avoid transplant rejection. However, these medications put the patient at risk for infections or developing cancer from the decreased function of the immune system.

Patients must take immunosuppressive medications daily for the rest of their lives. Skipping doses places the patient at high risk for organ rejection. Medication may be funded through insurance, Medicare, or Medicaid. If financial problems arise, the patient can consult a rehabilitation nurse case manager for suggestions about other possible sources. The patient should never stop taking medications without physician instructions specifically to do so.

Immediately after transplant, massive doses of immunosuppressive medications and steroids are given to prevent rejection. As time passes, the doses will be tapered until the patient may be weaned from the steroids entirely; a small maintenance dose of immunosuppressive medications, such as cyclosporin, may be all that is required. However, the dose is determined individually. The physician will determine the best possible dose for each patient after monitoring the patient's response to the medications.

Even though patients take the prescribed medications faithfully, the organ still may be rejected. If signs and symptoms of rejection appear, the doses of medications will be increased to attempt to reverse the rejection. Once rejection is reversed, the patient will once more be weaned from the medications (if possible) until the patient can return to a daily maintenance dose.

7. What about the increased risk for cancers?

Immunosuppressive therapy decreases the vigilance of the immune system in detecting and destroying cancers. Nurses should encourage patients to be screened regularly for cancer as appropriate for their age group or individually as scheduled by their physician. Patients also should notify their health care providers if suspicious signs or symptoms occur and should seek medical advice immediately. The seven warning signs of cancer follow the mnemonic CAUTION. See Box 17-2.

Box 17-2. Seven warning signs of cancer

- **C**hange in bowel or bladder habits
- **A** sore that does not heal
- **U**nusual bleeding or discharge
- **T**hickening or lump in or out of body
- **I**ndigestion or trouble swallowing
- **O**bvious changes in a wart or mole
- **N**agging cough or hoarseness

---

8. What happens if the kidney is totally rejected?

If the kidney is rejected and the immunosuppressive therapy is unsuccessful, the patient must return to dialysis. Patients may become eligible for another transplant; in that instance, the process is begun anew.

Key Points

- Waiting for a kidney to become available may be stressful for patients and families.
- Because of many diet restrictions before transplant, the patient is at risk for making poor food choices after transplant and will need education on appropriate dietary and fluid intake.
- Early detection of abnormal changes or symptoms ensures early treatment and may prevent rejection of the organ.
- Patients need to have a thorough understanding of the immunosuppressive medications and associated risks.

Internet Resources

National Kidney Foundation
http://www.kidney.org/

National Transplant Assistance Fund
http://www.transplantfund.org/

Bibliography

1. Holechek MJ: Nursing management: acute renal failure and chronic kidney disease. In Lewis SM, Heitkemper MM, Dirksen SR, editors: *Medical-surgical nursing: assessment and management of clinical problems,* ed 6, St Louis, 2004, Mosby.
2. Huether S: Alterations of renal and urinary tract function. In McCance KL, Heuther SE, editors: *Pathophysiology: the biologic basis for disease in adults and children,* ed 4, St Louis, 2002, Mosby.

Chapter 18

Cardiac Rehabilitation

Sandra H. Faria

1. **Why is cardiac rehabilitation important to a patient with heart disease?**

   Much of the cost of coronary artery disease (CAD) in the United States is due to temporary or permanent disability. The American Heart Association recommends that most persons with CAD undergo cardiac rehabilitation after being diagnosed with CAD. Cardiac rehabilitation programs focus on increasing cardiac capacity through exercise and educate the population on risk factors such as diet modification, tobacco and alcohol cessation, and management of cardiac drugs. These interventions help to prevent complications of CAD and improve patient outcomes after acute heart injury.

2. **How long does a cardiac rehabilitation program last?**

   Typically a cardiac rehabilitation program consists of three phases and encompasses 36 weeks.
   - Phase I relates to exercise in the hospital that is done for most patients after being diagnosed with CAD. The other two phases of cardiac rehabilitation relate to the outpatient setting.
   - Phase II occurs during the immediate outpatient period. Phase II usually is initiated within 2 to 3 weeks after hospital discharge.
   - Phase III occurs after the patient has been stabilized and does not need the continuous monitoring of an electrocardiogram. This phase usually lasts for 6 months to 1 year.

3. **Where might a cardiac rehabilitation program be held?**

   Cardiac rehabilitation programs may be in a community health setting, a major medical center, or a local hospital or may be offered as self-directed home programs.

4. **Who are candidates for cardiac rehabilitation?**

   Candidates for cardiac rehabilitation include
   - Survivors of myocardial infarction
   - Individuals with stable angina

• Patients who have undergone a coronary artery bypass graft surgery or percutaneous transluminal coronary angioplasty
• Patients with congestive heart failure

Studies have found that of the candidates who qualify for cardiac rehabilitation, particularly women, nonwhites, and elders, only a minority of individuals actually participate in the program.

5. What are referral and adherence characteristics?

Studies for years only used men as participants. Only recently studies were expanded to examine women, nonwhites, and elders. Eligibility rates compared with referral rates continue to show that males more frequently are referred and elders are seldom referred. Adherence rates tend to be higher in white men.

6. Do most cardiac patients attend cardiac rehabilitation programs?

The American Heart Association recommends that all patients with stable CAD attend cardiac rehabiliation, but few patients actually attend. A large percentage of the patients who begin cardiac rehabilitation drop out of the 6-month program before completion.

7. Why do patients drop out of the program?

The dropout rate is attributed to many reasons, including lack of insurance, denial of health problem, the use of home exercise machines, and excessive distance to the cardiac rehabilitation site.

8. What are mental health advantages of cardiac rehabilitation?

Research has shown that patients who undergo a cardiac rehabilitation program have dramatic improvement in depression, energy level, and exercise capacity. Cardiac rehabilitation improves social adjustment and functioning. The stress management and relaxation techniques learned are effective in lowering levels of self-reported emotional distress.

9. Many individuals who have had heart problems are afraid that the problem may happen again if they exercise or if they have sex. Does cardiac rehabilitation provide information and guidance for these individuals?

The cardiac rehabilitation programs include supervised exercise so that patients can increase exercise activity at their own rate and so that they are monitored as they do so. The patients also are instructed about activities in which they may be involved as they progresses in the program. Sexual activities, as with other exercise activity, are usually safe if the patients build up their tolerance and stop if chest pain develops. The patients receives information and guidance for sexual health as an integral part of the programs.

10. Are there standards for cardiac rehabilitation programs and professionals who teach them?

Several professional and governmental organizations have developed standard competencies for professionals in cardiac rehabilitation. The organizations also have developed program standards. By using these standards, the program can maintain its quality regardless of the setting in which it is located.

The competencies required of cardiac rehabilitation professionals include
- Needs assessment
- Goal setting
- Planning and implementing interventions
- Outcome evaluations

11. What kind of professionals make up the cardiac rehabilitation team?

Usually, the team consists of a medical director, a program coordinator, and a registered nurse. Other members of the team may include social worker, physical therapist, clergy, respiratory therapist, dietitian, mental health professional, pharmacist, and vocational rehabilitation counselor. The nurse's role may vary, but consistently the role consists of coordination and education of the patient and family. Taken together, members of a team have advanced practice knowledge about
- Cardiovascular disease
- Current intervention strategies
- Educational goals, methods, and tools
- Health psychology
- Nutrition
- Exercise physiology
- Emergency procedures
- Rehabilitation principles
- Care for patients with comorbid conditions
- Use of over-the-counter supplements used by patients

12. What are the general principles guiding a cardiac rehabilitation program?

The cardiac rehabilitation program usually starts a few days after the cardiac event. Cardiac testing can provide information about risk to patients and determines their need for further medical treatment, their exercise tolerance, and level of safe exercise with supervision. The individual patient risk, medications, types of exercise, and specific therapeutic exercises are factors in the beginning prescriptions for exercise training. Box 18-1 presents general principles.

> **Box 18-1.   General principles for exercise training in cardiac rehabilitation**
>
> - Patient and family are active participants in the program.
> - Early assessment using exercise testing is repeated and used to determine medical regimen.
> - Individual prescriptions for exercise training are used to enable the patient to obtain maximum function. The approach to assessment, planning of interventions, and evaluation of risk factors and psychosocial and occupational status is interdisciplinary. These assessments and evaluations are completed and communicated to the team and patient/family.

13. What is the first phase of cardiac rehabilitation?

The first phase of cardiac rehabilitation is the inpatient phase. In this phase, physical and psychological consequences of the cardiac event are limited for the patient who is still hospitalized. This phase may last from a few days for a patient with no complications to 2 weeks if other pathological conditions are involved.

The major components are
- Assessment for risk
- Early ambulation
- Physical activity
- Education of the patient and family

14. What kinds of exercise may be encouraged in phase 1?

The treadmill exercise test or "stress test" usually is done. The results of this test are correlated with other factors to form an individualized risk level (high, low, or moderate) that is used in the long-term treatment plan. Other modalities for exercise tests include the graded exercise test, stationary cycling, or arm crank ergometry. Adapted equipment may be used for patients with disabilities.

15. What kind of family assessment is done in phase 1?

Because patients and their family are included as part of the team in cardiac rehabilitation, assessment of the patient and family for stressors and coping ability is important. Variables in the assessment are
- Existing knowledge base
- Readiness to learn (motivation)
- Learning needs
- Patient and family goals
- Patient and family energy for learning
- Presence of support systems
- Time for learning
- Potential for understanding

16. **What are therapeutic goals during phase 1?**

The therapeutic goals for phase 1 include risk reduction, intensive monitoring, and early diagnosis and treatment of problems and complications. Conditioning or reconditioning and preparation for reentry into the community are also major concerns.

17. **What are some criteria for termination of an exercise session?**

Even though exercise may be a prescribed activity, complications still may occur. A patient should stop exercising if any of the signs or symptoms depicted in Box 18-2 occur.

Box 18-2. Criteria for ceasing an exercise session

- Fatigue
- Dizziness
- Symptoms of angina
- Drop in heart rate >10 beats/min
- Change in cardiac rhythm
- Nausea
- Drop in blood pressure >10 mm Hg
- Dyspnea
- Rise in heart rate >20 beats/min for myocardial infarction patients (or number determined by previous exercise testing)
- Rise in blood pressure more than the amount determined by previous exercise testing

---

18. **What are the areas of education in phase 1?**

Education in phase 1 focuses on the patient and the family, who must be made to feel a part of the team. The rehabilitation nurse introduces them to the disease condition and the treatment regimen and interventions and shares information about monitoring, wound care, chest pain, and other appropriate cardiac information. The nurse gives specific guidelines for activity, medications (prescription and over the counter), diet, tobacco use, activities of daily living, and follow-up care. The nurse also addresses preparatory information about when to return to work, sex, activity advancement, and lifestyle modifications. The nurse stresses the importance of ongoing monitoring of the patient status and addresses any questions or concerns.

19. **When does phase 2 occur?**

A patient will require close observation in phase 2 during the first 2 to 3 months after discharge. Patients will have supervision and will be monitored (telemetry) as they follow their prescribed exercise regimens. Phase 2 is the period when the patient and family will have the greatest adjustment in their lives. They may have much anxiety and develop fears about the condition. Ideally, a patient will have access to a cardiac rehabilitation program and will enroll and attend. The program will give the patient a team of individuals with which to interact during this period.

20. **What are the important areas to assess during phase 2?**

The rehabilitation nurse gives attention to areas to maintain the patient's quality of life. The nurse assesses the patient and family for signs of anxiety, depression, or other behaviors that prevent them from returning to a normal life. The nurse examines the patient's self-esteem because the patient must adjust to lifestyle changes. Many patients seem to feel that they have lost their sense of control over their lives. The quality cardiac rehabilitation program provides for psychosocial and physical needs. Any concerns or worries which the family has will be addressed. Learning needs are addressed, and interventions are planned to meet these needs.

21. **What is involved in phase 3 of the cardiac rehabilitation program?**

Phase 3 begins about 3 months after the cardiac event if the patient has no complications. Phase 3 is similar to phase 2 for a patient who has progressed smoothly. Patients continue to exercise with supervision, but at this point they do not have to be monitored (telemetry).

22. **What are therapeutic plans during this phase?**

In addition to cardiac care, other areas of importance are social support, emotional support, coping enhancement, and counseling and anxiety reduction. An important thing for the rehabilitation nurse to do at this point is to encourage patient/family enrollment and participation in a support group. Online support groups are available for patients and families who have computer access.

23. **Some sources/individuals describe phase 4 of a cardiac rehabilitation program. What is phase 4?**

Phase 4 is the maintenance of a healthy cardiac lifestyle. This phase is lifelong. Patients usually return to work and other normal life activities. It is important that patients know that they should not overextend themselves. Sometimes workplace assessments are done to evaluate patients' ability to return to work. Important areas to consider for returning to work are health status and exercise tolerance.

24. **What are some areas of concern during this lifelong phase?**

Altered role performance and social isolation are the major areas of concern at this phase. The patient must accept lifelong lifestyle changes and reentry into the community, and sometimes the patient has problems doing this. Home-based exercise programs are sometimes available if needed. The patient and family need to make arrangements with the primary care provider and cardiac rehabilitation team to discuss advance directives and do-not-resuscitate orders.

25. Is evaluation important in a cardiac rehabilitation program?

Evaluation is important. Two levels of evaluation are process and outcome. Process evaluation is the judgment and documentation of the rehabilitation process (including behaviors and activities). Outcome evaluation provides a way to judge and document the overall effectiveness of the cardiac rehabilitation program. One example of outcome evaluation is to determine whether the patient has lower cholesterol levels than those at entry into the program.

Key Points

- Cardiac rehabilitation program interventions help to prevent complications of CAD and improve patient outcomes after acute heart injury.
- Candidates for cardiac rehabilitation include individuals who have or have had any of the following: myocardial infarction, stable angina, coronary artery bypass graft surgery, percutaneous transluminal coronary angioplasty, or congestive heart failure.
- Research has shown that patients who undergo a cardiac rehabilitation program have dramatic improvement in depression, energy level, and exercise capacity.
- A cardiac rehabilitation program consists of three phases that involve rehabilitation professionals and a fourth phase that is lifelong in which the patient maintains a healthy cardiac lifestyle.

Internet Resources

American Heart Association
http://www.americanheart.org/

American Association of Cardiovascular and Pulmonary Rehabilitation
http://www.aacvpr.org/

Bibliography

1. Brewer L, Phillips BR, Boss B: Cardiac and cardiovascular rehabilitation. In Hoeman S, editor: *Rehabilitation nursing: process, application, & outcome,* ed 3, St Louis, 2002, Mosby.
2. Durnbaugh T: Gerontologic considerations. In Lewis SM, Heitkemper MM, Dirksen SR, editor: *Medical-surgical nursing: assessment and management of clinical problems,* ed 5, St Louis, 2000, Mosby.
3. Easton K: *Gerontological rehabilitation nursing,* Philadelphia, 1999, WB Saunders.
4. Murrock CJ: The effects of music on the rate of perceived exertion and general mood among coronary artery bypass graft patients enrolled in cardiac rehabilitation phase II, *Rehabil Nurs* 27(6):227-231, 2002.
5. Robinson-Smith G, Pizzi ER: Maximizing stroke recovery using patient self-care self-efficacy, *Rehabil Nurs* 28(2):48-51, 2003.

Chapter 19

Pulmonary Rehabilitation

Sandra H. Faria

1. **What are the basic components and focus of pulmonary rehabilitation programs?**

   All pulmonary rehabilitation programs have four basic components: exercise training, education, psychosocial/behavioral intervention, and outcome assessment. The rehabilitation program focuses on the major areas of concern for patients with pulmonary disease: ineffective airway clearance, ineffective breathing patterns, and impaired gas exchange.

2. **What health care professionals compose the pulmonary rehabilitation team?**

   Most pulmonary rehabilitation programs have a team of health care providers. This team may include a medical director, respiratory therapist, nurse, physical and occupational therapist, and exercise physiologist.

3. **Where might a pulmonary rehabilitation program be located?**

   Programs may be located in hospitals, outpatient, or home settings according to individual monitoring, cost, or access needs.

4. **What kind of subjective assessment should the rehabilitation nurse obtain from the patient?**

   A detailed assessment of the three most common respiratory-related complaints (dyspnea, cough, and activity intolerance) and a history of symptoms and smoking behavior are essential to plan care.

5. **What is the Borg CR10 Scale?**

   Dyspnea, or difficulty breathing, is described in many ways. Dyspnea may be called shortness of breath, suffocating, or chest tightness. The Borg CR10 Scale rates perceived exertion. The scale rates the intensity of dyspnea at rest or during physical activity. Patients point to the number on the scale that best describes the intensity of their breathlessness. The scale ranges from 0 (no breathlessness at all) to 10 or 11 (extremely strong) or 12 (absolute maximum). Chronic dyspnea contributes to functional disability.

6. Why is assessment of subjective data about a cough important?

The body uses a cough to clear the airway of mucus and protect against aspiration. A cough can be acute or chronic, productive or dry. A cough may be associated with other symptoms. Therefore questioning the patient about how the cough developed is important. If the cough is productive, the nurse should assess the sputum for thickness, color, odor, and blood.

7. What should the nurse find out about the patient's history of smoking?

The nurse should find out at what age the patient began smoking. The nurse should assess the type and amount of tobacco used (cigarettes, pipe, snuff) and whether the patient still smokes. Whether the patient has attempted to quit and reasons for continuing to smoke or not smoke are also good information questions to ask. The nurse also should attempt to ascertain whether the patient is ready to attempt a pulmonary rehabilitation program.

8. What information about the patient's activity should the nurse obtain?

Activity intolerance is a key subjective finding for patients who may begin a pulmonary rehabilitation program. Patients will usually complain of shortness of breath on exertion. They will complain of getting tired easily. The dyspnea is typically the reason they cannot continue with activity.

9. What key objective assessment data should the rehabilitation nurse obtain?

The nurse should
- Inspect the patient for any signs of respiratory distress. If obstructive disease is present, the inhalation/exhalation ratio may be abnormal (expiratory phase is prolonged).
- Look for any increase in anteroposterior diameter of the chest.
- Evaluate the rib cage for deformities that may cause breathing problems. Deformities that may cause restrictive defect include kyphosis or scoliosis. The nurse should observe the nail beds for cyanosis.
- Palpate for tenderness, crepitation, and respiratory excursion and for tactile fremitus.
- Percuss over the lung fields for abnormal sounds.
- Evaluate diaphragm location and excursion.
- Auscultate the chest area for normal breath sounds and listen for any abnormal or decreased sounds.

10. **What kinds of diagnostic tests may be done on a patient with pulmonary disease?**

Diagnostic tests include
- Pulmonary function tests to determine whether airflow problems exist (Table 19-1)

Table 19-1.   Pulmonary function tests

Test	Description
Vital capacity	Maximum amount of air exhaled from the point of maximum inspiration
Forced expiratory volume (FEV$_1$)	Volume of air exhaled during the first second of forced vital capacity
Functional residual capacity	Volume of air in the lungs at the end expiration position after a normal breath
Residual volume	Volume of air in the lungs after maximum exhalation
Total lung capacity	Total volume of air in the lungs after maximum inhalation

- Arterial blood gas analyses to detect acid-base abnormalities
- Pulse oximetry to reflect oxygenation of the tissues in a noninvasive manner
- Radiological studies to determine the presence of air or abnormal growths in the lungs

11. **Why are nutritional therapies important for the patient in pulmonary rehabilitation?**

The patient with pulmonary disease uses a tremendous amount of energy, lean body mass, and muscle to breathe. Therefore nutritional assessment becomes imperative in a pulmonary rehabilitation program. A thorough assessment of nutritional status includes laboratory tests, a measurement of height and weight, and a history of food intake.

Indications of malnutrition include a loss of at least 10% of normal body weight, visible muscle wasting, gastrointestinal symptoms lasting for more than 2 weeks, decreased ability to function (activities of daily living [ADL]), and edema. Patients should increase their consumption of calorie-rich foods, use dietary supplements, and begin a regimen of vitamin and mineral supplements. Overweight patients are referred to a dietitian to plan a healthy nutritional plan for good lung health and overall good health.

12. **Is dental health important for the patient with pulmonary disease?**

Dental care and oral hygiene are important because infections/bacteria in the mouth may lead to bacterial growth that spreads to the respiratory tract.

Pulmonary patients need to avoid respiratory infections. Infections tend to cause further lung damage in many patients and can lead to pneumonia and life-threatening illness. Therefore good dental hygiene reduces the number of microorganisms in the oral cavity, thus decreasing the risk for inhalation of these organisms into the respiratory tract.

13. **Why is patient and family education important in a pulmonary rehabilitation program?**

Education can promote changes in behavior and increase the patient's participation in self-learning. Box 19-1 presents areas of teaching.

Box 19-1.   Areas of education in a pulmonary rehabilitation program

- Anatomy and physiology
- Pathophysiology of lung disease
- Breathing training
- Energy conservation
- Medications
- Exercise guidelines
- Oxygen therapy
- Respiratory and chest therapy techniques
- Psychological factors such as coping, panic, and stress management

---

14. **Many patients with respiratory disease who enroll in pulmonary rehabilitation programs have "ineffective airway clearance." What does this involve and what kind of information is shared with the patient and family?**

Ineffective airway clearance means that patients cannot clear effectively the secretions in their airway; therefore the airway becomes obstructed. Many times the volume of secretions is so large that the person has trouble coughing effectively. The mucus may be too thick to cough up easily. Many times the respiratory muscles are weak, and this causes a hindrance to an effective cough. Lean muscle mass and nutritional status are factors that influence respiratory muscle strength. Patients with respiratory disease may have intermittent times when they experience ineffective airway clearance. Immobility further contributes to this problem. Teaching for the patient and family includes
- Measures to help with secretion removal, such as forcing fluids to keep mucus thin
- Avoiding milk because it thickens secretions
- Staying as active as possible so that no further muscle mass is lost
- Compressing a pillow against the chest wall to provide support for coughing

15. **What are the goals for caring for the patient with ineffective airway clearance?**

Box 19-2 presents several important goals to keep in mind when caring for patients with ineffective airway clearance.

Box 19-2.   Goals in caring for the patient with ineffective airway clearance

- Maintain a patent airway (priority).
- Master techniques to assist in producing an effective cough.
- Mobilize secretions.
- Maintain adequate hydration and humidification.
- Provide a nutritional diet.

---

16. **What is evidence of respiratory infection?**

If the mucus becomes discolored (yellow, brown, green) and if the patient becomes febrile, dyspneic, or disoriented, the physician should be notified immediately. Antibiotics will be ordered for the infection.

17. **What are nursing interventions for airway clearance problems?**

Most patients can be managed for airway clearance problems without invasive measures, but the nurse needs to recognize the need for artificial airway placement or intubation. All caregivers (including family) must know care measures to help the patient to maintain an open airway. Hydration measures are vital and include forcing fluids, monitoring fluid status, and teaching the family the importance of cleaning humidifiers to prevent bacterial growth. Nebulizers deliver medication through fine mist droplets that are inhaled into the lungs. The nurse should assess the patient for overhydration and should teach the family how to clean the nebulizer to avoid bacterial infection. The nurse can share techniques such as controlled cough (hold one's breath for several seconds and then cough 2 or 3 times) or huff cough (cross arms just below rib cage, take a deep breath while leaning forward and exhale sharply while whispering the word "huff" several times to keep the glottis open) with the patient and family to assist airway clearance. Deep breathing exercises help to mobilize secretions.

18. **What is the advantage of the patient's using the incentive spirometer?**

The incentive spirometer assists efforts for lung inflation. The spirometer lets the patients visually see how much airflow they can produce. These devices are inexpensive, and patients do not normally need assistance with them.

19. What does chest physiotherapy involve?

Chest physiotherapy is useful in patients who have ineffective airway clearance. The therapy involves chest percussion, chest vibration, and postural drainage. These techniques help loosen secretions so that the patient can expel them.

20. What drugs are important for the patient with ineffective airway clearance, and how are they administered?

One recommendation is that anyone with respiratory disorders receive a vaccine against pneumonia. Expectorants often are prescribed for the patient to assist in coughing up secretions. For the patient with emphysema and asthma, the goal is to decrease airflow obstruction and inflammation in the airway. β_2-Agonists are the treatment of choice for bronchodilation. Inhaled medications are preferred because the desired affect can be achieved with lower doses than when the drug is given systemically. Inhaled steroids may be added according to the treatment plan. Metered-dose inhalers should be used with a spacer device if the patient can manage the timing and coordination. The spacer device allows the droplets to be suspended long enough for the carrier molecule to evaporate, leaving the smaller molecule of drug to be carried deep into the lungs. However, if the patient uses a dry powder inhaler, such as Advair, the patient cannot use spacers. Antibiotics may be ordered for the patient when respiratory infection is evident. The use of peak flow meters for self-monitoring are recommended with written patient goals for treatment. Most commonly used is the red, yellow, green system for monitoring and treating asthma and bronchospasm. For the guidelines, visit **http://www.nhlbi.nih.gov/guide-lines/asthma/index.htm.**

21. What are the clinical manifestations of a respiratory infection?

Box 19-3 presents the manifestations of a respiratory infection.

Box 19-3.   Manifestations of a respiratory infection

- Mucus becomes discolored (yellow, brown, green)
- Fever
- Dyspnea
- Disorientation

---

22. When the patient cannot cough effectively, suctioning may be required. What are the key points to remember when suctioning the secretions from the intubated patient?

The most important point is to use sterile technique. The nurse does not want to introduce any bacteria into the patient's airway that is not already there. Therefore sterile technique is a must. The nurse should wash his or her hands before the procedure. The patient should hyperventilate with an ambu bag for five breaths before suctioning.

The nurse should not activate the suction until the catheter is in place in the airway and then should apply suction only while removing the catheter and should remove the catheter in less than 10 seconds. Suctioning the airway removes oxygen also, so the patient may become hypoxic. The nurse must watch for arrhythmias (especially premature ventricular contractions) and hyperventilate or preoxygenate the patient before suctioning each subsequent time. Suctioning also stimulates the patient and may increase intracranial pressure. If the nurse knows the patient has compromised intracranial pressure from a condition such as brain tumor or hydrocephalus, the nurse may delay subsequent suctioning a few minutes until the intracranial pressure has had time to return to normal. The nurse should suction the mouth last and discard the catheter afterward.

23. What are nursing interventions for the patient who has a tracheostomy?

Patients who cannot be weaned from the ventilator or cannot cough effectively to get rid of secretions may receive permanent tracheostomies. If the tracheostomy has a cuff, the nurse should suction the oropharynx before deflating the cuff. The nurse should perform tracheal care frequently to keep the tracheostomy tube clean. Providing humidity via a tracheostomy collar with a heated jet nebulizer prevents complications arising from dry, crusty secretions. Communication is a problem for the patient with a tracheostomy, so a plan needs to be made for facilitation of alternative methods of communication.

24. What information should the nurse teach to the family/caregiver of the patient with an artificial airway?

Box 19-4 provides basic information families and caregivers need about artificial airways.

Box 19-4. Education for caregivers of patients with artificial airways

- Care of the inner cannula is an important concept for the family to learn.
- Emergency phone numbers should be evident and displayed prominently in the home.
- Proper humidification is essential.
- Adequate amounts of fluid intake help to liquefy the patient's secretions.
- The patient and family should be cautioned to protect the tracheostomy opening from water or inhalation of foreign substances.

---

25. What is an ineffective breathing pattern?

Ineffective breathing pattern means that the respirations in the patient are inadequate to meet the oxygen demands in the body. Dyspnea and fatigue are the major symptoms described by patients with ineffective breathing patterns.

26. The patient may have alveolar hyperventilation or hypoventilation. What are the definitions of these conditions?

Alveolar hyperventilation occurs when hyperventilation (breathing too fast and deep for an extended period) causes the P_{CO_2} to fall below 35 mm Hg. Hyperventilation may result from anxiety or it may occur in a high altitude environment.

Hypoventilation (not breathing in enough air/oxygen) occurs if a person has a neurological condition or severe pulmonary disorder causing an inability to expand the lung adequately to acquire adequate oxygen and eliminate carbon dioxide. The P_{CO_2} is greater than 45 mm Hg, and the P_{O_2} is less than 60 mm Hg.

27. What are "obstructive defects"?

Obstructive defects are pulmonary conditions in which airflow is obstructed. Chronic obstructive pulmonary disease (COPD; emphysema, asthma, or chronic bronchitis) may cause this problem. In severe COPD the person may experience chronic hypoventilation (because of obstructed airway); thus hypercapnea (increased CO_2 level) becomes chronic also.

28. What are "restrictive defects"?

Restrictive disorders are characterized by decreased compliance of the lungs or chest wall or both. Pulmonary function tests are used to differentiate between restrictive and obstructive disorders. Restrictive disorders usually are classified as intrapulmonary or extrapulmonary. Extrapulmonary causes include chest wall problems in which the chest cavity/lung is restricted in movement; thus the person develops hypoventilation because of the inability to expand the chest/lungs. The restriction may be due to muscle weakness, which alters chest movement, or decreased compliance (movement) of the lungs and chest wall. The extent of the chest wall muscle/lung involvement depends on the pathological nature of the disorder. Other extrapulmonary causes of restrictive lung disease include central nervous system causes (brain injuries or narcotic/barbiturate use) and neuromuscular system disorders (myasthenia gravis or muscular dystrophy).

Intrapulmonary causes may include disorders of the pleura (pleurisy, pleural effusion, pneumothorax) or disorders of the parenchyma (atelectasis, pneumonia, or pulmonary fibrosis).

29. Can a patient have obstructive and restrictive disorders?

The patient with cystic fibrosis typically has obstructive and restrictive disorders. The thick secretions experienced in cystic fibrosis lead to obstructive disorder. The patient typically has thick mucus, infection, inflammation, and injury of the lung tissue. This injury can lead to fibrosis and progressive deterioration of the lung. Thus this restrictive condition compounds what was originally obstructive disease.

30. What are the subjective data obtained from patients with ineffective breathing patterns?

Patients feel like they cannot get their breath; thus dyspnea is the chief complaint that they describe. They also may complain of fatigue. Sleep pattern alterations (such as sleep apnea) also may be a problem, so they may complain of excessive sleepiness or loud snoring.

31. What objective data might the nurse obtain relevant to ineffective breathing patterns?

The nurse should look for signs of dyspnea (unusual postures to help breathing, use of accessory muscles) or changes in mental state (confusion or agitation are early signs of hypoxia). Pursed lip breathing or abdominal breathing may be signs of ineffective ventilation. Breath sounds may be decreased and reveal signs of obstruction (wheezing). Obesity often makes the condition worse. Pulmonary function tests (discussed previously) will indicate abnormalities and assist in diagnosis of the abnormal breathing pattern.

32. What are the rehabilitation goals for the patient with ineffective breathing patterns?

A major goal that can be accomplished through the pulmonary rehabilitation program is an increase in the patient's activity level. Supervised exercise that is increased slowly will let patients safely increase their level of endurance. Having supervision and consultants available at the rehabilitation program decreases patients' anxiety level and makes them feel more secure. This decrease in anxiety is another major goal. Other goals include
- Fewer complaints of dyspnea with activity
- Adequate breathing pattern during sleep
- Overall ventilation patterns that are more normal

33. What types of ventilation techniques might help the patient with an ineffective breathing pattern?

Pursed lip breathing may benefit the patient with ineffective breathing pattern. Breathing retraining to use pursed lip breathing or diaghragmatic breathing may help by relieving symptoms of breathlessness. These techniques usually assist the patient to have more effective ventilation. Pursed lip breathing is the technique of breathing slowly through puckered lips. Diaphragmatic breathing is especially useful in the partially paralyzed patient to strengthen the diaphragm. Studies have shown this technique to be ineffective in patients with COPD. The technique involves focusing on movement of the diaphragm and using abdominal muscles to breathe.

34. What is the benefit of exercise for the patient?

Exercise training is a basic part of any pulmonary rehabilitation program. Building up patients' ability for activity results in their having reduced dyspnea with exertion. Patients with COPD find that dyspnea is reduced remarkably with exercise training involving the upper arm. Lower extremity training with regular walking or treadmill use assists patients to perform ADL with less dyspnea.

35. What is respiratory muscle training and why might it be done?

Respiratory muscle training involves use of a device that generates high airway pressure with inspiration and normal airway pressure with expiration. Therefore the patient works hard during inspiration but relaxes a bit with the normal expiration. Research is needed to delineate the role of this training and the specific benefits it may bring to the patient.

36. Energy conservation is important to patients with respiratory disorders. What are some energy conservation techniques?

The best energy conservation technique for the patient with a respiratory disorder is to use breathing techniques in coordination with movement or activity. The patient may inhale before the activity and then slowly exhale while performing the activity. In addition, movement of the arms away from the chest can assist the chest to move during inspiration during an activity. Another tip is for patients to put their hands on their hips as they inhale while performing ADL. These techniques may help ventilation to be more effective so that the patients do not tire so easily.

37. What are ventilatory support devices?

Ventilatory support devices are noninvasive devices that mechanically move the chest wall by pushing on the anterior chest, abdomen, or back. These devices are especially helpful for paralyzed patients. The most frequently used devices are rocking beds and pneumobelts. The rocking bed uses gravity and the pressure of the abdominal contents to apply and remove pressure in an alternating manner on the diaphragm. This change in pressure in the thoracic cavity assists with ventilation. A pneumobelt is an inflatable bladder worn inside a corset that applies pressure on the abdomen. The belt is most effective when the patient is sitting upright.

38. What if none of the noninvasive ventilatory devices works adequately to assist the patient to breathe?

If noninvasive devices do not assist ventilation adequately, mechanical ventilation is the next step. The respiratory therapist inserts an endotracheal tube or tracheostomy tube and applies and sets the mechanical ventilator to ensure maximum performance of the lungs.

39. Can a mechanical ventilator be used in the home?

Yes, mechanical ventilators can be used in the home. Usually, mechanical ventilators for home use are more compact than the ones used in a clinical setting. Some ventilators are mounted on motorized wheelchairs and have enough suction and oxygen supply to last about 3 hours. These ventilators may be powered by electricity, but a backup system must be available in case of power outage. Home support services require a multidisciplinary approach. Respiratory therapists, nurses, and home health aides are part of the team. Physical therapists, occupational therapists, social workers, and dietitians also are important in the rehabilitation process for these patients.

40. What if the patient is ready to be weaned from the ventilator?

Weaning from a ventilator is the long-term goal for any patient who is mechanically ventilated in the health care facility or in the home. Weaning devices are available to help assist weaning of the patient with as little anxiety and as few problems as possible. Weaning parameters usually include criteria such as presented in Box 19-5.

Box 19-5. Ventilatory weaning parameters

- Inspiratory muscle strength
- Vital capacity
- Respiratory compliance
- Airway resistance

An index one may use in rehabilitation settings to measure readiness to wean is the rapid shallow breathing index. This index measures respiratory rate and tidal volume ratio in a 1-minute period using a T-piece while the patient is off the ventilator. The threshold for weaning is usually 1 to 5 breaths per minute. If the breathing is faster and more shallow, patients usually are not weaned successfully. T-pieces, continuous positive airway pressure, and positive pressure support are also useful to wean the patient from the ventilatory support.

Sometimes the weaning must be very gradual. The patient must be monitored closely for signs of respiratory distress. Continuous oxygen saturation levels are monitored. The patient must be given continuous emotional support because this time is stressful to the patient who has depended on a ventilator to breathe.

41. What is impaired gas exchange?

The normal lung functions to exchange oxygen and carbon dioxide between the alveoli and the capillaries. When this exchange fails to happen normally, impaired gas exchange occurs. Impairment can happen in a patient with a variety of lung conditions. Patients who have impaired gas exchange also have ineffective breathing patterns and ineffective airway clearance.

42. What are the signs/symptoms of impaired gas exchange?

The patient may experience confusion, restlessness, irritability, hypercapnea, changes in respiratory rate and depth, and inability to move secretions. Other symptoms may be acute shortness of breath and dyspnea on exertion or at rest. The arterial blood gas values will be abnormal, indicating a problem with gas exchange.

43. What are goals for the patient with impaired gas exchange?

The major goal is to improve ventilation and oxygenation. Other goals include
- A more normal mental status
- Ability to have a normal sleep pattern
- Increased ability to conserve energy
- Improve ADL abilities so that activities may occur without dyspnea

44. What effect does positioning have on the patient with impaired gas exchange?

Having the patient lean forward and rest arms on the thighs or on an overbed table may assist with the feelings of breathlessness. If the patient is in bed, moving side to side promotes ventilation and skin integrity. The head always should be elevated in the patient with a pulmonary disease because patients breathe more easily in an upright position.

45. When might oxygen therapy be used?

Intermittent use of oxygen can relieve the feelings of breathlessness and is considered a major part of the pharmaceutical management of the patient. Oxygen therapy does not treat the underlying problem but decreases the cardiac workload. Long-term oxygen therapy often is prescribed for patients with severe hypoxemia. The condition necessitates the use of oxygen at home. Medicare and most third-party reimbursements will authorize use of oxygen in the home if the P_{O_2} level is less than 55 mm Hg or the oxygen saturation level is less than 88%.

Key Points

- The four basic components to all pulmonary rehabilitation programs are exercise training, education, psychosocial/behavioral intervention, and outcome assessment.
- The Borg CR10 Scale can provide an objective assessment of the patient's dyspnea.
- Nutritional assessment is critical for pulmonary patients because of the tremendous amount of energy expended in breathing.
- Regular dental care and good oral hygiene are important for reducing the risk of respiratory infection.
- Major areas of concern for patients with pulmonary disease are ineffective airway clearance, ineffective breathing patterns, and impaired gas exchange.
- Oxygen therapy is considered a major part of the pharmaceutical management of the patient.

Internet Resources

American Association of Cardiovascular and Pulmonary Rehabilitation
http://www.aacvpr.org

American College of Chest Physicians
http://www.chestnet.org

American Thoracic Society
http://www.thoracic.org

American Lung Association
http://www.lungusa.org

Bibliography

1. Berry JK, Johnson JH, Ploeg KV: Respiration and pulmonary rehabilitation. In Hoeman S, editor: *Rehabilitation nursing: process, application, & outcome,* ed 3, St Louis, 2000, Mosby.
2. Lindell KO, Van Sciver T: Obstructive pulmonary disease. In Lewis SM, Heitkemper MM, Dirksen SR, editor: *Medical-surgical nursing: assessment and management of clinical problems,* ed 5, St Louis, 2000, Mosby.
3. Rooyackers JM, Berkeljon DA, Folgering HT: Eccentric exercise training in patients with chronic obstructive pulmonary disease, *Int J Rehabil Res* 26(1):47-49, 2003.

Chapter 20

Burn Rehabilitation

Susan R. Bulecza

1. **Are there national standards and guidelines for burn nursing practice?**

   Yes, the American Burn Association has developed "Guidelines for Burn Nursing Practice," and the Nurse Advisory Council of the Burn Foundation of Philadelphia has developed "Standards of Burn Nursing Practice."

2. **When does rehabilitation begin for a burn-injured patient?**

   Rehabilitation for a burn-injured patient begins the first day of injury. Initially, the goals of care are related to survival and minimizing loss of function. Once the patient has stabilized, goals of care focus on restoration of optimal wellness within the limitation of injury.

3. **What are the physiological concepts important in burn nursing care?**

   Physiological concepts important to burn nursing care are
   - Burn process: relates to type and extent of burn, any trauma, and nutritional status
   - Wound healing: relates to grafting and healing of wounds and donor sites
   - Mobility and function: relates to range of motion, positioning, and activities maintaining and restoring movement
   - Scarring: care activities focus on minimizing contracture and scarring
   - Early complications: care activities focus on minimizing complications such as edema, deep vein thrombosis, and cellulitis
   - Ongoing complications: care activities focus on reducing the risk of other complications such as neuromuscular problems, sensory impairment, and fragile skin throughout the healing and rehabilitation process.

4. **What is the most common type of burn injury?**

   Thermal burns are the most common type of burn injury. The mechanism of injury is due to exposure to flames, steam, frostbite, or hot liquids. The length of time the body is exposed to the mechanism of injury and its intensity correlates to the severity of the burn.

5. **What is the most destructive type of burn?**

Electrical burns are the most destructive. Although skin injury from an electrical burn is usually minimal, internal injury can be severe and extensive. The voltage, type of current, length of contact, and tract of the current influence the severity of the burn. Another unique characteristic of an electrical burn is that it will have a small entrance wound and a large exit wound.

6. **What are the two most important factors determining the rehabilitation course?**

Extent of skin loss and depth of the burn are the main factors that determine the rehabilitative course. The greater the skin loss, the more complex rehabilitation becomes. Significant skin loss affects the ability of the skin to maintain its many physiological functions such as protecting the body from infection and temperature regulation, and has negative effect on psychological health because of perceived identity loss and self-esteem. The severity of burn depth increases the need for grafting, risk of function loss, secondary complications, and prolonged healing. Rehabilitation nurses must know not only where the patient is in the healing process but also the circumstances of initial injury.

7. **How is severity of burn injury determined?**

Several assessment methods are used to determine the severity of burn injury. The rule of nines is one of the most common. Extent of injury is determined by visualizing the body as a grid with 12 sections, with each section representing 9% of surface area, except for the perineum, which is 1% (Figure 20-1). The more sections involved in the injury, the greater the severity. Another method is the Lund-Browder classification, which uses specific body surface area percentages correlated with age. The American Burn Association also has a method for classifying burn injury known as the Classification of Burn Severity. This scale takes into consideration extent of burn, location and type of burn, age, and depth.

8. **How should nursing interventions be focused during skin healing?**

Nursing interventions should focus on protecting fragile skin, reducing skin dryness, reducing itching, and protecting the skin from sun exposure. Lotions are effective in reducing skin dryness. However, the type used must contain components of water and lipid to enhance absorption and reduce evaporation. The nurse should avoid using lotions with lanolin and cocoa butter because they may cause irritation or contact sensitization. Reduction of dryness also can reduce itching. Itching is a major problem with healing skin, and the subsequent scratching can disrupt grafts and donor sites. Systemic antihistamines and topical antipruritic and anesthetic agents can help to reduce itching. Lotions with menthol or camphor are also useful. Nurses should not use topical benzocaine because of allergy potential. Because of potential hyperpigmentation and sunburn, the patient should avoid exposure to direct sunlight for at least 6 months.

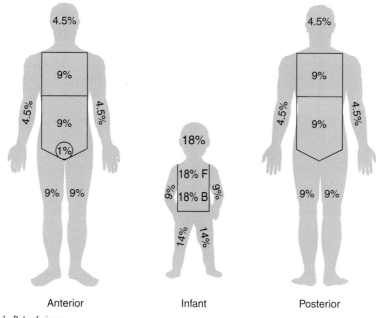

Figure 20-1. Rule of nines.

The patient should wear appropriate clothing, hats, and sunscreen with a minimal sun protection factor of 15 when exposed to sunlight.

9. **Because pain management is a major component of burn care, what is important for the nurse to know?**

Pain is a constant issue throughout burn recovery. Pain may be lifelong depending on the burn injury. Partial-thickness burns cause severe pain because sensory fibers are still intact; whereas full-thickness burns cause little, if any, initial pain because sensory fibers are destroyed. Most patients experience both types of burns. Appropriate pain management is critical to ensure optimal healing. Inadequately managed pain can influence physiological and psychological well-being. Pain type and intensity changes over the course of healing from acute injury-related pain resulting from therapy activities such as stretching and increasing range of motion to the healing of disrupted tissue such as contractures, peripheral neuropathies, and scaring. Procedures also induce pain. Therefore frequent and ongoing pain assessment using pain scales is essential. Narcotics are used most often for burn pain management and are effective. However, narcotics frequently are underused because of misperceptions associated with addiction. In addition to pharmacological management, comfort measures and relaxation techniques are helpful adjuncts in reducing pain. Coordination of therapy, planned rest periods, and anticipation of medication needs also contribute to reducing pain.

10. **Why is adequate nutrition important?**

Adequate nutrition is important for wound healing and to counterbalance the hypermetabolic state created from the stress response generated by the burn. Patients often start rehabilitation having suffered profound weight loss, decreased muscle mass, and significant protein depletion. Supplements of protein and calories frequently are needed to counterbalance these negative effects. Vitamin and mineral supplements are needed as well to enhance wound healing. Ongoing daily assessment of nutritional status is necessary to ensure that needs are met. Assessment should include calorie and fluid intake, weight, bowel and bladder functions, appropriate laboratory results including albumin and lipids levels, manual dexterity, mental status, pain level, type of foods consumed, swallowing, chewing, taste ability, and percent of meals consumed.

11. **What are the nutritional requirements for a burn-injured patient?**

Because the burn injury creates a hypermetabolic state for the patient, the patient will require an average of 5000 calories per day. The goal for the patient should be to lose no more than 10% of preburn weight. Box 20-1 presents the calculation for caloric requirements.

Box 20-1.   Calculation for caloric requirements in a burn-injured patient

To calculate accurately caloric requirements for a patient with a 20% or greater total body surface area (TBSA) burn, the nurse can use the following formula:

$$(25 \text{ kcal} \times \text{kg of body weight}) + (40 \text{ kcal} \times \% \text{ TBSA burn})$$

To ensure accurate caloric intake and prevent overfeeding throughout the healing process, the nurse needs to recalculate caloric requirements at least every 2 weeks.

12. **Should patients actively participate in wound care?**

Whenever possible and appropriate, patients should participate actively in wound care because this provides them with some measure of control. Participation may be as simple as allowing the patient to decide the time of care or as involved as the patient removing the dressing. Active participation by the patient allows for enhanced patient education, increased awareness of progress, and improved goal attainment.

13. **Why is it important for the rehabilitation nurse to know skin-grafting procedures and donor site care?**

Often a significantly burned patient may require additional procedures well into the rehabilitation phase for things such as contracture release or covering slow-to-heal areas. Also, a patient who needs multiple grafts may need to wait for the donor site to heal in order for a graft to be obtained, thereby prolonging grafting. The rehabilitation nurse must treat surgical procedures, regardless of how many the patient has had previously, as the first one each time. Consequently, the nurse should know what a skin graft is, the type of graft needed, and what it entails for this patient; pain management; identification of the donor site; and postoperative care of donor and graft sites.

14. Why is ongoing pulmonary assessment important?

Ongoing pulmonary assessment is important for several reasons. First, the patient could have suffered an inhalation injury to the respiratory tract that could have resulted in limited pulmonary function. So the nurse must understand what the patient's functional ability is and whether supplemental oxygen is required to maintain optimal function. Second, many of the procedures such as grafting are done using general anesthesia, which requires good postoperative respiratory care such as coughing and deep breathing to reduce complication risks.

15. When is a burn-injured patient considered ready for intensive rehabilitation?

The burn-injured patient can be considered ready for intensive rehabilitation when the majority of wounds have been grafted or have new skin cover and the patient is mobile enough to leave the bed for therapy.

16. What types of rehabilitation may a burn-injured patient need?

Types of rehabilitation include
- Mobility and gait training
- Self-care and daily living activities
- Muscle strengthening
- Scar management
- Skin care
- Counseling

17. Why are early ambulation and progressive mobility important?

Early ambulation is important to reduce the risk of clot formation, pneumonia, musculoskeletal deterioration, and contractures. Additionally, progressive mobility reduces edema and venous stasis, enhancing healing. However, ambulation must be a progressive process for those patients who have had prolonged bed rest so that they are able to adjust adequately to the position changes.

18. What is heterotopic ossification?

Heterotopic ossification is the deposition of bone in muscle fibers around joints in patients who have experienced trauma, and the condition is believed to be due to metabolic changes. The process creates a contracture or ankylosis.

19. **Who is most at risk for developing heterotopic ossification?**

A patient who has upper extremity full-thickness burns greater than 20% total body surface area is predisposed to develop heterotopic ossification. Heterotopic ossification manifests as pain in the affected joint with loss in range of motion. Elbow, hip, and shoulder joints are the most commonly affected. Nerve entrapment and neurological loss also may occur. Any forceful movement of the joint exacerbates pain and should not be done.

20. **Are neuropathies common in burn-injured patients?**

Yes, moderate to severely burned patients are at risk of developing neuropathies. The incidence of occurrence is between 15% and 29%.

21. **What is the main way to reduce hypertrophic scarring?**

Compression therapy is the main treatment for reducing and preventing hypertrophic scarring. The patient wears custom-fitted compression devices or garments 24 hours a day, starting as soon as wounds are closed, for as long as 1 to 2 years. Type of device or garment used depends on the type and extent of the wounds. Extensive education for the patient and family regarding these garments is necessary to ensure compliance. These devices or garments can be removed only for hygiene and skin care. For the nurse to assess the skin thoroughly whenever the garments are removed to guarantee skin integrity and absence of infection is important. Before discharge from the acute rehabilitation facility, the patient and family are taught to do this assessment daily.

22. **Should splints be used with burn patients?**

Splints may be necessary in some cases to maintain soft tissue joint structure length. However, caution is advised so as to avoid prolonged immobilization and tissue fibrosis. Dynamic splints used for joint stretching or a functional splinting with on/off scheduling may be helpful to maintain stretching.

23. **Who is responsible for the psychological recovery of the burn-injured patient?**

The entire health care team is responsible for the psychological recovery of the patient. Although ongoing psychological counseling for the burn-injured patient from a psychologist or psychiatrist is important, the other team members have a role as well. Because the nurse is often the team member who interacts with the patient the most, the nurse must stress the long-term benefits of psychotherapy in the recovery process, to deal not only with the depression that often accompanies these injuries but also the physical and emotional pain of treatment. The nurse also needs to address spiritual concerns. These concerns are generally not religion-specific but are more global questioning by the patients such as why they survived, why they suffered the injury, and not others. Interventions by the nurse such as active listening, referral to a spiritual counselor, or imagery can be helpful in the patient's healing process. The nurse must remember that many of the psychological concerns may not manifest fully until the patient begins to reenter into the family and community environments and begins fully to realize the extent of disfigurement and disability.

Key Points

- The American Burn Association and the Nurse Advisory Council of the Burn Foundation of Philadelphia have developed standards and guidelines for the care of burn-injured patients.
- Rehabilitation begins the first day of injury.
- Important physiological concepts to know are the burn process, wound healing, mobility and function, scarring, early complications, and ongoing complications.
- The greater the skin loss and more severe the burn depth, the more complex rehabilitation becomes.
- The rule of nines and Lund-Browder classification are methods for determining burn severity. Pain management is a major component in recovery.
- Adequate nutrition is important for wound healing and to counterbalance the hypermetabolic state created from the stress response generated by the burn.
- Early ambulation and mobility are important factors to reduce complications and enhance healing.
- The entire health care team is responsible for the patient's psychological recovery.

Internet Resources

American Burn Association
http://www.ameriburn.org/

Burn Prevention Foundation
http://www.burnprevention.org/

Burn Support Groups Database
http://www.burnsupportgroupsdatabase.com/

Alisa Anna Ruch Burn Foundation
http://www.aarbf.org

Bibliography

1. Dowling L: Advanced practice nurses' knowledge and assessment of nutrition, unpublished thesis, Tallahassee, 2003, Florida State University.

2. Latarjet J, Choinere M: Pain in burn patients, *Burns* 21 (5):344-348, 1995.

3. McCollom PL: Restoration after burn injury. In Hoeman SP, editor: *Rehabilitation nursing: process, application, & outcome,* ed 3, St Louis, 2001, Mosby.

4. Regojo PS, Wright C: A holistic approach to burn rehabilitation. In Derstine JB, Hargrove SD, editors: *Comprehensive rehabilitation nursing,* Philadelphia, 2001, WB Saunders.

Chapter 21

Orthopedic Rehabilitation

Jeanne Flannery and Sharon A. Aronovitch

1. **Why does phantom limb pain occur following removal of a diseased limb?**

   Phantom limb pain is the patient's perception of pain in the limb that has been amputated. Phantom limb pain results from the patient's brain having been "programmed" to receive sensations from the limb, and now the remaining nerves continue to generate impulses to the same somatosensory cortical region. This pain (sensation) can subside in a short period of time or last indefinitely. Pain can be elicited by touching the opposite limb or head, smoking cigarettes, or angina. Defecation, urination, or sexual intercourse is more likely to elicit pain related to leg amputation.

2. **What can be done to relieve phantom pain?**

   Phantom pain, which is pain that has persisted longer than 6 months after amputation, should be treated with nonpharmaceutical modalities first, such as biofeedback, a transcutaneous electrical nerve stimulation unit, heat, cold, therapeutic touch, massage, aroma therapy, ultrasound, acupuncture, and hypnosis. These modalities help the patient to focus on the activities rather than the pain. If all else has failed, only then should neuroleptics such as gabapentin (Neurontin) or analgesics be used. Surgical revision of the stump may be considered as a therapeutic strategy.

3. **Why is the positioning of abductor pillows following hip surgery so important?**

   The abductor pillow is used to ensure that the repaired hip does not dislocate through hip flexion, adduction, or rotation. The pillow is placed so that the wider end is located at the ankles and the narrower end is located just above the knees. The abduction pillow needs to be fastened in place with Velcro straps while the patient is in bed, during repositioning of the patient in bed, and initially during transfer from the bed to chair. Once the patient has learned how to maintain proper alignment of the repaired hip, the patient can discontinue use of the abductor pillow.

4. **What are the most common surgical complications following repair of a fracture?**

The most frequent complications following repair of a fracture are deep venous thrombosis (DVT), pulmonary emboli, and fat emboli. Patients with fractures of the hip need to be assessed for DVT and pulmonary emboli routinely. Nearly 70% of the patients undergoing hip surgery will be treated for DVT. Modalities for prevention of DVT include use of epidural anesthesia, anticoagulants, sequential compression devices, and early ambulation.

The incidence of pulmonary emboli following hip surgery is about 20%. Modalities for preventing pulmonary emboli are similar to those used to prevent DVT following hip surgery.

Patients with multiple fractures, fractures of the long bones, and closed fractures are more likely to develop fat emboli as a complication. The hypothesis is that fat molecules are released from the bone marrow into the blood following the severe injury. Preventive care for these patients includes early immobilization of the broken bone(s), proper splinting, and minimal manipulation of the fracture. Though the percentage of fat emboli is small (less than 10%), the patient needs to be assessed for this potential complication. The patient may manifest one or more of the following signs and symptoms: an increased respiratory rate (tachypnea), temperature greater than 103° F, subtle changes in behavior or mental status, petechiae on the anterior chest and axilla lasting a few hours, and laboratory abnormalities such as thrombocytopenia and a sudden drop in hematocrit.

5. **What potentially fatal occurrence may result from fractures of long bones and pelvis, multiple trauma, or arthroplasty of the hip or knee?**

Fat embolism syndrome may occur when fat globules are released from the bone marrow and travel through the bloodstream to the lungs or cerebral circulation. Twenty percent of cases are fatal, and death can occur within 30 minutes. Box 21-1 lists the symptoms of fat embolism.

Box 21-1.   Symptoms of a fat embolism

- Hypoxia
- Tachypnea
- Tachycardia
- Petechiae
- Fever
- Lipuria
- Chest pain
- Altered mental status
- Restlessness
- Confusion
- Lethargy
- Transient ischemic attack or stroke

6. What is the difference between skin and skeletal traction?

Traction typically is used to treat fractures of the long bones, though it also is used to manage minor fractures of the lower spine, muscle spasm, separation of the pelvic girdle, cervical spine fractures, and dislocation and fractures of the upper arm.

Skin traction is a force applied to the skin using tape, boots, or splints applied directly to the skin and is intended for short-term use until surgical intervention or placement of skeletal traction. Traction weights for skin traction are 5 to 10 pounds that assist in skeletal alignment, reduction of the fracture, and reduction of spasms to the injured site.

Skeletal traction is usually in place for longer periods of time to realign injured bones and joints. Skeletal traction requires the surgeon to insert a wire or pin into the bone, partially or fully, to align the injured bone. The weight for skeletal traction ranges from 5 to 45 pounds. Countertraction, which is the patient's own body weight, is necessary for either traction to be effective.

7. Why do some patients require external fixators for repair of a fracture?

An external fixator is used to stabilize a complex open fracture using a metal frame and pin system. Most pelvic and long bone fractures are placed in an external fixator.

8. Do patients with an external fixator require special nursing care and patient education?

External fixators provide an excellent source of entry for microorganisms into the skin. The nurse should assess pin sites at least every 8 hours for signs of infection (i.e., exudates, erythema, tenderness, and pain). The nurse also should assess pin sites for pin loosening, which can cause a local wound infection. The patient/family will be managing the care of the fixator for weeks to months and therefore will need to learn all aspects of the care the rehabilitation nurse is providing. The patient may require home care, and the rehabilitation nurse will make this referral.

9. Why should the nurse monitor the neurovascular status of a patient who has had orthopedic surgery?

A complication called compartment syndrome (palpable tightness of the muscle compartment indicating serious edema that may lead to hypoxia or anoxia of the tissues and cellular death) possibly may occur following a complex fracture injury or as a result of a cast, splint, or circumferential dressing. Compartment syndrome can occur in as little as 6 to 8 hours following an injury and can result in permanent loss of function in the injured extremity. The nurse must assess the patient for adequate circulation distal to the injury, surgical site, or cast. The assessment includes evaluation of skin color, temperature, capillary refill, distal pulses, sensation, and the patient's ability to move the part.

10. **What is a halo vest and how does the nurse care for the patient?**

The halo vest actually supports the halo apparatus used to stabilize a cervical spine injury. Pins are placed into the patient's skull and are attached to rods connected to the vest. Pin care is provided to the skull pin sites using a variety of cleansing solutions (e.g., normal saline, wound cleaners, alcohol swabs, and hydrogen peroxide). The patient is able to ambulate with this device. Nursing care includes assistance with some of the patient's activities of daily living such as dressing and personal hygiene. The patient should be lying on the bed when the skin is cleaned underneath the vest. The patient can wear a split white T-shirt between the skin and the vest to prevent sweating and skin irritation. The nurse assesses skin at the time of cleansing for signs of injury related to pressure from the vest on soft tissue located over the body prominences. The nurse must remember the patient is not able to turn the head; so all communication to the patient should be conducted facing the patient. Patients must be taught to ambulate with this brace because the weight of it may cause them to be off balance and tip from side to side.

11. **How should the nurse or family take care of a patient with a new cast?**

The new cast should be supported with the flat of the hands or on a pillow to avoid creating indentations in the wet cast that might cause pressure on the underlying tissue, and the extremity should remain elevated on pillows while the cast dries to avoid excessive swelling. The following strategies facilitate drying of the cast:
- Absorbent material can be placed beneath the cast.
- The cast can be exposed to air. A fan used to circulate the air in the room will speed evaporation.
- The patient can be turned frequently, if the cast is a body or leg cast.

12. **Once a cast is dried, how should care be given to the patient?**

- The nurse or family should always inspect the edges of the cast to make sure any rough edges are not poking into the patient's skin.
- Taping the edges of the cast might be necessary to protect the skin and prevent tissue injury (petalling).
- The nurse or family should inspect the patient's skin directly below the edges of the cast for erythema, edema, and irritation.
- The nurse should instruct the patient to report any noticeable odor, drainage, or pain that could indicate infection.
- When providing skin care, one should use creams and lotions sparingly so that the moistened skin does not stick to the cast material.
- Neurovascular assessments of the casted limb are to be completed every hour for the initial 24 hours following the application of a cast and then every 4 hours unless the physician orders otherwise.
- The rehabilitation nurse should instruct patients to notify them if pain under the cast occurs or the portion of the limb distal to the cast swells or loses sensation.

- The nurse must caution the patient not to insert objects under the cast (like coat hangers) to scratch itchy skin.

13. What factors slow bone healing?

Many factors, including the patient's age, health status, and nutritional level, affect the healing process of bone. If healing is prolonged or inadequate, the major orthopedic factors to consider are poor immobilization and approximation of the fracture. The ends of the bones may heal, but there may be nonunion of the fracture. The only solution to such a problem is open reduction surgery with the use of orthopedic appliances such as wires, plates, and screws, and a long rehabilitation period of non–weight bearing. Even surgery does not guarantee that the ends will heal together. Therefore to provide the best treatment and environment for healing broken bones is paramount.

14. Which orthopedic disorder is the leading cause of disability in the United States?

Arthritis has the distinction of being the leading cause of disability in the United States and affects more than 43 million persons; annual costs to care for them are more than $15 billion. Osteoarthritis is the most common type of arthritis, accounting for 40% of the cases. This type is called degenerative joint disease and usually affects persons age 50 and older.

15. What are the risk factors for osteoarthritis?

Box 21-2 lists risk factors for osteoarthritis.

Box 21-2. Risk factors for osteoarthritis

- Age (greater than 50 years)
- Congenital factors
- Obesity
- Joint trauma
- Repetitive joint overuse
- Mechanical stressors
- Prolonged immobility
- Joint hypermobility
- Peripheral neuropathy

---

16. What are the disabling symptoms of osteoarthritis?

The disabling symptoms of osteoarthritis include
- Deformity
- Localized pain, increasing with activity

- Morning stiffness
- Loss of joint motion
- Contractures
- Loss of function
- Asymmetrical joint involvement

17. How does rheumatoid arthritis differ from osteoarthritis?

Rheumatoid arthritis involves inflammation of symmetrical joints and, if unchecked, can involve all the joints in the body, causing nearly total immobility. The inflammation involves not only joints but also connective tissue and can produce systemic involvement, particularly in pulmonary, cardiac, vascular, hematological, and ophthalmological organ systems. Rheumatoid arthritis is an autoimmune disorder common among women 20 to 50 years old.

18. What surgery is used most commonly to relieve pain and correct joint deformities?

Arthroplasty, or joint replacement with ceramic or metal prostheses that may be cemented or noncemented, is used most commonly to relieve pain and correct joint deformities. About 70% of the hip and knee replacements are for osteoarthritis. Joints in the hand are more frequently replaced because of rheumatoid arthritis.

19. What is the most common early complication of hip replacement?

Hip dislocation (more commonly posterior) is the most common problem, occurring in about 2% of cases within the first 8 weeks. Box 21-3 list the symptoms of hip dislocation.

Box 21-3.   Symptoms of hip dislocation

- Change in length of the leg (shorter)
- Change in position of the leg (turns inward)
- Neurovascular impairments
- Acute groin pain
- A popping sound
- Bulge at the hip
- Inability to move the leg

---

20. In what circumstance is the use of the continuous passive motion machine recommended?

Continuous passive motion frequently is used after knee arthroplasty to increase flexion and reduce the incidence of postoperative knee manipulation. This early passive movement is thought to enhance healing and tissue remodeling and to reduce joint effusions and associated pain. The goal of 90 degrees of range of motion within 2 weeks is reached more rapidly with the use of continuous passive motion than without it, but ultimately no differences have been seen among patients with and without the therapy. Continuous passive motion does not replace the extensive exercise program but serves as adjunctive therapy.

21. What is a contracture?

Three types of contracture are
- **Arthrogenic:** resulting from damage to the cartilage, synovium, or joint capsule, commonly occurring with arthritis, but may be caused by infection or trauma. This type of contracture frequently occurs in shoulder, hip, spine, and knee joints and affects all directions of joint movement.
- **Soft tissue:** resulting from damage to the periarticular, subcutaneous, and cutaneous tissues, usually caused by burns. Range of motion is limited in just one direction.
- **Myogenic:** resulting from shortening of muscle tissue from inflammation, degeneration, trauma, or neurological abnormalities, which cause collagen replacement for muscle fibers. The limb is held in a flexed position.

22. How are contractures treated?

Contractures need to be prevented, if at all possible, through active and passive range of motion, proper alignment, and prescribed exercises. However, if severe contractures develop, the treatment is ultrasound (heat) and sustained stretching.

23. What methods are used to provide sustained stretching?

Serial casting provides sustained stretching. Immediately after stretching, a well-padded cast is applied to the joint. The cast is replaced every 2 to 3 days after more stretching and skin care. Ultimately, the cast is left in place for up to 5 days at a time. This approach works well on foot, knee, and elbow contractures.

Dynamic splinting provides dynamic tension to sustain stretching. The splint is molded to the limb, but with a stretched position, and is padded. The splint is attached with Velcro straps. A schedule is created that allows on/off times around the clock. The splints frequently are remolded to increase the stretch gradually, and the time spent in the splint gradually is increased as tolerance builds.

24. What are orthoses?

Orthoses are external rigid supports in the form of a brace or a splint designed to improve function or provide stability.

25. How does an orthosis assist in the rehabilitation of a patient with stroke?

An orthosis can permit independent ambulation by preventing foot dragging, loss of balance, and falls. A short leg brace with an attached shoe is applied to the lower leg on the patient's affected side. The brace extends to just below the knee and prevents the ankle from pronating (as the foot plantar flexes) by raising the toes during walking and directing the heel back to the floor.

26. What is the purpose of long leg braces?

Long leg braces, also called knee-ankle-foot orthoses, provide stability at each joint to permit standing. A hinge at the knee can be locked for support, or when unlocked, permits the knee to bend for ambulation. Generally, crutches or a walker is needed to provide additional support. Without adequate upper body strength, ambulating with long leg braces for any distance may require an excessive amount of energy.

27. What causes osteoporosis?

Osteoporosis (porous bone) results when bone resorption (osteoclasts) is more rapid than bone formation (osteoblasts). Deficiencies in calcium and vitamin D intake or metabolism, genetic predisposition, estrogen deficiency, low weight and body mass index, history of prior fractures, white race, being female, advanced age, inactivity, high caffeine intake, use of corticosteroids, excessive use of alcohol, and tobacco smoking contribute to the risk. Osteoporosis is 5 times more common in women, and particularly those who are postmenopausal. This metabolic disease manifests as a reduction in quantity and quality of bone, with alterations in bone cell functioning and decreased skeletal strength. Patients with osteoporosis often have postural abnormalities, decreased mobility, and pain. These symptoms may be due to spontaneous vertebral, hip, or rib fractures.

28. What rehabilitative measures are available for osteoporosis?

Patients with osteoporosis may be treated pharmacologically with drugs such as alendronate (Fosamax) to increase bone mineral density and with calcium supplements of 1500 mg per day. Weight-bearing exercise is encouraged but with caution not to flex or put torque on the spine to prevent placing stress on skeletal structures or to cause fractures. Pain generally can be managed with non-steroidal analgesics so that the patient can exercise. Exercise improves strength, coordination, balance, agility, and mobility, which helps reduce risk of falls.

29. What is heterotopic ossification?

Heterotopic ossification is the calcification of subcutaneous and periarticular tissues (formation of bone in a body part that does not normally produce bone). The hip is most frequently involved. Following brain or spinal cord injury, about 20% of patients have heterotopic ossification by 3 months after injury. The manifestations include limited range of motion, pain, erythema, and swelling in the affected limb, and laboratory tests may show an elevated serum alkaline phosphatase level. The condition is painful and irreversible; therefore as soon as the bone deposits mature, typically in 12 to 18 months, surgery can be done to increase range of motion.

Key Points

- Phantom limb pain results from the patient's brain having been "programmed" to receive sensations from the limb.
- Embolism is a potentially fatal complication following a fracture.
- Major factors that can slow bone healing are poor immobilization and approximation of the fracture.
- Arthritis is the leading orthopedic cause of disability.
- Osteoporosis is 5 times more common in women, especially those who are post-menopausal.

Internet Resources

American Academy of Physical Medicine & Rehabilitation
http://www.aapmr.org/

American Physical Therapy Association
http://www.apta.org

National Osteoporosis Foundation
http://www.nof.org

Bibliography

1. Conner L: Caring for people with musculoskeletal disorders. In Luckmann J, editor: *Saunders manual of nursing care*, Philadelphia, 1997, WB Saunders.
2. Fried KM, Fried GW: Immobility. In Derstine JB, Hargrove SD, editors: *Comprehensive rehabilitation nursing*, Philadelphia, 2001, WB Saunders.
3. Kotch MJ: Nursing management of the patient with an orthopedic disorder. In Derstine JB, Hargrove SD, editors: *Comprehensive rehabilitation nursing*, Philadelphia, 2001, WB Saunders.
4. Marek JF: Trauma to the musculoskeletal system. In Phipps WJ, Monahan FD, Sands JK, and others, editors: *Medical-surgical nursing: health and illness perspectives*, ed 7, St Louis, 2003, Mosby.
5. McKenzie LL: In search of a standard for pin site care, *Orthop Nurs* 2:73-78, 1999.
6. Nettina SM, Mason G, editors: *Lippincott's pocket manual of nursing practice*, St Louis, 1997, Mosby-Year Book.
7. Ruda SC: Nursing management: skeletal problems. In Lewis SM, Heitkemper MM, Dirksen SR, editors: *Medical-surgical nursing: assessment and management of clinical problems*, ed 5, St Louis, 2000, Mosby.
8. Sims GL, Olson RS: Muscle and skeletal function. In Hoeman SP, editor: *Rehabilitation nursing: process, application, & outcomes*, ed 3, St Louis, 2002, Mosby.

Chapter 22

Diabetes Rehabilitation

Mary Beth Vickers

1. What is the goal of diabetes management?

The goal of diabetes management is the prevention and amelioration of acute and chronic complications through good glycemic control.

2. Why should diabetes be a major concern of rehabilitation health care professionals today?

Diabetes is the sixth leading cause of death in America and the major cause of disability from disease in the United States (American College of Endocrinology, 2002). About 18.2 million persons in the United States have diabetes. Although an estimated 13 million persons have been diagnosed, 5.2 million more persons are estimated to have diabetes but are unaware that they have the disease (National Diabetes Statistics, 2003).

3. Is the prevalence of diabetes expected to increase?

The prevalence of diabetes in the United States is increasing in tandem with that of obesity, which often precedes diabetes. The implications for public health are enormous, given the high mortality and morbidity and economic costs associated with this disease and the increased incidence of obesity, in adults and children. New cases are diagnosed per year in 1.3 million persons aged 20 years and older.

4. What is the cost associated with diabetes?

According to recent data from the American Diabetes Association, the total cost of diabetes care in 1997 was $88.2 billion. In 2002 the National Institute of Diabetes and Digestive and Kidney Diseases reported total direct and indirect costs of diabetes are $132 billion annually in the United States.

5. Does any particular group of individuals develop diabetes?

Diabetes occurs more frequently in individuals who have a family history of diabetes, are obese, have a history of gestational diabetes, and are of a certain racial/ethnic group, which may include Native American, Hispanic American, African American, Pacific Islander, and Asian American.

6. **What are some acute and chronic complications of diabetes?**

Acute complications include insulin shock, diabetic coma, and diabetic ketoacidosis and occur in type 1 diabetes. Hyperosmolar hyperglycemic nonketotic syndrome occurs in type 2 diabetes. Chronic complications include microvascular and macrovascular complications such as long-term damage associated with dysfunction and failure of various organs, including the eyes, kidneys, nerves, heart, and blood vessels.

7. **What is the leading cause of death in individuals with type 2 diabetes?**

Cardiovascular disease is the leading cause of death in individuals with type 2 diabetes and accounts for more than 50% of all deaths. Hyperglycemia, a major cardiovascular risk, often is associated with diabetes, as is obesity. Renal failure (chronic and acute) is also a common complication that leads to death of diabetic patients.

8. **Why is it important for health care professionals to pay attention to elevated blood glucose levels in an acute, subacute, or long-term care setting?**

Diabetes often remains undiagnosed until the onset of other medical problems, when hyperglycemia may be found incidentally. In a 1998 study of 1034 consecutively hospitalized adult patients at an inner-city teaching hospital, after excluding patients who were admitted for a primary diagnosis of diabetes, 38% of all hyperglycemic medical patients and 33% of hyperglycemic surgical patients had undiagnosed diabetes at the time of admission. Mean glucose concentration in these patients was 299 mg/dl. Not only is this fact immediately relevant for the medical and surgical management of these patients, but over time, hypoglycemia leads to other health care complications, thus spiraling health care costs.

9. **What factors should be used to assess glycemic control in an effort to prevent long-term complications of diabetes?**

In addition to the routine daily assessment of blood glucose, glycemic control should be assessed primarily by periodic measurement of hemoglobin A_{1c} (HbA_{1c}) levels and secondary assessments should include regular measurement of the fasting preprandial and postprandial glucose levels.

10. **What is the hemoglobin A_{1c} test?**

The glycated hemoglobin test, more commonly referred to as the hemoglobin A_{1c} test, is a measure of the amount of glucose bound to hemoglobin molecules within red blood cells.

11. **Why is HbA_{1c} considered the gold standard for measuring glycemic control?**

Because red blood cells have a life span of about 90 days, measuring the amount of glucose bound to hemoglobin can provide an assessment of average blood sugar control during the 60 to 90 days before the test, which provides a long-term snapshot of effective or ineffective management of diabetes.

12. How often should a patient with diabetes have HbA$_{1c}$ measured?

Because the test results give feedback on the previous 2 to 3 months, having an HbA$_{1c}$ test done every 3 months gives pertinent data regarding the average blood sugars. If a patient has the HbA$_{1c}$ level measured only every 6 months, 3 months' worth of data that could be used to manage diabetes is missed.

13. What are the symptoms of hyperglycemia?

Symptoms indicative of hyperglycemia include polyuria, polydipsia, weight loss, polyphagia and blurred vision. Additionally, impairment of growth and increased susceptibility to infections may accompany chronic hyperglycemia associated with diabetes.

14. When is a clinical diagnosis of diabetes made?

A diagnosis of diabetes is made when symptoms such as polyuria, polydipsia, and unexplained weight loss are present, and a casual (random) plasma glucose concentration is equal to or greater than 200 mg/dl. *Casual,* or *random,* is defined as any time of day without regard to time since the last meal. Diagnosis also can be confirmed when a fasting plasma glucose level is equal to or greater than 126 mg/dl or when a 2-hour plasma glucose is greater than or equal to 200 mg/dl during an oral glucose tolerance test (American Diabetes Association, 2003).

15. What are some common errors that occur in managing the blood glucose levels when the patient must be admitted to the hospital?

The physician often does not always consider the patient's and family's input before prescribing the management plan. Box 22-1 presents common errors.

Box 21-1. Common errors in managing blood glucose levels for a hospitalized diabetic patient

- The outpatient regimen for diabetes often is continued unchanged.
- The outpatient regimen is withdrawn entirely on admission.
- Sliding scales often are overused.
- Intravenous insulin infusions often are underused.

The patient must be a partner in the changes required temporarily because of physiological stress, change in diet and activity, and new disease processes.

16. **What are some concerns/problems with the use of sliding scales to control blood glucose levels in the acute or subacute setting?**

    Sliding scales often are used as the sole means of insulin coverage instead of, or along with, longer-acting insulins. When used alone, without long- or intermediate-acting insulin preparations, sliding scales of short-acting, or rapid-acting, insulins may lead to peaks and valleys of systemic insulin supply, leading to erratic glucose control.

17. **When are sliding scales useful in the hospital setting?**

    Sliding scales can be useful to introduce a basal insulin analog or to evaluate a patient's initial response to insulin. Additionally, sliding scales can be justified in patients who are receiving parenteral nutrition, in whom each 6-hour period is similar to the last. Otherwise, use of sliding scales as the sole form of insulin coverage is usually inappropriate and strongly discouraged (Metchick and others, 2002).

18. **Why should blood sugar levels be managed in a rehabilitative setting?**

    Blood glucose levels greater than 200 mg/dl increase the patient's risk for infection and skin breakdown, impede the healing process, and contribute toward issues related to bladder function, gastrointestinal upset, and blood pressure management. Uncontrolled glucose levels also increase the incidence of tissue damage, leading to complications such as renal disease, retinopathy, neuropathy, and peripheral vascular disease.

19. **Why is maintenance of good glycemic control in diabetic patients who have peripheral vascular disease important?**

    Control of hyperglycemia ameliorates delayed wound healing, common in persons with diabetes who have peripheral vascular disease. Speculation on the underlying mechanism has focused on high glucose–induced activation of NF-κB–inhibited endothelial cell migration. Other conditions that may impede wound healing include malnutrition, vasoconstriction, and use of corticosteroids and tobacco products.

20. **Why is the rehabilitation nurse case manager's role critical with a diabetic patient following discharge from the acute or subacute setting?**

    The rehabilitation nurse case manager's role is critical in providing oversight of the diabetic treatment regimen; coordinating cost-effective, quality health care services; and providing the patient and family with information regarding meal planning, blood sugar management, and medication administration. The case manager's role is also essential to instill the importance of adhering to an often complex treatment regimen to avoid additional complicating factors and consequences such as further disability or even death.

21. Why is it important for health care professionals in any setting to understand the relationship between diabetes and cardiovascular disease?

Diabetes increases the risk of cardiovascular complications and mortality in patients with established cardiovascular disease. Patients with diabetes with no history of heart disease have the same risk for future cardiovascular death as nondiabetic patients with a history of myocardial infarction. Additionally, patients with diabetes have not experienced the reduction in mortality rates that recently has been observed in nondiabetic persons. Given this and the prediction of an increase in the prevalence of diabetes, the importance of diabetes as a cardiovascular risk factor is expected to increase substantially.

22. Why is it common to have a high number of diabetic patients in a rehabilitation setting?

One of the complications of diabetes is macrovascular disease. Additionally, diabetes mellitus is the leading cause of lower extremity amputations (LEAs) in the United States, accounting for about 50% of all nontraumatic LEAs. Studies indicate that among persons with diabetes, the rate of LEA is more than 40 times that for persons without diabetes (Centers for Disease Control, 2003). Additionally, in a 1998 report, of 4245 hospital admissions of patients with diabetes, 1.2% had a primary diagnosis of peripheral vascular disease, infection, and neuropathy or ulceration, which accounted for 2.1% of all hospital admissions. Following surgery and hospitalization for LEA, patients are transferred to a rehabilitative setting, where they remain until they have reached their maximum level of functioning.

23. What are some Internet resources that rehabilitation case managers can provide to their diabetic patients to assist them in obtaining information regarding this debilitating chronic disease?

Please see the Internet Resources box for a list of online resources to which the rehabilitation nurse case manager can direct diabetic patients for information on diabetes.

 Key Points

- Direct costs of diabetes are estimated at $50 billion per year in the United States.
- Long-term damage from diabetes causes dysfunction of eyes, kidneys, nerves, heart, and blood vessels.
- Diabetes often remains undiagnosed until the onset of other medical problems.
- Hemoglobin A_{1c} is considered the gold standard for measuring glycemic control; testing every 3 months gives a clear picture.
- Diabetes can be diagnosed when fasting plasma glucose level is equal to or greater than 126 mg/dl or a casual plasma glucose level is equal to or greater than 200 mg/dl.
- Diabetes is the leading cause of lower extremity amputations in the United States.

Internet Resources

Indian Health Service
http://www.ihs.gov/MedicalPrograms/Diabetes

National Diabetes Education Program
http://www.cdc.gov/diabetes/projects/ndeps.htm

National Institute of Diabetes and Digestive and Kidney Diseases
http://www.niddk.nih.gov

American Diabetes Association
http://www.diabetes.org

Juvenile Diabetes Foundation International
http://www.jdf.org

National Diabetes Information Clearinghouse
http://www.diabetes.niddk.nih.gov/health/diabetes/ndic.htm

Bibliography

1. American College of Endocrinology: American College of Endocrinology consensus statement on guidelines for glycemic control, *Endocr Pract* 8:5-11, 2002.
2. American Diabetes Association: Pre-diabetes description, 2003. Retrieved June 23, 2003, from http://www.diabetes.org/main/application/commercewf
3. Centers for Disease Control: Diabetes public health resource, 2003. Retrieved June 23, 2003, from http://www.cdc.gov/diabetes/faqs.htm#sources
4. Courtney L, Gordon M, Romer L: A clinical path for adult diabetes, *Diabetes Educ* 23:664-671, 1997.
5. Hirsch IB, Paauw DS: Diabetes management in special situations, *Endocrinol Metab Clin North Am* 26:631-645, 1997.
6. Hu F, Stampfer M, Haffner S, and others: Elevated risk of cardiovascular disease prior to clinical diagnosis of type 2 diabetes, *Diabetes Care* 25:1129-1134, 2002.
7. Malmberg K, Ryden L, Hamsten A, and others: Mortality prediction in diabetic patients with myocardial infarction: experienced from the DIGAMI study, *Cardiovasc Resusc* 34:248-253, 1997.
8. Metchick L, Petit W, Inzucchi S: Inpatient management of diabetes mellitus, *Am J Med* 113:317-323, 2002.
9. National Institute of Diabetes and Digestive and Kidney Diseases: *National diabetes statistics fact sheet*, Bethesda, MD, 2003, US Department of Health and Human Services, National Institutes of Health.
10. Sawin CT: Action without benefit: the sliding scale of insulin use, *Arch Intern Med* 157:489, 1997.
11. Van Den Berghe G, Wouters P, Weekers F, and others: Intensive insulin therapy in critically ill patients, *New Engl J Med* 345:1359-1366, 2001.

Chapter 23

Traumatic Brain Injury Rehabilitation

Jeanne Flannery

1. What is traumatic brain injury (TBI)?

Traumatic brain injury is a traumatic insult to the brain that could produce changes in the individual spanning every aspect of being: physical, cognitive, emotional, social, vocational, psychological, and spiritual. The patient's and family's roles, goals, expectations, and relationships may be changed. Recovery is a process that requires commitment from all the family and collaboration with a team of health care providers for an extended period of time: in severe injuries, for a lifetime.

2. How great is the problem of TBI?

Traumatic brain injury is so great that it has been called "the silent epidemic." Statistics are a low estimate, at best, because the reporting system nationally is not consistent. Multiple variables exist even among the reported cases, such as
- How the injury is defined
- Diagnostic codes used
- Emergency room visits accounted for
- Physician office follow-ups reported
- How severity is measured
- Cause of death stated accurately

Box 23-1 provides some of the best estimates available of the enormity of the problem of TBI in the United States.

3. What are the risk factors and causes of TBI?

Persons between 15 and 24 years of age are at greatest risk, and males are twice as likely to incur TBI as females. Persons younger than 5 and persons 60 years or older are at moderate risk, mainly from falls. Among those 65 and older, 11% of the TBIs from falls are fatal. Gunshots are 4 times as likely to be the cause of TBI in minority races. Hispanics and blacks have an incidence of TBI almost 3 times greater than the average rate (2.75 and 2.92, respectively), and TBIs are more likely to result from assault. Child abuse accounts for 64% of infant TBIs.

Motor vehicle accidents rank first among causes of TBI, regardless of ethnicity (50%). From 33% to 50% of all TBIs are estimated to be related to consumption of alcohol. Because alcohol/drug screening is not done routinely in assessment

---

Box 23-1.   Scope and significance of traumatic brain injury

- 2 million traumatic brain injuries (TBIs) annually
- 50,000 die before reaching a medical facility
- 1,000,000 are treated in emergency room or outpatient facilities
- 300,000 are admitted to the hospital
- 80,000 to 90,000 have long-term disabilities or are in a coma
- 2000 remain in a persistent vegetative state
- 5.3 million Americans are living with permanent disabilities
- 50,000 children sustain TBIs from bicycle injuries
- 400 of these children die
- 1.6 million persons are reported to have TBI, but care, if any, is unknown
- Lifetime cost for a patient with severe TBI is more than $4 million
- Costs to the United States annually exceed $48 billion for TBIs
- Every 5 minutes one person dies and another is disabled from TBIs

---

of patients with TBI, the estimate is low. Falls represent 21% of the causes; violence causes 12% (mostly from firearms); and sports and recreation account for 10% of TBIs.

4. How are TBIs classified?

Traumatic brain injuries are classified according to
- Mechanism of injury
- Glasgow Coma Scale (GCS)
- Type of injury
- Location of injury
- Primary or secondary injury

5. What are the mechanisms of injury in TBI?

Traumatic brain injury is caused by an external force delivered to the brain. The force can be direct contact, acceleration-deceleration, and rotational. In acceleration-deceleration the head moves in a straight line and receives the impact (coup), with the solid skull moving away more quickly than the soft brain tissue, causing the brain to be pushed against the area struck. The brain then reverses motion away from the impact, shearing (opposite but parallel sliding motion), pulling apart (producing tension), and finally compressing (pushing together) against the dural folds and solid bony prominence on the opposite side of the already stationary skull (contracoup).

Rotational injuries twist the brain within the rough interior of the skull. A rotational injury produces tension and shears tissue, as well as stretches the brain momentarily at the foramen magnum. This devastating force causes diffuse axonal injury with no apparent gross focal lesions.

Direct contact injuries occur from a moving object striking the stationary head. This injury, depending on the force, causes local effects extending from as little as a scalp laceration to skull fracture, extradural hematoma, contusions, and cerebral lacerations or as much as intracerebral hemorrhage.

Traumatic brain injuries can be open or closed. Open injuries result from direct impact and cause compound or perforating skull fractures in which the skull is distorted or indented. Dural tears, cerebral contusions, and lacerations can occur, and infection is a major threat.

Closed injuries have no break in the skull and meningeal barriers and no communication between the intracranial and external environment. These injuries may produce no abnormalities on radiological evaluation, yet they are just as serious as those that do.

6. How is the GCS used to classify TBI?

Table 23-1 depicts the GCS and classification.

Table 23-1.   Classification of traumatic brain injury with the Glasgow Coma Scale

Glasgow Coma Scale

Eye opening (E):	Verbal response (V):	Motor response (M):
• Spontaneous, 4	• Oriented, 5	• To voice, 6
• To voice, 3	• Confused, 4	• To painful stimulus, 5
• To pain, 2	• Inappropriate words, 3	• Withdraw, 4
• None, 1	• Incomprehensible words, 2	• Abnormal flexion, 3
	• None, 1	• Abnormal extension, 2
		• None, 1

Classification	Clinical features
GCS: 13-15, mild	Loss of consciousness: none to <20 minutes; no structural damage; may have amnesia, confusion, chronic headache
GCS: 9-12, moderate	Loss of consciousness; contusion or diffuse axonal injury; confusion
GCS: 3-8, severe	Coma duration 6 hours or greater; incomplete recovery from structural damage

Note: Score is E + V + M (maximum for each component being 4, 5, and 6, respectively); range is 3 to 15. Documentation should indicate the three components to the score. The scoring is not accurate when the patient is intubated or has a tracheostomy, has a spinal cord injury, or lateralizes.

7. What are the types of TBI based on pathophysiology?

Traumatic brain injury is categorized into focal or diffuse types. Table 23-2 presents injuries that comprise each type.

Table 23-2.   Focal and diffuse types of traumatic brain injury

Example	Description
Focal (almost 50%)	
Contusion (moderate to severe)	Bruising of the cortex of the brain (parenchyma) usually occurs in the frontal and temporal lobes.
	Bruising to deeper structures occurs, such as to basal ganglia, corpus callosum, and thalamus with petechial hemorrhages, surrounded by hypodense brain edema.
	Does not form a hematoma; hemorrhage disperses into tissues from 1 ml to more than 50 ml.
	Pia-arachnoid remains intact.
Laceration (more serious)	Traumatic tearing of the cortical surface of the brain occurs, including the pia mater (burst lobe).
	Occurs usually in frontal and temporal lobes and may be concurrent with contusion.
	Hemorrhage will occur.
Hemorrhage	Commonly occurs following blunt injury.
	May occur with minor injury, with or without a fracture, or from serious avulsion.
	Forms hematomas in potential spaces.
Epidural hematoma	Accounts for 1%-2% of all traumatic brain injuries (TBIs) and 20%-30% of all hematomas.
	Bleeding into epidural space occurs between the dura mater and skull.
	Bleeding is usually arterial, commonly the middle meningeal artery.
	Herniation is a potential complication without early operative intervention.
Subdural hematoma	Most common type and occurs in 10%-20% of all TBIs.
	Has the highest mortality rate.
	Occurs bilaterally in 15%-20% of cases.
	Classified into three types:
	• Acute: presents within 48 hours after a significant injury; high mortality
	• Subacute: occurs 48 hours to 2 weeks after a moderate injury
	• Chronic: occurs 3 weeks to several months after a low-impact injury; often bilateral; more frequent in older adults and chronic alcoholics
Intracerebral hematoma	Caused by penetrating injuries, deep depressed fractures, and diffuse axonal injury.
	Develops deep within the hemispheres and is surrounded by edema.
Subarachnoid hemorrhage	Occurs with severe TBI.
	May extend to intraventricular hemorrhage.
	Blood collects in the arachnoid space between the arachnoid and pia mater meninges.

Table 23-2. Focal and diffuse types of traumatic brain injury *continued*

Diffuse	
Concussion (mild)	Temporary axonal disturbances occur. No loss of consciousness occurs. Dysfunctions in attentional and memory systems occur. Classified into three grades of mild concussion: • Grade 1: dazing with recovery in less than a minute and no amnesia • Grade 2: retrograde amnesia that develops after 5-10 minutes, extending only a few minutes before injury • Grade 3: confusion, retrograde and posttraumatic amnesia that persists several minutes
Concussion (classic)	Transient diffuse cerebral disconnection from the brainstem reticular activating system occurs with microscopic bruising, but causes no structural defect. Classified as grade 4: immediate loss of consciousness, lasting less than 6 hours; retrograde and posttraumatic confusion (may last hours to days); amnesia; chronic headache and deficits in executive functions (may last weeks to months). May be accompanied by focal pathology.
Diffuse axonal injury	Is the major neuropathological process of brain injury. Shearing of axons; damage to small blood vessels occurs, with subcortical white matter, deep brain structures, and brainstem most frequently disrupted. Varies in degree from mild to severe: • Mild: coma 6-24 hours; 8% • Moderate: coma longer that 24 hours, but no brainstem signs; has incomplete recovery • Severe: usually primary brainstem injury; death or severe disability Mortality is 33%; 33% have severe disabilities or persistent vegetative state. Does not show microscopic damage on computed tomography.
Diffuse hypoxic-ischemic injury	Is a consequence of severe sustained increased intracranial pressure, respiratory, and cardiovascular compromise. Results in diffuse neural loss. Hippocampus, basal ganglia, and cerebellum are most vulnerable to lack of oxygen.

8. **What do the classifications of primary, secondary, and tertiary TBI mean?**

These classifications describe the pathological events that occur from the initial insult, the biochemical changes, the complicating processes initiated at the time of injury that lead to further intensive neural destruction later, and increased intracranial pressure (ICP) which, because the cranium is unyielding, worsens the status of the injury. Figure 23-1 depicts the relationship among the injuries.

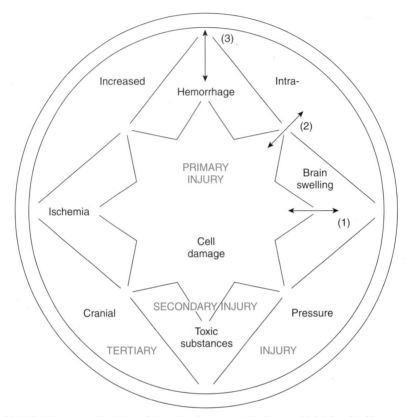

Figure 23-1. Model for stages of head injury. *Primary injury* is represented by the open-sided eight-pointed inner star. Direct cellular damage may be to neurons, glia, and vessels. *Secondary injury* is represented by the four-pointed open star. Each point depicts a mechanism of secondary injury: hemorrhage, brain swelling (caused by cerebral edema or increased cerebral blood volume), toxic substances (caused by inadequate clearance of metabolic wastes, deranged metabolism, or exogenous substances), and ischemia (caused by insufficient oxygen and glucose, and metabolic factors). *Tertiary injury* is represented by the closed circle. Tertiary injury is from increased intracranial pressure. The system is closed to the outside because the cranium cannot expand. The *open spaces* in the stars and the bidirectional arrows indicate the openness of the system. Arrow 1 indicates that primary injury can lead to secondary injury and vice versa. The same is true for arrow 2 between the primary injury and tertiary injury, and arrow 3 between the secondary injury and the tertiary injury. Positive feedback from tertiary injury produces intensified primary and secondary injuries. If uncontrolled, death of the patient results. (Data from Barker E, editor: *Neuroscience nursing: a spectrum of care,* ed 2, St Louis, 2002, Mosby; and Hickey JV: *The clinical practice of neurological and neurosurgical nursing,* ed 5, Philadelphia, 2003, Lippincott Williams & Wilkins.)

9. **What damage is included in primary brain injury?**

Initial injury destroys cell bodies and damages axonal projections so that with swelling, immediate loss of axonal transport occurs. Dynamic acute neural death continues over a 4-hour period with biochemical destruction of the damaged axons. This destruction continues for several days.

10. What does secondary TBI involve?

The process included in this complication includes events presented in Table 23-3.

Table 23-3. Secondary injury in traumatic brain injury

Event	Result
Axonal failure of aerobic glycolysis	Cellular acidosis
Failure of adenosine triphosphate production	Na^+-K^+ failure:
	• Intracellular K^+ leaks out.
	• Extracellular Ca^{2+}, Na^+, and H_2O move into cells.
Capillaries become permeable	Adhesion of leukocytes to capillary walls, creating blockages
	Reduction of lumen because of swelling
	Increased ischemia
Excitotoxicity from widespread release of excitatory amino acids (glutamate and aspartate)	Cellular swelling and disintegration
Release of free radicals (superoxide, hydroxyl, hydrogen peroxide, singlet oxygen, nitrous oxide)	Damage of cells, disruption of cell membranes through lipid peroxidation that spreads to other cells, perpetuating neural death
Ischemia precipitates coagulopathies	Disruption of the blood-brain barrier and vessel damage
Increased vascular permeability	Cerebral edema
	Decreased cerebral blood flow
Hypermetabolic state	Increased use of oxygen and glucose in an already deprived condition
	Slowed protein synthesis

11. What is tertiary brain injury?

Tertiary brain injury results from increased ICP, no matter what the primary injury or the location in the head. The four secondary mechanisms depicted in Figure 23-1 are cumulative from the cascade of events: hemorrhage, brain swelling, ischemia, and toxic substances, which lead to increased ICP. The system is open; therefore tertiary injury reflects back on primary and secondary injury, worsening all. Without intervention, the system closes within the unyielding cranium, and positive feedback results in the patient's death.

12. What is brain swelling?

Brain swelling is an increase in volume of the brain that can result in increased ICP, mass effect, and herniation syndromes. Brain swelling may be due to an increase in bulk weight of the brain (tumor), cerebral blood volume (congestive brain swelling), or an increase in water content within the brain (cerebral edema). Three types of cerebral edema are

- **Vasogenic edema:** most common; occurs when autoregulation is lost and the blood-brain barrier is disrupted; occurs predominantly in white matter
- **Cytotoxic edema:** increase in intracellular fluid derived from plasma, predominantly in gray matter; cells can no longer function
- **Interstitial brain edema:** increase in cerebral spinal fluid pressure within the ventricles or hydrocephalus leads to periventricular white matter edema

13. What is postconcussion syndrome?

Postconcussion syndrome may develop immediately after the patient becomes oriented after injury or within a few days. The complaints may persist for months. Generally, complete clearing of the majority of symptoms occurs within 6 months. These symptoms include

- Headache
- Visual disturbances
- Nervousness
- Dizziness
- Confusion
- Gait abnormalities
- Poor memory
- Decreased information processing
- Decreased attention span
- Decreased concentration
- Increased sensitivity to noise

However, as late as 1 year after injury, another cluster of symptoms may emerge, including

- Insomnia
- Forgetfulness
- Irritability
- Depression
- Anxiety
- Fatigue

Patients may have difficulty working, attending school, or fulfilling their role responsibilities satisfactorily because of a combination of these problems. Lack of extensive sick leave may even lead to loss of jobs. Often patients and families have not been prepared for such sequelae; and when the injury was so minor that hospital admission was probably not required, a connection between the injury and the myriad of difficulties may not be made. Relationships may even be in jeopardy because neither party knows that a physiological explanation exists for the changes in behavior.

14. What methods of prevention should rehabilitation nurses enhance?

Certainly research has supported that seat belts reduce injury severity. Nurses also should include use of seat belts in assessment and then provide information about them, for follow-up reinforces their value. The same procedure applies to helmets for children on skateboards, skates, scooters, and bicycles, and all patients riding all-terrain vehicles and motorcycles. In states where helmet laws do not exist, the responsibility of nurses is even greater to provide safety information.

Nurses can participate in the national Think First program that is provided in high schools, often with drivers' education classes. Materials are available for any age child or teenager, and a fairly graphic film is impressive. The film discusses additional protective strategies in contact sports and driving and stresses no drinking and driving.

There can never be too many volunteers; and if nurses can include young persons who have sustained a TBI who are interested in helping prevent injuries in others, the influence of their visit can be impressive.

15. Can the GCS be used to evaluate the patient's cognitive functioning status?

No, the GCS is used to evaluate arousal only in the early postinjury period when the patient's level of consciousness is impaired. Once the patient has sleep-wake cycles, can move, and can speak, the tool will have maximized its usefulness and the nurse will need to assess the patient differently. Rarely is GCS used outside of emergency departments and critical care units.

16. What is available for the nurse to use to assess cognitive functioning in a patient with low responsivity that does not require special training?

For more than 30 years a tool developed at Rancho Los Amigos Hospital in Downey, California, has served to provide a cognitive level for such patients. However, little research has been done with the use of this instrument, and the format allows subjectivity. The LOCFAS (Levels of Cognitive Functioning Assessment Scale; Flannery, 1993), which is derived from the Rancho Scale, has been researched extensively and serves well for patients with diffuse axonal injury; can be used by nurses with no training; does not require patient partici-pation for assessment; does not take extra time in the busy nurse's schedule (can be done during regular care); and is a single-behavior format so that it is more of an objective assessment. This tool is in Appendix 1.

17. What is likely to be the picture of clinical recovery from severe TBI?

Patients with a severe TBI have a disruption in their arousal system; therefore they are in coma that lasts days to weeks. As they emerge from coma, there is a pattern of recovery. At first the patient has no movement and no response to any stimuli, and the eyes are closed. Then the patient has generalized movements or abnormal posturing. Then, as awareness begins, the patient has nonpurposeful movement, wakefulness, and fleeting attention. The patient then responds locally to stimuli, tracks objects, and may follow simple commands inconsis-tently. Unless the speech center has been disturbed focally, the voice may return at this point, although words are not purposeful.

No way exists to predict how long the patient will remain in any level. In some cases, recovery is progressive and change can be seen each day. In others, the patient may reach Level 3 (just described) and remain there for years.

With progression the patient becomes confused and agitated. The patient can achieve and maintain little attention to external stimuli. Posttraumatic amnesia remains; the patient is disoriented; verbalization is confused and is often confabulated. The profound attentional deficits preclude the patient's being able to focus or to perform requested tasks, answer questions, or think. The patient has no insight as to the situation, cannot reason, is extremely distractible, and is intolerant of even routine care. Aggressiveness, combativeness, labile behavior, plunging from hyperactivity to hypoactivity and back again, and disinhibition of behavior are likely. The patient is still totally dependent in bowel and bladder management as well.

The patient may be able to improve to the point that evolving independence begins. Moving through Levels 5 to 8, the patient gradually regains orientation and the ability to provide self-care with gradually decreasing cueing, monitoring, and direction. The disinhibition, motor restlessness, agitation, and lability probably will persist, but to a lesser degree. Frontal lobe damage or the associated complex connections may leave deficits in executive functions and create social problems as well. These areas include
- Information processing
- Initiation
- Planning
- Execution
- Regulation of behavior

Resulting problems are
- Disorganized thought processes
- Impaired motivation
- Lack of insight
- Inaccurate self-appraisal
- Limited planning skills
- Lack of impulse control
- Disinhibition
- Perseveration
- Easy frustration
- Irritability
- Stress intolerance

Finally, patients recognize their own problems and limitations and can learn compensatory strategies to work around them. Although some physical deficits still may be present, the cognitive, behavioral, and psychosocial issues are what interfere with the patient's social interactions, personal relationships, and vocational pursuits. This phase lasts for an extended period of time, at best, and may be lifelong. The patient and family become frustrated and lose hope over time, without support. This is a challenging stage of recovery.

18. **Why is nutritional assessment paramount when the rehabilitation nurse first receives the patient with TBI?**

Because TBI is one of the most stressful events the human body endures, the physiological stress response is intense and pervasive. Blood glucose levels become high and remain elevated, without insulin drip intervention, and protein catabolism is high, leading to negative nitrogen balance. The patients are essentially in starvation but worse because they are not readily able to mobilize fat stores; therefore they do not enter a conservation stage, as a normal person would who is starved, and protein losses are much greater. These patients can lose enough nitrogen to reduce body weight by 15% *each week*. For example, a 200 pound 17-year-old who lifted weights and was on the football team may lose 30 pounds per week following TBI and look weak and emaciated by the time he is transferred to an acute rehabilitation facility.

Even though the patient will have required enough energy to support this massive stress response to equal 4000 to 6000 kcal per day, such an amount is not provided for several reasons. A jejunal feeding route is preferred because it avoids gastric intolerance but maintains the integrity of the intestinal mucosal lining. The patient's system cannot tolerate the volume or the concentration of tube feeding that would be necessary to provide so many calories. Secondly, measures to reduce the stress response are taken so as to reduce the caloric need. Additionally, research supports that overfeeding leads to complications such as hypertonic dehydration, hyperlipidemia, hepatic fatty degeneration, azotemia, metabolic acidosis, refeeding syndrome, and hyperglycemia, which worsens the brain injury. A more reasonable approach is taken with providing around 35 kcal/kg per day, which would be a little more than 3000 kcal for the patient described, based on weight on admission.

Thus by the time the rehabilitation nurse receives this patient, because of the continued stress response, the patient is likely to have
- Body weight less than normal (may exhibit loss of 30 pounds or more)
- Protein depletion
- Muscle wasting
- Weakness
- Negative nitrogen balance
- Elevated basal metabolic rate
- Decreased ability to use ketones (absent ketonuria)
- Elevated glucose use

Therefore a comprehensive nutritional assessment is paramount to determine the best dietary regimen for the patient. Even a slight degree of any of these manifestations should be considered serious and should be addressed specifically to hasten the reparative phase of the stress response and initiate weight gain and strength development.

19. **What type of problems are expected following TBI?**

Box 23-2 gives a partial list of most common problems expected following TBI.

Box 23-2. **Impairments following traumatic brain injury**

- Impaired arousal and attention
- Impaired short-term memory
- Impaired cognitive functioning
- Impaired learning
- Impaired affect
- Impaired expressive and receptive communication
- Impaired sensory integrity and perception
- Impaired balance and anticipatory reactions
- Impaired motor function (including mobility, vision, speech)
- Impaired autonomic nervous system
- Impaired respiratory function
- Altered muscle elastic properties

---

20. **What is persistent vegetative state?**

In some TBIs the patients never achieve progress beyond the level of arousal that occurs at Level 2, in which there are sleep-wake cycles. The brainstem function is intact, but without evidence of cortical function. Patients may have minimal spontaneous motor activities and may track minimally, but without response to verbal stimulation. Patients who remain vegetative for 3 months without improvement rarely achieve independence. Patients must have remained in this state for a year after the injury has stabilized before "persistent" can be attached as a descriptor.

21. **To predict outcomes of TBI, what does the nurse need to consider in addition to the myriad of variables that relate to the type, location, severity, and complications of the TBI?**

The nurse also must consider preinjury factors such as those presented in Box 23-3.

Box 23-3. **Preinjury factors associated with positive rehabilitation outcomes of traumatic brain injury**

- Motivated
- Persistent
- Creative
- Good academic history/level of education
- History of achievement

Box 23-3. Preinjury factors associated with positive rehabilitation outcomes of traumatic brain injury *continued*

- Strong support systems (family/friends)
- Good social relationships
- Well-adjusted personality
- Strong ego, self-esteem
- Good vocational skills
- Good interpersonal skills
- Intelligent quotient >120
- No learning disabilities
- No history of hyperactivity
- No substance abuse history
- No criminal history
- No behavioral problems history
- Good motor skill development
- Good general health and physical fitness
- Moderate age and body type

22. **What two types of factors, external to the patient, that are present after injury can influence the patient's recovery?**

Social factors and environmental factors are important. Examples of these are in Box 23-4.

Box 23-4. Postinjury social and environmental factors

Social Factors
- Family's support capabilities
- Family's adjustment
- Family's and friends' reaction
- Ability to reintegrate into avocational activities

Environmental Factors
- Treatment settings
- Quality of room/housing
- Expertise of health care providers
- Attitudes of health care providers
- Equipment available
- Staffing of facilities
- Specific needed facilities available

23. **Because cognitive Level 4, confused-agitated, is the level a patient must be for eligibility to be admitted in most acute rehabilitation facilities, how can the patient be managed best, once admitted?**

With the patient in this agitated state, the best approach is to allow the patient the most freedom in which the patient still can be safe. If the patient has physical deficits, a Craig or Vale bed can be used that allows the patient the ability to stand without the danger of falling out of bed and yet confines the patient within the padded walls, over which the patient can see. The patient has space to move about (king-size mattress on the floor) safely.

If the patient has greater physical stability, a sitter should be hired who has been trained to care for the agitated patient. The patient then can be permitted to roam free, accompanied by the sitter. Without confinement, the patient can expend energy, be content, and still be safe. The two interventions to avoid, if at all possible, include physical restraints and medications (chemical restraints). With physical restraints patients become intensely focused on getting loose and may harm themselves in the attempt. With medication strong enough to subdue the agitation, the effect often is cognitive slowing and interruption in the rehabilitation process.

24. **How does the rehabilitation nurse design the management plan for the patient who has impaired cognition?**

The nurse, along with all the related disciplines that provide care for the patient, can readily determine the cognitive level through the use of LOCFAS (see Appendix 1) and can establish interrater reliability over time and situations. Once the cognitive level is determined, each discipline has certain short-term objectives that are discussed with the team for each week. All disciplines work to support all goals, not just their own. Nursing has a basic management plan that is based on the patient's capabilities at each of eight cognitive levels. The plan includes for each cognitive level
- The expected general behaviors
- The expected linguistic behaviors
- The goal and methods of facilitation
- Interventions, including communication
- Family education and support

(Please see Appendix 3 for the entire plan.) This collaborative effort is generally interdisciplinary. Specialized facilities may have cross-training among disciplines, allowing for a transdisciplinary approach.

25. **Aside from cognitive impairment, what are the two most frequent disabilities following TBI?**

The two most frequent losses are mobility and prehension (grasping). At the *disability* level, the nurse must determine whether the *impairment* can improve or cannot improve. Note: Accurate assessment of an impairment does not mean that it can be fixed. If not, assistive devices can be used and compensatory strategies can be taught. Additionally, modification of the environment often is needed to prevent a *handicap* (refer to Chapter 1, question 13 for review of terms).

26. How does the combination of cognitive deficits and physical disability affect outcomes?

Patients with higher-level physical skills and low-to-moderate–level cognitive functioning are more likely to be handicapped by society—directly by their family and friends. Because they look and move normally, expectations often are set too high for them cognitively, which sets everyone up for failure. Patients with low-level motor skills and higher-level cognitive functioning often are judged based on their appearance and are not expected to function at the level of which they are capable. With devices to compensate for physical deficits, these patients do well in adjusting and going on with their lives. Persons must be taught not to leap to conclusions about the capabilities of a patient just because of physical impairments or, conversely, not to expect too much of a patient because of little or no physical impairment. Accurate assessment of cognitive functioning can provide the appropriate starting place for the rehabilitation nursing management plan (Appendix 3).

27. When is it appropriate to try to teach a new task to the patient with TBI?

The patient who is at Level 5 or below has severe short-term memory deficits and a short attention span, inability to initiate, and inability to complete a task without cueing. Furthermore, the patient cannot separate current occurrences from long-term memories, and therefore confabulates. The patient is unlikely to be able to remember the beginning of the sentence by the time the nurse reaches the end. With patience, time, and positive reinforcement, this patient can *relearn* but cannot yet assimilate enough information to learn a new thing. For example, the patient who has forgotten the names of objects can relearn them. Likewise, the patient can relearn how to tie a shoe or the things to look for to tell whether a shirt is on frontward. These learning tasks use first, declarative memory or "knowing that," and second, procedural memory or "knowing how," but they retrieve and refresh memories, not create new ones.

When the patient progresses to higher cognitive levels, the patient can learn new tasks, and for the nurse to initiate teaching is appropriate. The teaching episodes must be short, introducing small components at a time, with much repetition, strong encouragement and reinforcement, and patience.

For declarative memory tasks, depending on the location and severity of the injury, the patient may never be able to achieve the goal without help. For this reason many aids have been developed to assist patients to be more independent. Patients are taught the compensatory strategies for the specific goal they need to accomplish. For example, if remembering the names of persons is necessary to be able to return to work, then that one task is addressed intensely. The patient learns exactly how to address individuals to acquire the needed information in a voice-activated tape recorder. The patient then can enter the data in an organized pocket notebook or personal digital assistant so that the next time the patient hears the name, the patient can access the file. Many ways exist for the patient to compensate, and the task the patient is taught is not the name, but the technique for storing the name in a retrievable file that replaces the poorly functioning memory file.

28. What is the effect of TBI on the patient's family?

The stress and disruption of family function can be overwhelming. The amount of time and effort the patient will require erodes the family's quality of life. The caregiver essentially has the burden of care and responsibility on top of all the other roles that must be filled and may get no relief from it day in and day out. Research has shown that in about 3 years of enduring such upheaval, the family structure begins to disintegrate. Health care providers need to be sure that the family joins a support group to be able to discuss and validate the many dilemmas that they face. When the caregiver is the mother, concerns arise regarding who will take care of the brain-injured child if something happens to her. If the patient was 17 when injured and now is 37, the mother is, perhaps, between 55 and 77 years old. With excellent care, the patient will surely outlive the mother. Another concern is about financial resources and how long they will last with such a consistent drain on them. The nurse needs to guide the mother to establish with the family how the patient will be managed and then arrange with an attorney the legal documents that support decisions, such as durable power of attorney and trust.

29. Is depression a problem among patients with TBI?

Yes, patients who recover to the level where they can appreciate what they can no longer do and who they used to be may face depression. Although the suicide rate is low, patients need to be treated for depression and to be monitored for suicidal ideation. Depending on the preinjury coping skills and the support they receive after injury, patients may be unable to accept their cognitive deficits, their psychosocial failures, and social isolation and manage their lack of impulse control.

30. Is there a risk of substance abuse in patients with TBIs?

Yes, a particular risk exists among those patients who are young or who had preinjury habitual use of drugs or alcohol. Because the risk is known, substance abuse resources and discussions are incorporated early in the rehabilitation program. Programs such as Alcoholics Anonymous and Narcotics Anonymous cannot be used without modification for the patient's cognitive level. Families need to be included in this education so that they do not inadvertently become enablers.

Key Points

- Traumatic brain injury is so extensive it is called "the silent epidemic."
- Every 5 minutes one person dies and another is disabled from TBI.
- Traumatic brain injuries are classified according to mechanism of injury, GCS score, type of injury, location of injury, primary or secondary injury, and cognitive functioning level.
- Diffuse axonal injury may show no gross abnormalities on radiological testing yet can be severe.
- Secondary injury worsens the damage caused by the initial insult through biochemical changes and complicating processes that began at the time of injury and lead to intensive neural destruction later.
- Tertiary injury is the damage that occurs from increased ICP, which without intervention can lead to death.
- Postconcussion syndrome may cause problems for up to a year after injury and yet the patient/family may never have been taught about it.
- The GCS is used to evaluate arousal.
- The LOCFAS is used to evaluate cognitive functioning.
- Patients emerging from coma follow a progressive pattern of recovery, but the length of time spent in any level is completely individualized.
- There is no evidence of cortical functioning in a patient who is in a persistent vegetative state.
- Preinjury personality, intelligence quotient, habits, skills, education, and relationships can influence a patient's recovery.
- Rehabilitation for a patient with TBI requires collaboration of an interdisciplinary team.
- The effect of caring for a patient with TBI can cause disintegration of the family in several years.

Internet Resources

National Institute on Disability and Rehabilitation Research
http://www.ed.gov/about/offices/list/OSERS/NIDRR

Neuroscience Center
http://www.neuroscience.cnter.com

Brain Injury Association, Inc.
http://www.biausa.org

Traumatic Brain Injury Information
http://www.tbiinfocenter.com

National Center for the Dissemination of Disability Research
http://www.ncddr.org

Bibliography

1. Baggerly J, Le N: Nursing management of the patient with head trauma. In Derstine JB, Hargrove SD, editors: *Comprehensive rehabilitation nursing,* Philadelphia, 2001, WB Saunders.

2. Blank-Reid C, Barker E: Neurotrauma: traumatic brain injury. In Barker E, editor: *Neuroscience nursing: a spectrum of care,* ed 2, St Louis, 2002, Mosby.

3. Flannery JC: Common neurologic interventions. In Burrell LO, Gerlach MJ, Pless B, editors: *Adult nursing: acute and community care,* ed 2, Stamford, CT, 1997, Appleton & Lange.

4. Flannery JC: Neurologic surgery & trauma. In Burrell LO, Gerlach MJ, Pless B, editors: *Adult nursing: acute and community care,* ed 2, Stamford, CT, 1997, Appleton & Lange.

5. Hickey JV: Craniocerebral trauma. In *The clinical practice of neurological and neurosurgical nursing,* ed 5, Philadelphia, 2003, Lippincott Williams & Wilkins.

6. Hickey JV: Management of the unconscious neurological patient. In *The clinical practice of neurological and neurosurgical nursing,* ed 5, Philadelphia, 2003, Lippincott Williams & Wilkins.

7. Winkler PA: Traumatic brain injury. In Umphred D, editor: *Neurological rehabilitation,* ed 4, St Louis, 2001, Mosby.

Chapter 24

Stroke Rehabilitation

Jeanne Flannery and Sue B. Pugh

1. What are the modifiable risk factors for stroke?

Box 24-1 presents the modifiable risk factors for stroke.

Box 24-1. Modifiable risk factors for stroke

- Hypertension (systolic blood pressure >140 mm Hg); risk factor second only to age
- Cigarette smoking
- Salt intake
- Obesity
- Elevated serum fibrinogen levels
- Diabetes
- Sedentary lifestyle
- Use of contraceptives with high doses of estrogen (if smoking is added and the person is 35 years old or older, the risk is 22 times higher than average)
- Hyperlipidemia
- Alcohol abuse
- Atrial fibrillation and other cardiac disease
- Use of cocaine

---

2. What are the nonmodifiable risk factors for stroke?

Nonmodifiable risk factors for stroke include
- Age (88% of stroke deaths occur in those 65 years old or older; risk more than doubles for each decade after age 55)
- Race (blacks have almost twice the risk and twice the mortality of whites)
- Male gender (57% of strokes are in men, but 62% of deaths are among women)
- Heredity
- Previous history of stroke or cardiovascular disorder

3. What are the chances of having another stroke after the first one?

About 10% to 18% of the 600,000 survivors of strokes each year will have a second stroke within a year. About 42% are at risk for another stroke in 5 years.

4. **Why is prevention of stroke so important to the health care industry?**

Prevention of stroke is important because someone has a stroke every 53 seconds, and someone dies from stroke every 3.1 minutes, and the cost to society is almost $50 billion per year. More than 4,600,000 persons are stroke survivors, and they represent about 75% of the patients in long-term care facilities, 60% in rehabilitation facilities, and 50% of hospitalized patients with neurological disorders.

5. **Why is early treatment so important?**

Stroke is divided into two main classifications: ischemic and hemorrhagic. Ischemic strokes account for 85% of all strokes and include thrombotic and embolic origins of occlusion.

Based on animal studies of precise time for progression from occlusion to infarct and research in human recovery that evaluated the time when circulation is reestablished after occlusion, recovery is time dependent.

When occlusion occurs, within 2 to 5 minutes of complete oxygen deprivation, neurons will die. This core area of cell death is called infarct. Immediately surrounding the infarcted area, a larger area of less ischemic tissue, called penumbra, exists. In this ischemic area the cells are stunned and cannot function electrically, but they are still alive because of collateral circulation. This low-flow perfusion causes extension of the original infarct if treatment is not provided immediately. The reason for extension of the infarct is that glucose continues to be delivered to this area without adequate oxygen, which produces anaerobic glycolysis, resulting in lactic acid buildup that kills cells. Additionally, with this low-flow perfusion, water that causes edema and white blood cells, platelets, and coagulation factors that slow circulation even further continue to be delivered to the area and contribute to tissue damage.

If reperfusion can be established within 90 minutes, the greatest amount of improvement in symptoms is seen within 24 hours and in outcomes at 3 months.

6. **What is reperfusion injury?**

When circulation is reestablished, acute inflammation of the ischemic tissue occurs. During reperfusion, neutrophils release proteases and oxygen free radicals that further damage the compromised but viable cells and cell membranes. The patient may experience new or identical symptoms of stroke after circulation is reestablished and therefore must be observed carefully.

7. **What is a transient ischemic attack?**

A transient ischemic attack (TIA) is an episode of ischemia producing focal symptoms that may last as little as 5 minutes or as long as 24 hours but will clear completely by that time. Transient ischemic attacks often are forewarnings of an impending stroke. A patient may have only one TIA before a stroke, or as many as 100. The time varies from hours to years before a stroke. The possibility also exists that a subsequent stroke never occurs. Because strokes occur in 75% of cases of TIA, prevention interventions through the modification of risk factors should be aggressive.

8. What is a reversible ischemic neurological deficit?

Reversible ischemic neurological deficit, also called a small stroke, is like a TIA except the signs persist longer than 24 hours. Signs resolve completely, usually by 48 hours.

9. What are the causes of an ischemic stroke?

Ischemic strokes can be embolic or thrombotic. An embolic stroke indicates that a clot, typically from a cardiac source, has dislodged and is occluding the cerebral vessel and causing the stroke. A thrombotic stroke is caused from a narrowing of the diameter of the vessel wall. Occasionally, ischemic stroke results from a combination of both.

10. What are the symptoms of ischemic stroke?

Symptoms may include sudden onset of weakness, paralysis, numbness or tingling on one side of the body. Dizziness, changes in coordination, slurred speech, and visual changes also may be symptoms of stroke. The most important symptom of stroke that differentiates these symptoms from other neurological disorders is the sudden onset aspect.

11. What about persons who complain of a severe headache?

Severe headache is associated with only 15% to 20% of strokes. Eighty-five percent of strokes are ischemic and are typically painless. The hallmark of hemorrhagic strokes is the sudden onset of a headache that is described as the worst headache of the patient's life.

12. What new treatment generated the name "brain attack?"

The drug alteplase (Activase) is used in the acute treatment of stroke. Alteplase is currently the only thrombolytic agent that is approved by the Food and Drug Administration to treat acute stroke. Because this medication must be administered within 3 hours of the first symptom of stroke, the public is being educated to treat a stroke like a heart attack and thus to seek treatment immediately. Thus the name for acute stroke is brain attack.

13. Do all stroke patients who arrive within 3 hours of their first symptom of stroke receive alteplase?

No, not all stroke patients receive alteplase. Inclusion and exclusion criteria exist. The most important initial diagnostic test is a computed tomography scan, which indicates whether the stroke is ischemic or hemorrhagic. If the patient has an ischemic stroke, then the patient meets the first criterion for inclusion. The patient must also arrive within at least 2½ hours of the first symptom, for the normal workup takes 20 to 30 minutes at the best institutions.

Box 24-2 lists other exclusion criteria besides cerebral or subarachnoid hemorrhage.

Box 24-2.   Factors that exclude alteplase therapy for stroke

- Current or recent use of anticoagulants
- Previous stroke within 3 months
- Major surgery within 2 weeks
- Rapidly progressing neurological signs
- History of bleeding within 3 weeks
- Recent myocardial infarction
- Seizures with stroke
- Pregnancy

---

14. What else can be done for the stroke patient during the acute phase?

Adequate perfusion is everything. Health care personnel should limit the use of blood pressure–lowering drugs to only those patients whose blood pressure is greater than 220/110. Autoregulation is impaired with a stroke, leaving neurons dependent on minute-to-minute supply of oxygen and glucose from systemic systolic blood pressure. Cerebral perfusion pressure and cerebral blood flow cannot respond to metabolic cellular needs but are maintained passively by the blood pressure. Because abnormal blood glucose levels and elevated body temperatures increase cellular metabolic demands, the nurse should maintain blood glucose levels less than 200 mg/dl and greater than 70 mg/dl. The patient's temperature should not be higher than 100° F.

15. When should blood pressure be lowered?

If a patient is going to receive alteplase, then the patient's systolic blood pressure should be lowered to 180 mm Hg, but no lower. As the brain tissue senses the loss of oxygenated blood, it increases blood pressure in an attempt to restore perfusion. Also, brain tissue that has been exposed to high pressure for an extended time will respond as if it were ischemic when blood pressure is lowered too much.

16. Why should blood glucose be maintained between 70 mg/dl and 200 mg/dl?

The recent research in stroke has found that patients with blood glucose levels greater than 200 mg/dl had worse outcomes than those patients with blood glucose levels less than 200 mg/dl. Available research used 200 mg/dl as the parameter, so lowering the glucose level to 180 mg/dl or even to more normal ranges possibly could be more beneficial, but this has not been determined yet.

17. Because high blood pressure is a risk factor for future strokes, when should the patient resume or initiate blood pressure medications?

With the benchmark length of stay in an acute care institution for stroke being 4 days, blood pressure management probably should not be started until after patients are discharged from the acute care hospital and have started intense rehabilitation.

18. To avoid another ischemic stroke, what is the recommended antiplatelet agent?

Research indicates that the best preventive medication for future stroke is aspirin. The specific dosage is still debateable, but newer research is indicating a dosage of 325 mg per day.

19. When should warfarin (Coumadin) be used for stroke prevention?

Warfarin is the recommended treatment for atrial fibrillation. Because atrial fibrillation is a common cause of embolic stroke, warfarin frequently is viewed as the medication to prevent future strokes. However, recent studies have indicated that aspirin is more effective in preventing future strokes, except in the population of patients with atrial fibrillation.

20. The American Heart Association advocates the use of lipid-lowering drugs to prevent heart disease. Does that apply to stroke too?

Yes, because stroke is a cardiovascular disease, patients at risk for stroke should take a lipid-lowering medication to assist in the prevention of stroke.

21. When should physical rehabilitation begin following acute stroke?

Physical rehabilitation should begin as soon as the patient is stabilized and while the patient is still in the acute care setting. Because patients will be living with any stroke-related impairment for the rest of their lives, rehabilitation nurses should begin helping them immediately to learn to adapt and regain as much function possible.

22. Are any particular impairments common to stroke?

Forty percent of patients have swallowing deficits (dysphagia) following stroke. Rehabilitation nurses should evaluate all patients for their ability to swallow safely. Just because a patient can speak does not mean that the patient can swallow. Nurses should assess swallowing before the patient attempts oral intake.

23. How should the rehabilitation nurse assess dysphagia?

Box 24-3 presents the observations the rehabilitation nurse should make to assess for dysphagia.

Box 24-3.   Dysphagia assessment

- Is the swallow evident by rise and fall of the Adam's apple (larynx)?
- Can the patient cough on demand?
- Does the patient use multiple swallows on a single mouthful?
- Are changes in voice identifiable after a swallow: gurgling, wet, hoarse, breathy?
- Is gag reflex weak or absent?
- Does the patient get short of breath during eating?
- Are breath sounds congested?

---

24. What nursing measures should the nurse use to assist the patient in swallowing?

Box 24-4 presents the measures that may help to prevent aspiration.

Box 24-4.   Measures to assist a dysphagic patient to swallow

- Position the patient sitting straight up with head placed slightly forward.
- Provide semisoft or soft foods and thickened liquids.
- Teach the patient to place food on the back of the tongue on the unaffected side.
- Teach the patient to sweep the affected side with the tongue to prevent trapping of food in the cheek.
- Provide a distraction-free environment during meals, so the patient will not try impulsively to swallow at the same time as talking or breathing.

---

25. How long following a stroke can a patient expect to recover?

In general, a patient typically recovers the majority of function in the first 90 days following stroke. However, a growing body of research indicates that persons with strokes can gain further function years after their stroke with some of the new rehabilitation techniques being studied.

26. What effect does stroke have on bowel and bladder function?

Bladder incontinence occurs in 75% of patients, but it generally clears within 3 to 6 months, for most within the first month. Some persons (15%) will experience the problem after 6 months. Bowel incontinence occurs in 31% of patients, but usually resolves within 2 weeks.

27. How does the rehabilitation nurse assist the patient with incontinence?

The rehabilitation nurse begins a strict bladder retraining regimen immediately, starting with every 4-hour straight catheterization and postvoid catheterizations for residual urine. Bladder scans and urodynamic studies evaluate bladder function. Medications to relax bladder muscles, such as oxybutynin (Ditropan), or to stimulate bladder contraction, such as bethanechol (Urecholine), may assist in control.

A bowel program prevents constipation by providing adequate fluids, daily administration of stool softeners, and administration of progressive stimulants such as milk of magnesia, cascara, bisacodyl (Dulcolax) tablets or suppositories, and oil retention enemas, if needed. A bowel movement is expected with no less frequency than every 3 days. Positioning in an upright position for evacuation at the same time every day helps. Diet is modified if diarrhea occurs.

28. How do patients with stroke on the right side of the brain differ in symptoms from patients with stroke on the left side of the brain?

Because of the unique organizational structure of the brain, with the right hemisphere functioning differently from the left to accomplish a global outcome, a stroke on one side produces considerably different deficits than a stroke on the opposite side.

Box 24-5 presents signs and symptoms of stroke on the right side of the brain, and Box 24-6 presents signs and symptoms of stroke on the left side of the brain.

Box 24-5.   Signs and symptoms of stroke on the right side of the brain

- Deficits in perception of nonverbal stimuli, such as sounds, voice intonation, and facial expressions
- Lack of inhibitions
- Spatial-perceptual deficits (position, distance, rate of movement, relation to self)
- Lack of voice control; talks incessantly, reads aloud fluently without comprehension; confabulates
- Inappropriate social behavior
- Short attention span
- Inability to think abstractly
- Poor judgment; lack of insight
- Impulsiveness, impatience
- Hemiparesis or hemiplegia of left side of the body
- Left homonymous hemianopsia (may not see past midline)
- Anosognosia (denial of affected side)
- Overestimation of abilities
- Apraxia (inability to use objects or words properly)
- Distractability
- Anxiety, frustration, fear of failure
- Difficulty performing any task with nonverbal directions
- Loss of appreciation of beauty: music, art
- Loss of recognition of places; becomes lost within and outside the home

Box 24-6.   Signs and symptoms of stroke on the left side of the brain

1. Aphasia
    a. Expressive (loss of vocabulary, perseveration)
    b. Receptive (cannot understand verbal directions)
    c. Global (combination)
2. Agraphia (inability to write)
3. Alexia (inability to read)
4. Acalculia (cannot solve mathematical problems)
5. Intellectual impairment
6. Short-term memory impairment; difficulty in learning
7. Depression, frustration, but plods with perseverance at tasks
8. Right hemiparesis or hemiplegia
9. Right homonymous hemianopsia (may not see past midline); difficulty distinguishing left from right

29. What nursing measures are specific for the patient with a stroke on the right side of the brain?

Box 24-7 presents nursing measures for the patient with a stroke on the right side of the brain.

Box 24-7.   Nursing measures for the patient with a stroke on the right side of the brain

- Decrease sensory stimuli.
- Do not use gestures with explanations.
- Move slowly, explaining movements.
- Remind patient of the condition (expects to be independent).
- Remind patient of affected side (ignores the existence of affected side); place patient in front of mirror to remind patient about tasks such as to straighten up, to dress affected limb, and to wash the affected side of the face.
- Name objects, places, and persons each and every time.
- Break tasks into simple, single steps.
- Explain what objects are for.
- Prepare family for outbursts and lack of inhibitions.
- Provide safety from impulsive movements with belts, side rails, and lap boards.
- Reorient patient to location.

30. What nursing measures are specific for the patient with a stroke on the left side of the brain?

Box 24-8 presents nursing measures for the patient with a stroke on the left side of the brain.

> **Box 24-8.   Nursing measures for the patient with a stroke on the left side of the brain**
>
> • Determine type of aphasia and devise alternative communication methods.
> • Speak slowly, using gestures, pictures, music, and visual stimuli.
> • Use simple one-syllable nouns and verbs and two-word sentences.
> • Approach patient within field of vision; remind patient to turn head to see beyond field of vision.
> • Use repetition to assist with learning impairment.
> • Provide praise support and motivating activities for patient to assist with depression caused by patient's disabilities.
> • Use pictures, objects, and gestures to help patient with loss of understanding of words.

31. Why do nurses without special rehabilitation education overestimate the capabilities of a patient with stroke on the right side of the brain?

Patients affected by stroke on the right side of the brain usually are outgoing, cheerful, and eager to try anything asked of them, and they believe they can do anything (because of anosognosia). Patients with a stroke on the left side of the brain may have worse motor impairment and look less able, but they generally recover more readily than patients with stroke on the right side of the brain.

32. What is constraint-induced movement therapy?

Constraint-induced movement therapy assists cortical reorganization through forced use of the affected limbs. The unaffected limb is constrained while repetitive exercises are done 7 hours a day, 5 days a week for 12 days. This intense activity increases neurocircuitry in the damaged motor cortex to almost double, often remediating the impairment.

33. What is the Bobath system of rehabilitation?

Bobath is a neurodevelopmental approach that relies on building on brain plasticity for the goal of relearning. Reprogramming can occur through specific positioning and patterned exercise. Recovery is linear, in a stepwise progression; therefore basic motions are stimulated until restored, and then they serve as foundation for the next level of functioning. For example, posture is corrected first through normal alignment to maintain normal tone. If tone is abnormal, positioning and passive stretching exercises must be continued until tone is normalized, before movements can be expected. The process is cyclical, for movement is necessary to function, which then affects posture.

34. What is spasticity?

Spasticity is a velocity-dependent hypertonic disorder. The faster the extremity is moved, the greater the tone and ultimate resistance in the muscles. Spasticity demonstrates an imbalance between inhibitory and excitatory mechanisms and occurs in 65% of stroke survivors. Flaccid paralysis at the onset of a stroke gradually becomes spastic paralysis as muscles regain tone. Patients with spasticity generally require 3 times as long in rehabilitation as those without spasticity.

35. What is included in treatment for spasticity?

Treatment of spasticity includes
- Maintenance of soft tissue length
- Prevention of or decrease in pain syndromes
- Appropriate motor training to eliminate unnecessary muscle force
- Development of motor control into effective function
- Encouragement of slow, controlled movements, such as sustained stretch
- Medications to reduce spasticity, such as baclofen (Lioresal), dantrolene sodium (Dantrium), or botulinum toxin (Botox)
- Prevention of habitual abnormal compensatory movement patterns

36. How is cognitive impairment manifested in the patient with stroke?

Cognitive impairment following stroke may include the problems presented in Box 24-9.

Box 24-9. Manifestations of cognitive impairment following stroke

- Loss of memory
- Short attention span
- Increased distractibility
- Poor judgment
- Inability to reason, calculate, or think abstractly
- Confusion, hallucinations, delusions
- Decline in flexibility
- Inability to perform more than one task at a time
- Delay in processing information
- Decreased ability to understand new ideas
- Abnormal interpretations of environment
- Inappropriate decision making and social behavior
- Disorientation
- Loss of inhibitions
- Altered step patterns

---

37. What hope lies in the future to improve outcomes from ischemic stroke?

Currently animal studies are ongoing to test a stroke vaccine. Thus far the results look promising in that when rats were given a middle cerebral artery stroke 5 months after being given the vaccine, the lesions were reduced by 70% compared with the nonvaccinated group. Neuroprotective strategies, such as the use of hypothermia (33° C), in combination with the use of intraarterial thrombolytic therapy (agent delivered directly to the clot), γ-aminobutyric acid agonists, calcium channel blockers, and free radical scavengers may soon reveal the right combination to improve outcomes.

38. Why is hemorrhagic stroke so important when it is so infrequent compared with ischemic stroke?

Hemorrhagic stroke results from a primary rupture of a blood vessel and accounts for 15% of all strokes. Important for all nurses to realize is that the mortality rate is high. About 6% of persons with hemorrhagic stroke die before reaching the hospital. Within 30 days of the event the mortality rate is twofold to sixfold higher than for ischemic stroke, causing death in 37.5% of the population. More than half of these patients die within the first 2 days.

39. How much blood lost from a ruptured cerebral artery produces the devastating massive hemorrhagic effect?

Because no extra space exists in the cranium with a normal brain, with normal cerebrospinal fluid, and normal cerebral blood flow, as little as 30 ml of blood can produce mass effect, creating midline shift, herniation, and ultimately death.

40. What are the causes of hemorrhagic stroke?

Intracerebral stroke results from rupture of a small, deep penetrating artery, forcing blood into the surrounding parenchyma, creating a hematoma. Generally, in 20% to 30% of patients the clot volume increases in the first 24 hours. The clot compresses adjacent cerebral tissue and displaces it. Cellular ischemia results, and cerebral edema develops, increasing intracranial pressure. Neurotoxicity can result from blood degradation and ischemia. A major hemorrhage can cause midline shift and herniation, with a mortality rate of 50%. These strokes are often a result of long-standing, poorly controlled hypertension frequently in an older person.

Subarachnoid hemorrhage results from bleeding into the subarachnoid space, most often caused by a ruptured cerebral aneurysm or arteriovenous malformation. Aneurysms rupture more commonly in women 35 to 60 years of age. The prognosis remains poor, even with technological advances, with only about one third recovering without major disability. Incidence in blacks is twice that of whites. The blood is forced into the subarachnoid space at the base of the brain (circle of Willis) and spreads into the basal cisterns. Pressure from surrounding tissue stops the bleeding, and a clot forms. The location of the clot interferes with cerebrospinal fluid flow and, along with the inflammatory response, creates cerebral edema.

41. How do symptoms of a hemorrhagic stroke differ from those of an ischemic stroke?

With a hemorrhagic stroke the person has a sudden, violent, explosive headache, classically described as "the worst headache of my life." Loss of consciousness may occur immediately, or a decrease in the level of consciousness may occur.

Vomiting, stiff neck, blurred vision, photophobia, and mild temperature elevation may result from meningeal irritation. Pupillary changes from pressure on cranial nerves III, IV, and VI may be present. Increased intracranial pressure may cause seizures, bradycardia, widened pulse pressure, and hypertension. All of these symptoms occur in addition to the stroke syndrome that likewise would be manifested in the ischemic stroke.

Key Points

- Someone dies from stroke every 3 minutes, and more than 4.6 million persons survive stroke; the cost annually is $50 billion.
- Strokes occur in 75% of patients with TIAs.
- Reversible ischemic neurological deficit is a small stroke; deficits completely resolve, usually by 48 hours.
- Eighty-five percent of strokes are ischemic and are typically painless.
- The patient's temperature must be maintained no higher than 100° F, blood glucose must be greater than 70 mg/dl and less than 200 mg/dl, and blood pressure should not be treated unless greater than 220/110 mm Hg. Blood pressure should be no lower than 180 mm Hg.
- Aspirin 325 mg daily typically is recommended to patients who have had an ischemic stroke to reduce risk of further strokes.
- The greatest amount of recovery from stroke occurs in the first 90 days.
- Patients with strokes on the right side of the brain appear to be able to do more than they are able and generally take longer to recover than patients with strokes on the left side of the brain.
- Mortality rate for hemorrhagic stroke is high; 6% of victims die before reaching the hospital, and greater than 50% die within 2 days.

Internet Resources

National Institute of Neurological Disorders and Stroke
http://www.ninds.nih.gov/index.htm

Post Stroke Help
http://www.poststrokehelp.com/

American Heart Association
http://www.americanheart.org/

American Stroke Association
http://www.strokeassociation.org/

National Stroke Association
http://www.stroke.org

Bibliography

1. Barker E: Brain attack/stroke management. In Barker EL, editor: *Neuroscience nursing: a spectrum of care,* ed 2, St Louis, 2002, Mosby.

2. Bartels MN: Pathophysiology and medical management of stroke. In Gillen G, Burkhardt AL, editors: *Stroke rehabilitation: a function-based approach,* St Louis, 1998, Mosby.

3. Flannery JC: Disruption of circulation in the brain and spinal cord. In Burrell LO, Gerlach MJ, Pless BS, editors: *Adult nursing: acute and community care,* ed 2, Stamford, Conn, 1997, Appleton & Lange.

4. Gatens C, Hebert AR: Cognition and behavior. In Hoeman SP, editor: *Rehabilitation nursing: process, application, & outcomes,* ed 3, St Louis, 2002, Mosby.

5. Hickey JV, Hock NH: Stroke and other cerebrovascular diseases. In Hickey JV, editor: *The clinical practice of neurological and neurosurgical nursing,* ed 5, Philadelphia, 2003, Lippincott.

6. Hinkle JL, Bowman L: Neuroprotection for ischemic stroke, *J Neurosci Nurs* 35(2):114-118, 2003.

7. Youngblood NM: Nursing management of the patient with a cerebrovascular accident. In Derstine JB, Hargrove SD, editors: *Comprehensive rehabilitation nursing,* Philadelphia, 2001, WB Saunders.

Chapter 25

Spinal Cord Injury Rehabilitation

Jeanne Flannery and Susan R. Bulecza

1. **What is the rehabilitation goal after spinal cord injury?**

   The rehabilitation goal after spinal cord injury is to minimize disability. Although this goal is simple and straightforward, the process to achieve it is complex, even daunting at times. To achieve maximum independence, the process requires a multidisciplinary team and a holistic approach. Patient interventions and education need to address all of the following areas:
   - Vocational
   - Psychosocial
   - Sexual
   - Functional skills and activities of daily living
   - Adaptive equipment and environmental adaptations and modifications
   - Health maintenance and physical needs
   - Recreation

2. **Where should a spinal cord–injured person receive rehabilitation to achieve optimal outcomes?**

   Because of the complexity of rehabilitation required for these patients, facilities that specialize in spinal cord rehabilitation or have large spinal cord rehabilitation components are best suited to achieve optimal outcomes. The United States has 16 rehabilitation facilities (see Box 25-1).

Box 25-1. Model Spinal Cord Injury System Centers

Model Spinal Cord Injury System Centers in the United States, which are sponsored by the National Institute on Disability and Rehabilitative Research, work together to demonstrate improved care, maintain a national database, participate in independent and collaborative research, and provide continuing education relating to spinal cord injury. Centers are currently located in the following states:

Continued

Box 25-1.   Model Spinal Cord Injury System Centers *continued*

Alabama
University of Alabama at Birmingham SCI Care System
University of Alabama at Birmingham
Spain Rehabilitation Center
1717 6th Ave South, Room 190
Birmingham, AL 35233-7330
(205) 934-3334

California
Regional Spinal Cord Injury Care System of Southern California
Rancho Los Amigos Medical Center
Los Amigos Research and Education Institute, Inc.
7601 E Imperial Hwy, HB 206
Downey, CA 90242-4155
(562) 401-7161
Northern California SCI System
Santa Clara Valley Medical Center
950 S Bascom Ave, Suite 2011
San Jose, CA 95128
(408) 295-9896

Colorado
Rocky Mountain Model Spinal Cord Injury System
Craig Hospital, Research Department
3425 S Clarkson St
Englewood, CO 80110
(303) 789-8306

Florida
South Florida SCI System
University of Miami School of Medicine
PO Box 016960, Mail Locator R-48
Miami, FL 33101
(305) 243-7106

Georgia
Georgia Regional Spinal Cord Injury Care System
Shepherd Center, Inc.
2020 Peachtree Rd, NW
Atlanta, GA 30309
(404) 350-7580

Box 25-1.   Model Spinal Cord Injury System Centers *continued*

Massachusetts
Special Projects and Demonstrations for Spinal Cord Injuries
Boston Medical Center
New England Regional Spinal Cord Injury Center
88 E Newton St, F-511
Boston, MA 02118
(617) 638-7358

Michigan
University of Michigan Model Spinal Cord Injury Care System
University of Michigan Health System
Department of Physical Medicine and Rehabilitation
300 N Ingalls, Room NI2A09
Ann Arbor, MI 48109-0491
(734) 763-0971

Missouri
Missouri Model Spinal Cord Injury System
University of Missouri—Columbia
Department of Physical Medicine and Rehabilitation
One Hospital Dr, DC046.00
Columbia, MO 65212
(573) 884-7972

New Jersey
Northern New Jersey Model Spinal Cord Injury System
Kessler Institute for Rehabilitation
1199 Pleasant Valley Way
West Orange, NJ 07052
(973) 243-6871

New York
Mount Sinai Model Spinal Cord Injury System
One Gustave Levey Place, Box 1240
New York, NY 10029-6574
(212) 659-9369

Pennsylvania
Thomas Jefferson University Hospital
132 S 10th St, 375 Main Bldg
Philadelphia, PA 19107
(215) 955-6579

Continued

Box 25-1.   Model Spinal Cord Injury System Centers *continued*

School of Medicine, University of Pittsburgh
3471 5th Ave, Suite 90
Pittsburgh, PA 15213
(412) 648-6654

Texas
Model Spinal Cord Injury System—Texas
The Institute for Rehabilitation and Research
1333 Moursund Ave
Houston, TX 77030
(713) 797-5946

Virginia
Virginia Commonwealth Regional Spinal Cord Injury System
Virginia Commonwealth University
Medical College of Virginia
Department of Physical Medicine and Rehabilitation
Box 980677
Richmond, VA 23298-0677
(804) 828-0861

Washington
Northwest Regional Spinal Cord Injury System
University of Washington, School of Medicine
Department of Rehabilitation Medicine
Box 356490
Seattle, WA 98195-6490
(206) 685-3999

---

3. **What are the main requirements necessary for a spinal cord–injured patient to achieve maximum independence?**

The three requirements are knowledge, ability, and attitude. Knowledge is important to empower the patients to develop self-reliance. A comprehensive assessment of the patients' physical abilities and problem-solving skills is critical for determining the patients' capacity for performing a task independently or having the autonomy to direct others in assisting them. Knowledge and ability often are achieved more easily than attitude. Developing an independent attitude often can be one of the biggest barriers patients and the rehabilitation team have to overcome. A natural tendency for those caring for patients is to allow a dependency attitude to develop in the patients. To counter this, those caring for the patients, even from the first day of injury, need to emphasize the patients' autonomy and responsibility in their own care. Often this is not easy for the nurse because it frequently requires a "tough love" approach, which minimizes the natural tendency of the patients to allow someone else to do a task for them because it is easier.

An example of a strategy rehabilitation nurses must use is when patients fall in attempting to transfer from wheelchair to bed. Instead of lifting them into bed, nurses might actually sit on the floor with the patients to convey a caring attitude but actually talk the patients through the steps for them to use to pull themselves back into the chair. The nurses will check the patients, allow them to rest, and then encourage them to attempt the transfer again. Should the patients be at home alone, they have to have the confidence that they can manage such an event independently.

4. **Is there an age-related pattern to traumatic spinal cord injury, and what is the most frequent cause of injury?**

Yes, the age group most often affected is individuals between 16 and 30 years old. Motor vehicle accidents followed by violent acts, such as gunshots, and falls are the most common causes. Typically, a young male involved in a motor vehicle accident is the most common patient. The rate of occurrence is 4 times greater in males than in females. Additionally, injuries occur more frequently on weekends and during the summer. This age group, particularly males, typically engages in more risk-taking behaviors, such as driving too fast (boats or cars), driving while using drugs or alcohol, diving into unknown bodies of water, and playing contact sports. Even when the rules are being followed, this group may be easily distracted, such as in turning to talk with friends in a car, or adjusting the radio while talking on the phone. They tend not to believe that accidents could happen to them.

5. **Does injury to a particular area of the spine more often produce spinal cord injury?**

Yes, injury to the cervical spine produces spinal cord injury about 40% of the time because of the poor mechanical stability of the cervical spine, making it more susceptible to injury. Injury to the more stable thoracic or thoracolumbar areas is less likely to produce spinal cord injury. Additionally, spinal cord injury often is associated with head injury. About one third of patients sustaining a cervical injury also have at least minor brain injury.

6. **Why is clarifying for the patient what a "bruised" spinal cord means important?**

Bruising indicates contusion, in which bleeding from the small blood vessels occurs within 30 minutes and may continue for hours as just the primary injury. Often a patient will interpret a "bruised" spinal cord to mean a temporary condition and that paralysis will go away once bruising resolves. However, this is often not the case. "Bruising" or hemorrhage in the spinal cord frequently results in permanent neurological damage. Because of the natural inflammatory response of the body, the process itself causes secondary injury beginning in minutes and extending for hours after the initial insult, furthering the destruction of neurons. This secondary damage is what creates most of the disability.

7. What does secondary injury of the spinal cord mean?

The primary injury that occurred on impact results in ischemia of the spinal cord because of disruption of neurons and the vascular supply, leading to necrosis of the neurons. The secondary injury is a process of self-destruction of the area extending beyond the initial injured site beginning within 30 minutes of impact and continuing for hours, perhaps even weeks. The inflammatory response resulting from the primary injury produces a cascade of events:

1. The hypoxia of the neurons in the gray matter causes the release of vasoactive agents and catacholamines:
   - Norepinephrine
   - Serotonin
   - Dopamine
   - Histamine
2. Vasoactive agents cause vasospasm and impede blood flow in microcirculation, which furthers ischemia and leads to necrosis.
3. Proteolytic and lipolytic cellular enzymes, protein kinases, and protein phosphatases are released from the injured cells and cause delayed swelling, demyelination of the axons, neuronal cell membrane damage, and necrosis of the cord.
4. Vascular trauma enhances the release of vasoactive agents and leads to increased vascular permeability, and swelling, which furthers ischemia.
5. Cellular energy failure causes a release of excessive excitatory neurotransmitters (such as glutamate, aspartate, and the amine acetylcholine) is widespread.
6. Excitatory transmitters (glutamate) cause membrane depolarization, opening the calcium channels and creating intracellular calcium influx into neurons and glia, which
   - Damages the cell membranes
   - Damages intracellular processes, including mitochondrial function, depleting cell energy
   - Intracellular sodium influx and potassium efflux, causing further cellular swelling
   - Activate phospholipases and proteases to generate oxygen free radicals:
     - Superoxide
     - Hydroxyl
     - Hydrogen peroxide
     - Nitrous oxide
7. Free radicals disrupt cellular membranes, dissolve microtubules, cause cell death, and lead ultimately to the further development of more free radicals.
8. Breakdown products from the initial injury also lead to the production of free radicals.

Inflammation also includes the healing process, but the complex process of healing itself can be further detrimental. The macrophages remove the debris, and astrocytes form scar tissue. This scar tissue prevents any regeneration and reconnection of the neuronal pathways.

8. **What can the nurse tell the family to clarify the physician's explanation that the degree of injury cannot be determined immediately?**

The nurse can explain that a natural process of inflammation occurs that is stimulated by the initial injury and can cause further damage. Depending on whether the patient was started on methylprednisolone therapy on arrival in the emergency room, the nurse may discuss that this therapy is an attempt to reduce as much of the secondary damage as possible. Otherwise, the nurse may need to approach the subject from the point that until reflexes return after recovery from spinal shock (complete loss of motor, sensory, reflex, and autonomic function below the level of injury), loss of function may seem worse than it may turn out to be. Spinal shock typically resolves, neuron by neuron, in 1 to 6 weeks. Because no research has found an effective way to control the secondary damage, to dwell on a possibly worsening condition is not appropriate. The shock to the family may be greater initially than to the patient if the patient has other injuries, pain medications, secondary surgeries, and many treatments. At least the acceptance that some change may occur in several weeks serves to provide a delay in the need to accept, wholly, the impact of this injury all at once, which can be devastating.

9. **What is meant by neurological return?**

Neurological return is defined as return of some or all voluntary motor function or sensation lost at time of injury and means that some degree of connection still exists between the brain and spinal cord below injury level. In contrast, return of spinal reflexes below the level of injury does not constitute neurological return but is simply resolution of spinal shock (the loss of all neurological function below the level of injury that gradually recovers spontaneously over 4 to 6 weeks). The majority of neurological return occurs during the first year after injury.

10. **Contrast complete and incomplete spinal cord injury.**

A complete spinal cord injury means total loss of sensory and motor function below the level of injury. Although most injuries do not result initially in complete severance of the cord, many become complete injuries from the secondary inflammatory damage that occurs within hours. Incomplete spinal cord injury means some degree of motor and sensory function (at least half of the muscles below the injury have a muscle grade <3 on a 5-point scale) remains below the level of injury; the lowest sacral segment (S2 to S4) is spared, which maintains bowel and bladder continence. The degree of injury cannot be determined fully until spinal shock resolves. The majority of spinal cord injuries probably have not more than 20% loss of function from the initial injury (based on extensive animal studies), but the injuries progress relatively unimpeded through secondary insult, causing extension of the injury and increased disability.

11. What is Brown-Séquard's syndrome?

Brown-Séquard's syndrome occurs when one side of the cord is damaged or sustains more damage than the other. Symptoms include loss of proprioception; loss of motor function, vibration, and deep touch on the same (ipsilateral) side as the injury; and loss of pain, light touch, and temperature sensation on the opposite (contralateral) side. Patients with this syndrome also may have spasticity below the injury level on the side of injury. This hemisection of the cord is commonly the result of a knife or bullet wound.

12. What is central cord syndrome?

Central cord syndrome occurs when the central portion of the spinal cord is injured (the area where the corticospinal tract fibers controlling the arms are located), leaving the peripheral areas of the cord intact (the area where the corticospinal tract fibers controlling the legs are located). This type of injury almost always occurs in the cervical area. Symptoms include upper extremity weakness that is greater than any weakness in the lower extremities. Total loss of function of the arms may occur, with normal below-the-waist function. This injury is difficult for patients and families to understand, and adaptation to the disability is challenging. Community reentry is particularly hard because the patient can walk. Persons do not realize how dependent this individual is with no ability to use the hands. In many cases sacral (S2 to S4) sparing occurs, leaving bowel/bladder function intact. This injury occurs more frequently in elderly persons in whom the spinal canal has narrowed because of arthritic changes.

13. What are conus medullaris and cauda equina syndromes?

Conus medullaris and cauda equina syndromes can result from injury to the sacral cord and lumbar-sacral nerve roots. Both syndromes result from a lower motor neuron injury and produce varying degrees of flaccid paralysis of lower extremities, areflexic bowel and bladder, and loss of sexual function. If the injury involves only cauda equina (horse's tail), which is the spinal nerve roots, recovery is possible because peripheral nerves can regenerate.

14. What are the physical effects of spinal cord injury?

The physical effects of spinal cord injury are
1. Autonomic dysfunction
   - Altered genital function
   - Impaired thermoregulation
   - Bradycardia and peripheral vasodilation
2. Hypotension
3. Orthostatic hypotension
4. Risk of deep vein thrombosis and pulmonary embolism
   - Autonomic dysreflexia
   - Gastrointestinal and urinary tract complications
   - Bladder and bowel incontinence

5. Skin breakdown
6. Skin infections
7. Sensory impairment
   • Pressure ulcers
   • Injuries from wheelchair, splints, or braces and friction or pinching
   • Burns
8. Voluntary motor paralysis
   • Risk for kidney stones from loss of calcium in bones not bearing weight
   • Muscle atrophy
9. Spasticity
   • Falls
   • Traumatic injuries
10. Heterotopic ossification
    • Loss of function of an innervated limb
    • Loss of wheelchair use because of inability to be positioned
    • Loss of control because of loss of function
11. Impaired breathing and coughing
    • Risk of atelectasis, pneumonia, and respiratory insufficiency
    • Risk of aspiration
12. Osteoporosis (risk for fractures)

15. Where is a spinal cord–injured patient most likely to develop heterotopic ossification, and how will it present?

Generally, heterotopic ossification only occurs below the level of injury, with the hips being the most commonly affected and the ankles and wrists rarely being affected. Heterotopic ossification occurs in about 20% of patients, usually within the first 12 weeks after injury.

Because of loss of sensation in affected areas, pain most likely will be absent. The first symptoms may be decreased range of motion and swelling in the affected limb. Warmth and redness also may be present in the affected area. Confirmatory diagnosis can be made with laboratory work; an elevated serum alkaline phosphatase level helps confirm heterotopic ossification. Because heterotopic ossification is not reversible, treatment focuses on preventing further progression. If limitation is severe, reconstructive surgery may be required. However, surgery cannot be performed until 12 to 18 months after diagnosis. The delay in surgery reduces the chance of recurrence.

16. What nursing interventions are appropriate for reducing the patient's risk of heterotopic ossification?

Nursing interventions appropriate for reducing the risk of heterotopic ossification are to
• Provide education to the patient and caregivers about heterotopic ossification and why the patient is at risk.

- Perform and teach caregivers to do range of motion exercises on all of the patient's joints daily.
- Increase patient's mobility as soon as possible.
- Position the patient properly in bed and wheelchair.

17. Are there prolonged cardiovascular effects from spinal cord injury?

Yes, because of the fact that most injuries occur at or above the thoracolumbar region, permanent disruption occurs between the brain and the sympathetic neurons that maintain normal cardiovascular reflexes. This condition often results in exercise intolerance or exercise-induced hypotension. Also, if the injury is cervical or high thoracic, venous return to the heart is reduced, which results in reduced stroke volume and cardiac output.

18. What is quad coughing and why is it important?

Because of the innervation of respiratory muscles at the cervical and thoracic levels, injury at either of these levels results in some degree of respiratory compromise. Therefore an assisted coughing technique, quad coughing, is necessary to help the patient clear secretions.

To perform quad coughing, the nurse places the patient in an upright sitting position or lying on the back. The nurse then places the heel of one hand under the xiphoid process and asks the patient to take several deep breaths. At that time the patient is to hold the breath for several seconds. Next, the patient is to cough while the nurse pushes in and up with the heel of her hand against the diaphragm in a quick thrusting motion. These steps may be repeated as many times as necessary to clear secretions.

19. What is autonomic dysreflexia?

Autonomic dysreflexia is a medical emergency. The condition generally occurs in 10% to 85% of individuals who have an injury at or above T6. Autonomic dysreflexia is thought to occur because of a lack of communication between the brain and sympathetic neurons in the thoracolumbar spine. When the afferent impulses cannot reach the brain, a mass stimulation of the sympathetic reflex (tightening blood vessels, causing the blood pressure to rise) and nerves below the injury is initiated. No inhibitory cerebral control can reach this area. If the high blood pressure is not controlled, it may cause a stroke, seizure, or death. Table 25-1 presents symptoms of autonomic dysreflexia.

20. What can cause autonomic dysreflexia?

Autonomic dysreflexia is caused by some type of noxious stimulus below the level of injury. Common causes include bowel or bladder distention, urinary tract infection, or bowel impaction. Other causes include certain medications,

Table 25-1. Symptoms of dysreflexia

Symptoms	Presentation
Initial symptoms	Increased blood pressure
	Bradycardia
	Sudden intense pounding headache
	Flushing and profuse sweating above level of injury
Other symptoms	Pallor and coolness below the level of injury
	Anxiety
	Piloerection (goose bumps)
	Blurred vision
	Cardiac arrhythmias
	Nasal congestion
	Visual field disturbances

lower limb muscle spasm, urinary calculus, pressure ulcers, lower limb injury or infection, uterine contractions, ingrown toenail, sudden change in room temperature, invasive diagnostic and therapeutic procedures such as digital stimulation for bowel training, or an operative incision.

21. **What should be done for the patient experiencing autonomic dysreflexia?**

The rehabilitation nurse should know the signs and symptoms of autonomic dysreflexia and act immediately because this is a medical emergency. Reduction of the triggering stimulus and quick management of increased blood pressure are key interventions so that complication risk is minimized. The rehabilitation nurse must teach the patient to recognize the signs and symptoms and to direct caregivers in the emergent care for himself or herself. The patient who is at home must know to tell anyone available what to do to lower the blood pressure and find the noxious stimulus and relieve it. The nurse should teach the patient to check for bladder distention or kinks in an indwelling catheter first and then to check for bowel impaction. The caregiver must elevate the patient's head and lower the legs and feet immediately to lower the severe hypertension to reduce the risk of cerebral hemorrhage or myocardial infarction. The caregiver should loosen any constricting clothing or devices and should check the blood pressure every 2 to 5 minutes. If the change in the patient's condition does not lower the blood pressure, the caregiver must obtain professional help. The caregiver must attempt to find the noxious stimulus and remove it if possible. If this has occurred before, the patient's physician may have provided a quick-acting antihypertensive for use as needed, such as nifidepine 10 mg, which the patient can bite and swallow.

22. What is a halo brace?

A halo brace is a device used to restrict cervical spine movement and stabilize the spine. The brace allows the patient some degree of mobility and independence. The components of a halo are the head ring, which attaches to the skull with pins, vertical metal rods that attach the head ring to the vest, and the plastic vest that has a sheep-skin liner to protect the patient's skin. The patient is measured before the halo is applied to ensure appropriate fit. The halo can be used after surgical cervical intervention or as the main therapy.

23. What complications should the rehabilitation nurse be aware of for a patient wearing a halo brace?

Pin sites are the areas where complications most often occur. These complications may include infection—which can lead to septicemia, osteomyelitis, or subdural abscess—and pin loosening, which can result in spinal destabilization. Frequent assessment of pins and pin sites, good pin site hygiene, and early treatment of infection can reduce the risk of complication significantly.

Skin under and around the vest portion of the brace is an area of frequent complication such as pressure ulcers and rashes. Frequent skin assessment, especially of bony processes, and hygiene that includes monthly vest-liner changes help maintain intact skin.

If a patient complains of pain related to the halo brace, the nurse should investigate further, for pain generally is not associated with normal wearing. Pain can be an indication of loosened pins, pin site infection, or excessive pressure from the vest.

24. What is Horner's syndrome?

Horner's syndrome results from the loss of function of the cervical sympathetic nerve supply and can be unilateral or bilateral in presentation. Horner's syndrome presents as miosis (pupillary constriction), ptosis, slight elevation of the lower lid, sinking of the eyeball, and loss of sweating (anhydrosis) on the side of the injury.

25. When might the nurse see Horner's syndrome in a spinal cord–injured patient?

The nurse may see Horner's syndrome if the patient has a partial transection of the spinal cord at T1.

26. What loss of function results from different levels of spinal cord injury?

Table 25-2 displays the loss of function according to levels.

Table 25-2. Loss of function according to level of spinal cord injury

Level of injury	Motor function	Sensory function
C1-C4	Quadriplegia No function from neck down	No sensation from neck down
C5	Quadriplegia No function from below upper shoulders down Can control head	No sensation below clavicles except deltoid, clavicle, and part of forearms
C6	Quadriplegia No function below shoulders and upper arms	No sensation below clavicles except deltoid, clavicle, arms, palms, and thumbs
C7	Quadriplegia No function in part of hands and arms; can extend wrists	No sensation below clavicle except most of arms and hands
C8	Quadriplegia No function in part of hands and arms Can control elbow, wrist, and finger extension and finger flexion	No sensation below chest and part of hands
T1-T6	Paraplegia No function below midchest Full function arms, hands, and shoulders	No sensation below midchest Full sensation above midchest including arms and hands
T6-T12	Paraplegia No function below waist Trunk muscles intact	No sensation below waist
L1-L3	Paraplegia No function in legs and pelvis except hip rotation and flexion and partial leg flexion	No sensation lower abdomen and legs except partial inner and anterior thigh
L3-L4	Paraplegia No function in part of lower legs, ankles, and feet; can extend knee	No sensation parts of lower legs, feet, and ankles
L4-S5	Incomplete paraplegia Motor control disrupted and varies with level of injury Bowel and bladder may be disrupted depending on injury level Intact with S2-S5 injury	Loss of sensation varies depending on level of injury

27. What level of independence can be expected for each injury level?

Table 25-3 displays the functional abilities possible, based on the level of spinal cord injury.

Table 25-3. **Degree of independence that can be achieved according to level of spinal cord injury**

Injury level	Functional abilities
C1-C4	Depends on ventilator
	Requires full assistance for activities of daily living (ADL)
C5	Requires adaptive mouth-operated tools/equipment and special computer technology for some degree of independence
	Requires full assistance for ADL
C6	Needs adaptive devices to use arms and requires motorized wheelchair
	May be able to assist with some self-care
	Requires full assistance for transfers
C7	Can independently perform some ADL
	Requires wrist splints for finger flexion
	Can use manual wheelchair with special handgrips
	May be able to drive modified vehicle
	May need assistance with transfers
C8	Able to shift position in wheelchair
	Uses wheelchair independently
	Performs ADL independently if in wheelchair
	Can grasp and release with hands
	Can perform bladder and some bowel care independently
T1-T6	Completely independent in wheelchair with full control of upper body
	Independent with bladder care and some bowel care
T6-T12	Completely independent in wheelchair and most self-care and ADL
L1-L3	Completely independent in wheelchair, self-care, and ADL
L3-L4	May be able to walk with braces
	Fully independent in wheelchair
L4-S5	Walk with braces
	Independent

28. **Because spasticity is a common problem for spinal cord–injured patients, what information and interventions are important for the rehabilitation nurse to know?**

If spasticity is going to occur, it will occur anytime between 4 weeks and 8 months after injury. Spasticity typically increases in intensity until about 2 years after injury. At that time, intensity tends to decrease. Arm flexors and leg extensors most often are affected. Spasticity can present problems in positioning the patient and in the patient's ability to participate optimally in rehabilitation activities. Spasticity requires appropriate management to reduce contracture risks.

The nurse must explain to the patient and family that spasticity is only a reflex response so that they do not misinterpret it as the return of normal voluntary movement. Treatment may include physical therapy and medications. Nursing interventions for reducing spasticity may include stretching exercises, applying resting splints, performing daily skin assessment, and protecting bony prominences.

29. Do spinal cord–injured patients experience pain after the acute phase?

Yes, pain after the acute phase is categorized as neuropathic pain and has three types: nerve root, phantom, or abdominal or lower extremity. Pain most often occurs during the first year and can affect any level of injury. Nerve root pain often occurs around the area at the level of injury. Phantom pain occurs below the level of injury and is described as sharp and burning. The cause of phantom pain is thought to be due to inappropriate signals from damaged nerves or abnormal uncontrollable signals from repaired nerves. Abdominal pain may be attributed to uterus, bladder, colon, or stomach distention. Because of the unknown cause of neurogenic pain, treatment is nonspecific. Thorough assessment is necessary to rule out possible causes or complications. Medication such as anticonvulsants or psychotropics may be prescribed to mitigate symptoms. The nurse must educate the patient about neurogenic pain and that it does not represent an acute medical problem.

For the nurse to attempt comfort measures in response to the patient's complaints is important. The patient may perceive that a particular part of the body needs adjusting because that is where the patient perceives the pain is. The patient may require small adjustments in position frequently regardless of the probability that it will not relieve the pain or even that the identified area is the actual source of the pain. For the nurse to acknowledge the patient's pain, accept it as valid, and attempt to relieve it is important to prevent frustration, anger, depression, hopelessness, and grief in the patient.

30. What are the goals of bladder and bowel management programs for spinal cord–injured patients?

The goals of bladder and bowel management programs are to
• Be safe, appropriate, and cost-effective and to minimize lifestyle disruption.
• Provide the patient with some measure of control and independence.
• Reduce the risk of complications.

31. What should be included in a bowel and bladder program?

Bowel programs should include proper food and fluid intake, appropriate medication use, and the use of techniques that stimulate reflexes and enhance peristalsis. Programs should be tailored to each patient's needs and abilities. The level of injury determines the type of bowel dysfunction. For example, a cervical injury or high thoracic injury produces the inability to feel the urge to defecate but maintains intact reflex activity. With a sacral cord injury in conus medullaris or cauda equina, there is no reflex and anal tone is lost; therefore no retention of stool occurs. The nurse must include the patient in the planning of programs to decide on preferred frequency and timing of elimination, to ensure optimal compliance, and to reduce complications. Once the timing is decided, the patient drinks the preferred oral stimulant, such as hot coffee or warm prune juice, at that same time every day. The use of a daily stool softener and an every-other-day suppository is a typical approach. Another variation adds a laxative on the second day with the suppository every third day. Digital stimulation of the anal reflex also may be required. The desire, ultimately, is that only the oral stimulant and then digital stimulation is required for a regular bowel movement. (Please refer to Chapter 11 for bladder program information.)

32. What is important for the rehabilitation nurse to know regarding prevention and management of pressure ulcers?

The rehabilitation nurse must understand how significant the problem of pressure ulcers is for the spinal cord–injured person. Eighty-five percent of all spinal cord–injured individuals develops a pressure ulcer at some point in their lives, and 7% to 8% of those that do develop an ulcer die from complications. Therefore development of a good program for prevention and management of pressure ulcers for each patient is important. The following elements should be included:
- Identification of contributing factors and associated risks that lead to pressure ulcer formation
- Elimination of any modifiable contributing factors, such as pressure relief on ischial tuberosities at timed intervals
- Assessment of the patient's skin and general condition, nutritional status, and possible pressure ulcer characteristics
- Prompt treatment and early intervention for identified pressure ulcers
- Prevention or management of complications including infection

33. How can the nurse assist the ventilator dependent–spinal cord injured patient to attain some measure of independence?

The nurse can assist the patient to attain some measure of independence by
- Identifying a method of communication that allows the patient to express needs and requests
- Providing education to the patient and caregivers on the patient's abilities and limitations
- Ensuring that the home environment has been adapted to accommodate ventilator equipment
- Collaborating with other health care team members to ensure that the patient and caregivers are trained to provide appropriate respiratory and equipment care
- Developing strategies with the patient that allows the patient some degree of control in respiratory care and helps the patient develop skills necessary to direct care
- Ensuring that the patient has the least restrictive equipment and optimal adaptive devices to allow maximum mobility and independence

34. **Should the nurse do cognitive assessments on spinal cord–injured patients?**

To do a cognitive assessment or have one done on all patients with cervical level injuries and on any patient in whom the type of trauma causing the spinal cord injury could have caused an injury to the head as well is appropriate. A cognitive assessment will assist in ruling out traumatic brain injury. Because minor brain injury sequelae are mild, the condition might go unnoticed at first unless directly assessed. Problems resulting from brain injury could slow or interrupt the patient's rehabilitation.

35. **How does spinal cord injury affect sexuality?**

Spinal cord injury affects sexuality in several ways. Often the physical capacity to perform sexually is altered greatly because of changes in function and motor movement. Not only does this alteration affect the patient's ability to be intimate with a partner, but also it can create logistical difficulties such as the presence of catheters and the mechanics of undressing. Social perceptions also influence the patient's sexuality in that society tends to view individuals with disabilities as sexless and without desires. Spinal cord injured individuals often view themselves as no longer desirable or sexually attractive to others. Therefore to address sexuality and sexual function during rehabilitation is critical. If the patient has a sexual partner, the partner should be included in discussions where appropriate and with the patient's permission. If the nurse does not feel comfortable initiating these discussions, the nurse should make a referral to a sex therapist to ensure that this area is addressed. For the female patient, birth control must be addressed because of complications of delivery and caring for a baby. A male patient may be able to provide his partner with a child, but health care personnel must provide counseling, education, and opportunity to discuss all the strategies and the responsibilities.

The rehabilitation nurse can use the PLISSIT model to discuss sexual concerns at the nurse's level of comfort with the patient. PLISSIT is an acronym for permission, limited information, specific suggestions, and intensive therapy.

36. **What are the goals for the sexuality component of rehabilitation for the patient with a spinal cord injury?**

The goals for the sexuality component of rehabilitation are
- The patient should be comfortable with his or her sexuality as a spinal cord–injured individual and understand that a fulfilling sex life is an appropriate goal.
- The patient should have a thorough understanding of how he or she functions physically and understand what adaptive devices may be needed during a sexual encounter.
- The patient should have an understanding of his or her fertility and ability to father or bear a child and any risk involved.
- The rehabilitation nurse must address the patient's psychosocial needs through appropriate referrals and counseling.

37. What is a resource that can assist with information and referrals for spinal cord–injured patients?

An excellent resource is the National Spinal Cord Injury Association Resource Center that provides referrals and information on spinal cord injury and related topics to health care providers, patients, and families. The center can be reached at 1-800-962-9629.

38. When should the nurse address community reentry?

The nurse should address reentry early in rehabilitation to ensure that physical environment adaptation and modifications can be done before the patient returns home; transportation needs can be identified and appropriate equipment obtained or modified; work environment modification can be identified or retraining planned; and personal care attendants can be hired and trained. The reentry plan may require the rehabilitation nurse to visit the home or workplace to assess for modification and adaptation needs and identify resources for the family to obtain appropriate equipment and financial assistance. The plan may include patient home passes that progress in length so that the patient and family feel comfortable and capable of meeting the patient's needs in the community environment. Reentry might progress in a pattern such as 2 hours during the afternoon, with no meal involved, and then 4 hours with a meal and probably an elimination process. After each visit the family spends time with the rehabilitation team members to work out problems. When the family is ready, an overnight visit is planned. This visit can occur after the patient and at least one family member have passed a performance test on the necessary competencies to keep the patient safe. The visit will involve bowel care, bathing, dealing with sleep, comfort, bladder care, meals, transfers, and lots of patience. The nurse must learn from the patient and the family, separately, their perception of success of the visit. All have much to learn. One might suggest a pass that includes a recreational outing to deal with difficult access, crowds, the problem solving needed for emergencies, and things such as incontinence in a public place.

Many components are involved just to prepare the patient and family for homecoming. Getting ready to return to work is another layer on top of going home. Adjustment is not easy, and counseling for all is necessary.

39. What is the current focus in spinal cord injury research?

Current research is focused on gaining a better understanding of the molecular and cellular changes that occur with spinal cord injury and the resultant outcomes so that better treatments can be developed to prevent or reduce a negative outcome. Also, research is being conducted in the area of cell replacement as a method to cure or heal spinal cord injury. Studies are ongoing in the search for neuroprotective agents that can prevent secondary injury. Cellular biofeedback studies to retrain cells to function in the absence of cerebral stimulation has shown beginning success in clinical trials.

Key Points

- For the patient to achieve maximum independence, the rehabilitation process requires a multidisciplinary team and a holistic approach.
- Injury to the cervical spine produces spinal cord injury more often than injury to other areas of the spine and more often is associated with head injury.
- The rehabilitation nurse must understand and be able to explain the difference between neurological return and return of spinal reflexes.
- The degree of spinal injury cannot be determined until spinal shock resolves.
- Autonomic dysreflexia always should be considered a medical emergency. Patients must be taught early to recognize symptoms and seek immediate treatment.
- Bowel and bladder management programs for spinal cord–injured patients should begin as soon as the patient is stable and should be individualized to the needs of the patient.
- Development of a good program for pressure ulcer prevention and management is imperative, for 85% of all spinal cord-injured individuals develop a pressure ulcer at some point in their lives, with 7% to 8% of them dying from complications.

Internet Resources

National Spinal Cord Injury Association
http://www.spinalcord.org/

Christopher Reeve Paralysis Foundation
http://www.apacure.com/

American Spinal Injury Association
http://www.asia-spinalinjury.org

International Spinal Cord Regeneration Center
http://www.electriciti.com/spinal/

Bibliography

1. Barker E: Neurotrauma: spinal cord injury. In Barker E, editor: *Neuroscience nursing: a spectrum of care,* ed 2, St Louis, 2002, Mosby.
2. Hickey JV: Vertebral and spinal cord injuries. In Hickey JV, editor: *The clinical practice of neurological and neurosurgical nursing,* ed 5, Philadelphia, 2003, Lippincott.
3. Mahoney D: Nursing management of the patient with spinal cord injury. In Derstine JB, Hargrove SD, editors: *Comprehensive rehabilitation nursing,* Philadelphia, 2001, WB Saunders.
4. Somers MF: *Spinal cord injury: functional rehabilitation,* ed 2, Upper Saddle River, NJ, 2001, Prentice-Hall.

Chapter 26

Immune System Disorders Rehabilitation

Jeanne Flannery and Susan R. Bulecza

1. How are all of the immune disorders connected to rehabilitation?

The common element for immune disorders is the disruption of the ability of the body to regulate and protect itself, which results in chronic disease occurrence and a need for adaptation. Nurses are key in helping patients modify and adapt their lifestyles to the necessary changes brought about by the disease so as to achieve optimal function and quality of life. There are many immune system disorders. Some of the disorders more commonly seen by rehabilitation nurses are discussed.

2. What impact does fibromyalgia have on society?

Fibromyalgia affects 5 million to 6 million persons in the United States and is one of the most common rheumatic syndromes. From 3% to 10% of the general population is affected, and the percentage increases with age. Fibromyalgia is more common among women, ages 20 to 50 and is 7 times greater in women than men. The difference more than doubles as women enter the 60 to 70 age range. About 20% of all visits to a rheumatology practice are related to this syndrome. This disorder results in more unemployment and work absenteeism than rheumatoid arthritis and osteoarthritis combined. This one factor alone costs more than $9.2 billion a year. The need for rehabilitation measures to improve this syndrome or to assist the patients to adapt to it is profound.

3. What causes fibromyalgia?

Fibromyalgia has been described for more than 90 years, yet the diagnosis was not established until 1990. Fibromyalgia is believed to be autoimmune in origin, yet the trigger is unclear. The disease may be a complication of hypothyroidism, or in men, sleep apnea, and may occur after a febrile illness. Fibromyalgia is known to be associated in more than 50% of patients with sleep disturbances. Disruption of stage 4, non–rapid eye movement sleep may cause the disease. Additionally, muscle microtrauma and neurotransmitter imbalance are strongly implicated as causative. An association with prior sexual abuse or domestic violence also exists. Furthermore, the belief is that fibromyalgia may result from referred pain amplification from deep structures, a pain-spasm cycle from repetitive stress to muscle, or reaction to a latent virus or bacteria. Fibromyalgia is associated with rheumatoid arthritis, systemic lupus erythematosus, polymyositis (chronic acquired inflammatory disorder of skeletal muscle), and polymyalgia rheumatica.

4. How can the pathophysiology of fibromyalgia be explained?

Several hypotheses of the pathophysiology of fibromyalgia have been proposed because it is not understood completely. The following are findings in those with fibromyalgia:

- Disorder of muscle energy metabolism (lower adenosine triphosphate and adenosine diphosphate levels, higher adenosine monophosphate levels, and changes in the number of capillaries and fiber area), but it is unknown why
- Inflammatory or immunopathological disorder of the muscle
- Generalized pain perception disorder (pain intolerance) as a result of central nervous system (CNS) functional abnormalities (lower blood flow in the thalamus)
- Neuroendocrine disturbance (adrenal hyporesponsiveness)
- Depressive disorder
- Serotonin disorder (chronic stress response may produce lower peripheral and central levels)
- Sleep disturbance

One theoretical model identifies the following cascade of events:

1. Identification of preexisting factors (serotonin receptors, endorphins)
2. Identification of precipitating factors (muscle microtrauma, deconditioning, sleep disturbance)
3. Assessment of resulting manifestations (pain, fatigue, depression)
4. Change in the somatosensory cortex and the hypothalamus regulation leading to an imbalance in neurotransmitters in the dorsal horn of the spinal cord, specifically
   - Decrease in serotonin
   - Decrease in endorphins
   - Increase in substance P
5. Development of increased cutaneous nociception
6. Development of increased sympathetic outflow
7. Development of increased muscle nociception
8. Resulting skin hypersensitivity
9. Resulting muscle contraction and deconditioning

5. How is the patient diagnosed with fibromyalgia?

The National Institute of Arthritis and Musculoskeletal and Skin Diseases has recommended a set of laboratory screening tests, because diagnosis of this syndrome is a diagnosis of exclusion. Generally, the diseases that are being ruled out will create abnormalities in some of the following tests:

- Complete blood count
- Erythrocyte sedimentation rate
- Alanine aminotransferase

- Total protein
- Albumin
- Globulin
- Alkaline phosphatase
- Calcium
- Phosphorous
- Glucose
- Blood urea nitrogen
- Electrolytes
- Creatinine
- Thyroid-stimulating hormone
- Urinalysis

These tests, if positive, indicate the possibility of one of the disorders that may have some similar manifestations that need to be ruled out. Specific tests can follow to identify that indicated disease. Some of the diseases that must be considered for ruling out include

- Rheumatoid arthritis
- Systemic lupus erythematosus
- Depression
- Human immunodeficiency virus (HIV) disease (neuropathy)
- Hypothyroidism
- Sleep disorders
- Polymyalgia rheumatica
- Polymyositis
- Metabolic myopathies
- Neuropathies
- Lyme disease
- Dysthymia
- Personality disorders
- Psychotic illness
- Cancer
- Parkinsonism
- Chronic fatigue syndrome

Additonally, a complete history and physical examination must be done, along with the Mini-Mental State Examination to rule out psychiatric disorders. The diagnosis cannot be made based on the findings from this examination alone. If the patient has experienced widespread pain in four quadrants for at least 3 months and has pain on palpation (with 4 kg/cm^2 of palpation pressure) of at least 11 of 18 identified bilateral tender points, fibromyalgia is considered as the diagnosis. The pain is considered regional rather than following a dermatomal or peripheral nerve distribution. In normal persons these points may be tender, but in patients with fibromyalgia they are hypersensitive. The points include

- Occiput
- Low cervical
- Trapezius
- Supraspinatus

- Second rib at costochondral junction
- Lateral epicondyle
- Gluteal region
- Greater trochanter
- Medial fat pad of the knee

6. What is the clinical presentation of the patient with fibromyalgia?

This disorder has no visible signs. However, in addition to the painful tender points, the patient may complain of
- Postexercise malaise
- Multiple joint pain
- Chronic headaches
- Impaired memory (recent recall), concentration, and problem-solving abilities
- Restless, nonrestorative sleep
- Chronic aching, burning, or gnawing pain focusing particularly around the posterior neck, shoulders, low back, and hips
- Chronic fatigue
- Irritable bowel syndrome
- Restless legs
- Menstrual irregularities
- Abdominal pain
- Sensitivity to extreme temperatures
- Muscle spasms
- Subjective numbness (paresthesias)
- Muscle stiffness, particularly in the morning
- Mental stress
- Loss of functional abilities

Furthermore, for the patient to report having consulted several specialists before the current visit about the vague symptoms is not unusual.

7. What medications can be helpful to the patient with fibromyalgia?

All treatment modalities are intended to help the patient cope with the chronic problem, but all are only symptomatic. Tricyclic antidepressants such as amitriptyline (Elavil) remain a standard order to increase rapid eye movement sleep, but research has indicated that after 3 months the effect is equal to a placebo. Cyclobenzaprine (Flexeril) may be used to relieve muscle spasms and improve morning stiffness. Imipramine pamoate (Tofranil-PM), another tricyclic antidepressant, potentiates serotonin and norepinephrine by blocking reuptake to treat depression. Fluoxetine hydrochloride (Prozac), sertraline hydrochloride (Zoloft), or paroxetine (Paxil), also selective serotonin reuptake inhibitors, can be used for depression. Opioids and cortisone are ineffective and should never be prescribed. Nonsteroidal antiinflammatory drugs and aspirin are used for pain but are generally ineffective. Vitamin supplements may be prescribed for well-being. Zolpidem (Ambien) is used only with severe cases of sleep disturbance when all other modalities have not helped. Clonazepam (Klonopin) also may be used for restless legs syndrome. Both of these drugs are habit forming and so should be used sparingly.

8. **What other measures can the rehabilitation nurse implement to assist the patient with fibromyalgia?**

Full-spectrum light therapy may be helpful to assist with depression and lack of motivation, particularly if used on arising. Exercise, including stretching exercises, swimming, and walking, and physical therapy are beneficial in reducing fatigue, aiding in relaxation, and improving overall conditioning. Complementary therapies such as tai chi, yoga, massage therapy, biofeedback, deep breathing, meditation, therapeutic touch, and guided imagery may be used to manage pain and enhance relaxation. Other comfort measures include heat from moist packs, hot shower, or whirlpool and acupressure and acupuncture. Because fibromyalgia has a known stress-related component, the nurse needs to be certain the patient acquires excellent stress-management strategies. Adequate rest is strongly encouraged because sleep is so disturbed. A healthful diet is necessary to provide strength and improve a sense of well-being. The nurse should encourage the patient to join a fibromyalgia support group.

9. **What are the goals of therapy for fibromyalgia?**

Because there is no cure for fibromyalgia, the goals are to manage symptoms, such as the restoration of sleep and the management of pain.

10. **What is the focus of the rehabilitation nurse's patient/family education?**

Teaching should include information about the disease. Additionally, all the treatments should be discussed in relation to their efficacy and which symptoms they should help. The nurse should address factors that disturb sleep. The topic requiring the most attention is the importance of exercise in the control of symptoms and improvement of well-being. The nurse should present the benefits of adopting a lifetime commitment to exercise to the patient. This may be a difficult concept to promote because the patient is in pain, is fatigued, and is depressed.

The nurse must use excellent listening skills and encourage the patient to discuss her or his selection of coping strategies. The nurse should not make any judgment against these strategies unless one is not safe. Traditional treatments are not effective; therefore the nurse should encourage the patient to try any modality that might provide relief from the symptoms. The nurse must teach the methodology of stress management to help the patient prevent exacerbation of symptoms.

Because patients probably have experienced the perception that persons do not believe them or discount the myriad of complaints, they may require reinforcement that they are not "crazy" through discussion of the many avenues health care providers need to use to reach a diagnosis. Anxiety is a frequent problem that may develop once the patient learns that the disease is only manageable, not curable, and that many therapies have little or no effect and the pain may never be relieved. If the anxiety is not relieved, the nurse should recommend psychological counseling.

The nurse should explain the importance of a fibromyalgia support group and provide information to contact the local group. Additionally, the nurse may need to explain the importance of alternative pain control modalities because medications do little to relieve pain. If the patient does not seem to accept these, the nurse should refer the patient to a pain clinic where strategies to cope with the pain are taught.

The rehabilitation nurse always should instill hope in future progress toward the management of the disease. Providing the patient with the address and phone number of the Fibromyalgia Network may empower the patient: 5700 Stockdalae Highway, Suite 100, Bakersfield, CA 95309, (805) 631-1950.

11. What is rheumatoid arthritis (RA)?

The incidence of RA is 2 to 4 persons per 100,000 annually. The disease is 2 times more prevalent in women than men, with diagnosis most often occurring between the ages of 40 and 70. Rheumatoid arthritis is a debilitating systemic autoimmune disorder, but the exact cause has not been determined. Infections and environmental factors are thought to trigger or play a role in the development of RA. Also, genetic factors, such as having the haplotype designation of HLA-DR4, may cause one to be more susceptible (60%). Individuals with RA produce an autoantibody (rheumatoid factor) that forms immune complexes with immunoglobulin G (IgG). The lymphocytic phagocytes attack the immune complexes, which creates a series of events within the inflammatory process in the joint. These events release lysosomal enzymes that destroy the cartilage and subchondral bone.

Rheumatoid arthritis is a chronic multisystem arthritis characterized by inflammation of the peripheral body joints, with associated effects in other body systems such as eyes, skin, cardiac, and respiratory. Additionally, many persons with RA are cold intolerant.

12. How is RA diagnosed?

Diagnosis of RA is complicated. Laboratory tests are generally not conclusive for RA in early stages of the disease, and onset of symptoms can be insidious and nonspecific. The American College of Rheumatology has defined criteria for classifying RA, but they are used only as guidelines for diagnosing RA in individual patients. To be classified as having RA, the patient must meet four of these seven criteria: morning stiffness for longer than 1 hour; arthritis of three or more joints; arthritis of hand joints; symmetrical arthritis; rheumatoid nodules over extensor surfaces or bony prominences; serum rheumatoid factors present in abnormal amounts; and radiological changes.

13. **What are the more common symptoms of RA?**

The most common symptoms of RA, included within the criteria for diagnosis, are
- Morning joint stiffness lasting longer than 1 hour and present for at least 6 weeks
- Three or more joints with soft tissue swelling and fluid and present for at least 6 weeks
- Symmetrical joint involvement (e.g., both hips) and present for at least 6 weeks
- Chronic pain

14. **What is the long-term cause of the disease?**

Although the course of RA can be categorized as long remission, intermittent, or progressive, the majority of patients diagnosed with RA have progressive cases. Joint destruction and disability are the outcomes for those with progressive RA.

15. **What are the nursing goals for patients with RA?**

The goals include
- Preventing loss of function and deformity
- Reducing pain
- Optimizing compliance with therapy

16. **How should nursing interventions be prioritized?**

Pain assessment and management should be a primary intervention for the rehabilitation nurse. Unmanaged pain can reduce significantly the patient's ability and willingness to participate in physical and occupational therapies. Pain also can reduce the patient's ability to perform activities of daily living independently and the ability to work or care for family members.

Another critical intervention is patient education. Because few of the patients are hospitalized initially, opportunities for patient education are few; therefore the nurse should maximize every opportunity. Education must include verbal and written information and return demonstration for exercises.

An excellent information resource for the health care provider and patient is the National Arthritis Foundation. The foundation has local chapters that may provide services such as support groups for patients and families, adaptive equipment loan programs, and information hotlines.

Given the multitude of purported cures and treatments for arthritis in the media, the nurse should assess carefully the patient's use of inappropriate therapies and the use of culture-influenced and herbal therapies. The nurse must provide education on any therapy that poses harm to the patient.

17. **How can joint damage be minimized?**

Because the amount of joint deformity correlates with the degree to which synovitis is controlled, patient compliance with the medication regimen is important.

In collaboration with the physical and occupational therapists, the nurse should teach the patient how to protect the affected joints and emphasize that stressing affected joints can increase damage and pain. Patients may feel that reducing the use of, or not using, the joint is giving in to the disease; therefore, the nurse needs to explain to the patient that reducing use or using adaptive equipment reduces destruction of the joint over time and is an appropriate strategy.

18. What are the rehabilitation goals for patients with HIV?

Fortunately, medical management has advanced to the degree that HIV now is considered a chronic immunodeficiency disease. For most HIV-positive patients who adhere to and respond to treatment, disease progression is reduced, allowing them a relatively symptom-free life. However, for patients whose disease process progresses, rehabilitation goals should focus on the following:
• Reducing neurological deficits and complications
• Maintaining cognitive and physical function
• Promoting independence within disease limitations
• Maintaining optimal nutritional status and intake
• Promoting a positive self-concept
• Minimizing the negative psychosocial impact of HIV

19. When may the rehabilitation nurse encounter patients with HIV?

Rehabilitation nurses most often will encounter patients with HIV when they have become symptomatic as a result of the many opportunistic infections. Many of these infections result in debilitation and loss of function. Patients may have one or more of these at a specific time. Therefore the nurse needs to understand the pathophysiology, progression, and resultant limitations of each patient and tailor interventions accordingly.

20. What is a common element in symptomatic patients with HIV?

Fatigue is a major problem for most patients with HIV, regardless of the cause. Therefore to provide the patient with education on ways to conserve energy, reduce stress, and the importance of adequate rest and sleep is critical. Ongoing assessment of the patient is important to ensure that fatigue is not hindering the patient's ability to eat, prepare, or obtain food, or perform activities of daily living. The nurse must assess nutritional status and intake continually to ensure optimal caloric consumption and that nutritional needs are met.

21. Human immunodeficiency virus can produce dementia. How does this occur?

Human immunodeficiency virus is able to cross the blood-brain barrier and infect directly the white matter in the CNS. The virus uses the same "unlocking" system it uses to enter T4 lymphocytes in the body because these microglia, oligodendrocytes, and astrocytes have the same "locking" system, the expressed

CD4 antigen, to which HIV can bind. The high-speed transmission of impulses among the parts of the brain is disrupted and thinking is slowed. Each cell that HIV has entered dies and cannot be replaced. Ultimately dementia results. This dementia occurs in about 10% of patients and may be among the first symptoms. This problem can be compounded by the many opportunistic diseases that can produce encephalopathy.

22. How can the rehabilitation nurse recognize HIV dementia?

Patients first may notice that their handwriting is deteriorating. They have motor speed slowing and difficulty with cognitive tasks. They will complain of and exhibit memory loss. A wide variation in the degree of impairment may occur within a day, going to confusion from lucidity. During times when the patient is thinking close to normal, the patient is likely to express extreme concern about the ability to maintain independence. The patient may experience improvement with increased efficacy of the retroviral treatment.

23. What is Guillain-Barré syndrome (GBS)?

Guillain-Barré syndrome is a debilitating autoimmune disorder of the peripheral nervous system that includes the spinal and cranial nerves. About 2 persons per 100,000 acquire this disease annually worldwide. The cause is uncertain; however, two microorganisms clearly have been implicated in some forms of the disease: cytomegalovirus and *Campylobacter jejuni* (25% to 40%). The majority (60% to 70%) of patients have a history of an acute infection within 2 weeks before the onset of GBS, such as upper respiratory infection, gastrointestinal illness, or pneumonia. Some persons may have received a vaccination with live virus, had surgery, received a transplant, or have a disease such as systemic lupus erythematosus, HIV, or Hodgkin's disease.

24. What is the pathophysiology of GBS?

The autoimmune response triggered by virus or other unknown factors attacks the myelin sheath on the peripheral nerves, which causes inflammation and edema. What causes the immune system not to recognize the myelin as "self" is unknown. Perhaps the viral infection caused some modification in the Schwann cells, which produce myelin, so they appear foreign.

When the T cells (lymphocytic macrophages) are influenced by chemokines (immune messenger chemicals), they squeeze between the cells creating vascular walls and migrate toward the targeted tissue. They recruit other lymphocytes, and the army of cells wages war on the myelin as if it were an enemy invader.

Because of tissue destruction, the inflammatory process is initiated, with production of more chemokines, more macrophages, and more destruction of innocent tissue occurring, stripping the nerves of myelin between the nodes of Ranvier.

The demyelination causes loss of saltatory conduction (action potential hopping from node to node), which results in slowed, disturbed, and dyssynchronous conduction, or complete conduction block. Furthermore, the inflammatory process actually may damage the axon beneath the myelin sheath, leading to nerve degeneration. This damage reduces the ability of muscles to respond in numbers and in strength and leads to a poorer recovery. The demyelination is patchy, with the antimyelin antibody generally attacking the anterior and posterior spinal nerve roots and the segmental peripheral nerves or, in about 50% of cases, the brainstem cranial nerves.

25. What is the presentation of a patient with GBS?

Generally, GBS begins with motor weakness that usually begins in distal lower extremities symmetrically. The patient experiences loss of deep tendon reflexes, and bladder atony occurs. The motor weakness progresses in intensity and continues to ascend. Weakness to total paralysis of the trunk, neck, face, and lower cranial nerves develops. The patient may have myoclonic jerks. When the diaphragm and intercostal muscles become involved (about 30% of patients), respiratory failure results; and the patient becomes ventilator dependent.

The most common cranial nerves to become involved include the facial (cranial nerve VII), producing inability to smile, frown, whistle, or suck through a straw; the glossopharyngeal (cranial nerve IX); vagus (cranial nerve X); spinal accessory (cranial nerve XI); and hypoglossal (cranial nerve XII). Problems with cranial nerves IX and X lead to inability to talk and swallow normally. Autonomic dysfunction (about 50% of patients) results from cranial nerve X involvement and includes tachycardia, arrhythmias, low cardiac output, hypotension/hypertension, facial flushing, diaphoresis, pulmonary dysfunction, ileus, urinary retention, poor venous return, and loss of sphincter control. Some of these disturbances may be life threatening.

Sensory changes produce distal hyperesthesias (tingling, burning), numbness, and decreased vibratory sense and proprioception. These symptoms tend to be located in a stocking and glove distribution and they do not progress or last for a long time. Nonetheless, they are disturbing to the patient.

About 25% of patients have pain. One type of pain is an extension of the hyperesthesias. The patient may scream when touched. The sheet may be intolerable. Even a breeze can cause the patient exquisite pain.

Another type of pain is symmetrical muscle aching or cramping more often in the large muscles, such as gluteal muscles, quadriceps, and hamstrings, and then lower leg muscles, back, arms. The pain tends to be worse at night, preventing sleep. Research supports that this type of pain is not neuritic. The pain is thought to be caused by muscle changes related to the neuropathy. The pain can be intense and may require a morphine drip for relief.

26. **The hallmark for diagnosing GBS includes what select group of symptoms?**

The rehabilitation advanced practice nurse should recognize GBS through the following set of symptoms:
1. Rapidly evolving, progressive, usually ascending
   * Paresthesias
   * Muscle weakness
   * Paralysis
2. Diminished or absent deep tendon reflexes

27. **What diagnostic studies are used to support the clinical diagnosis of GBS?**

Supportive studies include the following:
* Lumbar puncture to obtain cerebrospinal fluid (CSF): CSF has elevated protein, with normal count of mononuclear cells
* Nerve conduction studies and electromyography: slowing or blocked conduction velocities in motor and sensory nerves

28. **How does the clinical course of GBS progess?**

The clinical course of GBS has three stages in the majority of cases:
1. First stage: from onset to nadir (the point of greatest severity)
   * About 50% reach it in 1 week
   * About 70% reach it in 2 weeks
   * About 80% reach it by 3 weeks
   * Some continue to progress in weakness for 1 to 2 months
   * A small number have a fulminating type and reach nadir in 24 to 48 hours
2. Second stage, plateau: begins at point of stability in clinical course, but no recovery occurs. The period may last from 2 days to 4 weeks
3. Third stage, recovery: begins at plateau and continues until no further recovery occurs. Because recovery depends on remyelination and in axonal injury, regeneration of nerves, the process may take up to 2 years.

29. **What should the rehabilitation nurse know about prognosis when trying to provide support for the patient who has just started to show signs of recovery?**

The process of recovery will occur in descending order, with the last symptoms clearing first, if they can clear, reaching the distal legs last. About 80% of patients will have progressed to ambulation within 6 months. About 50% of patients will have minor deficits, such as diminished or absent tendon reflexes. Ten percent to 20% of patients will be left with persistent disability. During the recovery period, severe pain may persist and must be treated for rehabilitation to be tolerated.

The most common deficits that remain include weakness of the anterior tibial muscles, intrinsic muscles of the hands and feet, quadriceps, and gluteal muscles.

About 5% of persons die from the autonomic nervous system disturbance leading to cardiac, respiratory, and other systems failure.

30. What are the indicators of a poor prognosis?

The indicators related to poor outcomes include
• Rapid progression from onset to quadriplegia
• Respiratory failure leading to ventilator dependence
• High level of severity at nadir
• No improvement in 3 weeks following plateau
• Known *C. jejuni* infection in the prodromal period

31. What is the medical management of GBS?

Generally, two treatments work by reregulating immune function:
1. Plasmapheresis is the replacement of 100% of the patient's plasma with albumin and saline (up to addition of 30% more) to eliminate the mediators of the autoimmune response. A plasma exchange occurs every day for 5 days as a course. Access is generally through a central line, and the treatment is tolerated well. Transient hypotension is likely.

   More courses of treatment may be required if the patient relapses. No limit exists to the number of courses, and in some facilities exchanges simply are ordered daily until the patient is better. Each exchange may take from 3 to 7 hours, depending on the patient's size, weight, full plasma volume, and hematocrit (the lower the hematocrit, the higher the plasma volume).
2. Intravenously administered immunoglobulin usually is given for 5 days on a regimen of 0.4 to 2 g/kg per day. Venous access is adequate. The patient may experience headaches but usually tolerates the treatment well. A second course may be required.

In either case the treatment should begin immediately on diagnosis. If making the diagnosis takes longer than 2 weeks, intravenously administered immunoglobulin will not work. Steroids have no benefit.

32. For the patient who still is recovering from major deficits or who has permanent deficits, what are the goals for the rehabilitation nursing management plan?

The goals for rehabilitation of the patient with GBS are
• Assist in resolution of problems caused by respiratory deficits.
• Facilitate adaptation to dysphagia to prevent aspiration.
• Alleviate pain.
• Prevent pressure sores.
• Prevent muscle injuries while in a weakened state.
• Prevent contractures.
• Plan an appropriate exercise program that does not cause fatigue or overuse.
• Provide psychological support.

33. What nursing interactions are needed to meet rehabilitation goals?

1. Respiratory management
   - Vital capacity should be monitored frequently.
   - Pulmonary rehabilitation may be needed.
   - In older adults who become ventilator dependent, weaning is a goal but may be difficult.
   - Postural drainage and chest percussion can assist in removing secretions when muscles are weak for coughing.
2. Communication, swallowing
   - Weak oropharyngeal and laryngeal muscles may persist and require alternative methods for communicating.
   - Swallow evaluations are required to prevent aspiration.
   - Teach strategies in eating and drinking that guard against aspiration.
3. Psychological support
   - Accept that the patient may fear relapse or death (even if recovery is excellent).
   - Allow the patient to discuss concerns:
     - Immobility
     - Lack of control
     - Difficulty in communication
   - Empower the patient with input into his or her plan and as much control as possible with the schedule.
   - Refer patient/family to counseling when beneficial.
4. Alleviation of pain
   - Acknowledge neuropathic pain.
   - Use hot and cold therapy.
   - Use a cradle to keep sheet off of skin if hypersensitive.
   - Reposition frequently.
   - Provide massage.
   - Use complementary modalities, such as therapeutic touch, hypnosis, Reiki, or transcutaneous electrical nerve stimulation if the patient is interested.
   - Provide pharmacological interventions and evaluate effectiveness; if inadequate, collaborate with physician in modifications.
5. Safety for joints, muscles, and skin
   - Provide appropriate supportive and comfort surfaces.
   - Develop collaboratively a positioning program with therapists.
   - Develop collaboratively a range of motion program (positions chosen by the patient that ease pain may lead to shortened muscles or contractures).
   - Provide massage.
   - Follow prescribed stretching program.
   - Evaluate skin frequently.
6. Exercise program
   - Monitor patient to prevent fatigue.
   - Teach the patient how to follow the designed exercise program and assist him or her.
   - Remind the patient that fatigue may be a major concern for a year and to stop exercise at the first point of fatigue, muscle ache, or pain exacerbation.

- Monitor the patient to prevent overuse (may precipitate loss of function and overwork damage).
- Provide scheduled rest periods.
- Monitor the patient for abnormal sensations after exercise, such as tingling and paresthesias, indicating overuse.
- Prepare for future exacerbation (years after apparent full recovery) if the patient is expected to function at maximum effort.
- Teach the patient to contact a health care provider if recurrence of symptoms occurs (2% to 5% experience onset and pattern similar to original episode).
- Evaluate the patient for cardiovascular fitness, for GBS may have deconditioned the patient to such a degree that he or she cannot tolerate the therapy that the muscles can and may require a much slower program.
7. Adaptive equipment
- Most patients will require a wheelchair for several months.
- Various levels of walkers will be needed as strength returns.
- The most common residual weakness is in the calf and anterior tibial muscles that control dorsiflexion; therefore an ankle-foot orthosis often is required.
- If lateral ankle weakness persists (peroneal muscle), an ankle stirrup splint may be needed.
- Air splints may be used for knee instability, for this usually resolves and long-term equipment is not required.
- The rehabilitation nurse should assess the home to determine whether any other assistive equipment may need to be installed for the patient's safety.

34. What is multiple sclerosis (MS)?

Multiple sclerosis is the most common demyelinating disease of the CNS and the most common neurological disorder of young adults. The average age at onset is 30 years, with a range from infant to 50 years, though infants and children are not commonly diagnosed. The amount of evidence in children is considered to be small because of underdiagnosis.

Multiple sclerosis is an autoimmune disorder that probably is triggered by more than one factor. Exposure to a virus, or perhaps bacteria, is thought to create the response, but no one organism is believed to be responsible. When this exposure occurs in persons of a specific genetic predisposition, such as the HLA-DR2 group, the disorder may occur. Little is understood about its cause.

35. Who are those most at risk for MS?

Two main factors establish the risk for MS and work in tandem. Heredity is one factor, and an environmental trigger in genetically susceptible persons is another.
- Heredity is important. Those greatest at risk are Caucasians of western European lineage. Multiple sclerosis is rare in some races, such as black Africans

and Eskimos. Furthermore, 70% to 75% of cases are women 10 to 50 years of age, with the average age of onset at 30 years. Persons with a sibling with MS make up 5% of the cases. Fifteen percent of cases is composed of those who have a close relative with MS.

- Environment is important. A geographic pattern to prevalence exists. Areas farthest from the equator to the north have prevalence of 200 per 100,000. Worldwide, the greatest prevalence is in North America (Pacific Northwest, Great Lakes region, and Canada), Europe (Scandinavia, northern Germany, and Great Britain), Australia, and New Zealand, in areas farthest from the equator. No population living between latitudes 40° north and 40° south is at high risk. In this area, nearest to the equator, prevalence is 1 per 100,000.

Studies of these populations have indicated that if persons migrate before they are 15, they acquire the lower risk related to their new location; however, after 15, they carry with them their original high degree of risk, indicating how important an effect a cold climate seems to have. Perhaps another inherent factor exists, such as exposure to organisms that are more common in colder climates, or may be it is a lack of something, such as sunlight, that would strengthen the immune system during childhood. Much is still to be learned.

36. Why is MS important to rehabilitation health care providers?

About 350,000 Americans have been affected with MS during their most productive years, which has had a tremendous impact on our society. In little more than 8 years after diagnosis, irreversible disability occurs. The disability progresses, perhaps for 30 years, reducing quality of life and ultimately preventing employment. Individuals may become socially isolated because of immobility or embarrassing incontinence.

Direct costs for one person over a lifetime have been estimated at $2.2 million. This figure does not address the indirect costs, such as loss of income, or the intangible costs, such as family's providing care. Rehabilitation strategies may be the positive link that helps to hold the family together.

37. What is the pathophysiology of MS?

The autoimmune attack on the myelin sheath is mediated by B cells and T cells. Although a humoral component has been known to exist for more than 3 decades, the antigen to which the antibodies are directed has not yet been identified.

Synthesis of immunoglobulin increases in the CSF, particularly oligoclonal IgG. This may indicate lack of normal regulation of B cells. The antibody myelin/oligodendrocyte glycoprotein, or anti-HOG, has been found in 76% of patients with the progressive types of MS. T cells and B cells are present in the inflammatory plaques that are lesions at points of myelin destruction containing products of inflammation.

T suppressor cells (CD8) are reduced, permitting T cell activation. Myelin is destroyed directly by the T cells, which mistake the myelin or the oligodendrocytes for foreign cells, ultimately damaging the underlying axons irreversibly. The process is cyclical for a period of time, with myelin loss, followed by replacement of the oligodendrocytes, which replace the myelin, and myelin loss, until the oligodendrocytes are destroyed and myelin is no longer replaced.

38. How is the diagnosis of MS made?

No single test will confirm the diagnosis of MS; therefore diagnosis depends on history and physical examination. The diagnosis is based on neurological deficits in a patient age 10 to 50 that involve two separate sites in the CNS (usually white matter) and that occur at different times, separated by at least a month.

39. What diagnostic tests support the clinical diagnosis of MS with paraclinical evidence?

The following diagnostic tests support the clinical diagnosis of MS:
1. Magnetic resonance imaging (MRI): If at least four lesions (plaques) are greater than 0.6 cm and are located in the lateral periventricular or posterior fossa areas with demyelination, and perhaps brain atrophy, the test is considered positive (about 5% of patients with MS do not show lesions).
2. Evoked potentials: 85% of patients with MS have slow or absent visual evoked responses (nerve conduction measurement).
   - 67% of patients show positive lesions on brainstem auditory evoked responses.
   - 27% of patients show sensory abnormalities on somatosensory evoked responses, even though a clinical examination is normal.
3. Lumbar puncture: Lumbar puncture is done only when other tests are inconclusive. Cerebrospinal fluid will show elevated IgG levels, the presence of oligoclonal bands in 90% to 97% of MS cases, and elevated mononuclear cell (pleocytosis).
4. Electroencephalogram: The results may reflect the effect of plaques.
5. Positron emission tomography scan: Scan shows changes in metabolism and the presence of plaques.

40. How is the clinical course of MS described?

The four different types of MS each have a different clinical course. These types are
1. Relapsing-remitting
   - Most common (85% of patients start with this)
   - Symptoms last in excess of 48 hours and remit gradually
   - Partial to complete remission between attacks
   - Continuous over a period of 10 years with little increase in deficits
   - Progresses to secondary-progressive type in 50% to 70% of patients

2. Primary-progressive
   - Onset at older age
   - Spinal cord disease
   - Progressive course
   - Persistent deficits
   - Possible periods of improvement
3. Secondary-progressive
   - Begins as relapsing-remitting
   - Develops after 2 or more decades
   - Symptoms worsen progressively
4. Progressive-relapsing
   - Progressive course from the beginning
   - Progressive between attacks
   - Occurs in 5% of patients

41. How are the symptoms of MS described?

Generally the symptoms of MS can be related directly to a specific type of dysfunction, with the initial signs and symptoms cutting across all areas of cranial nerve, motor, sensory, cerebellar, neurobehavioral, and sexual dysfunction, along with fatigue. Initial signs and symptoms include
- Sensory loss (37%): useless hand syndrome, numbness
- Acute optic neuritis (36%): transient visual loss or blurred vision with a Marcus Gunn pupil (dilates with light instead of constricts)
- Motor dysfunction: weakness (35%), hand clumsiness, spastic paraparesis
- Paresthesias (24%): burning, tingling
- Diplopia (15%)
- Ataxia (11%)
- Vertigo (6%)
- Lhermitte's sign: electrical shock–like sensation shooting down arms, back, or legs
- Acute transverse myelitis
- Intolerance to heat (Uhthoff's sign: motor function declines after fever, hot shower or bath, exercise, or exposure to hot weather)
- Paroxysmal facial pain
- Spinal cord compression symptoms
- Sphincter disturbance

These symptoms may disappear in a few days or weeks but will recur, or other symptoms will appear. About half of patients will remain with no significant disability for 10 years or more.

42. What are the treatment goals for MS?

Multiple sclerosis has no prevention, no cure, and no way to prevent its ultimate outcome. However, the goals are to
- Enhance recovery from acute exacerbation
- Slow the natural course of the disease
- Manage the symptoms

43. Which pharmacological therapies are approved for modifying the disease course?

Currently the drugs used to modify the disease process are the "ABCs":
1. Avonex (interferon beta-1a)
   - Reduces rate of clinical relapses in relapsing-remitting.
   - Reduces development of new plaques on MRI.
2. Betaseron (interferon beta-1b)
   - Reduces rate of clinical relapses in relapsing-remitting and secondary-progressive.
   - Reduces development of new plaques on MRI.
   - Delays disability.
3. Copaxone (glatiramer acetate)
   - Reduces rate of clinical relapses in relapsing-remitting.
   - Reduces development of new plaques on MRI.

44. How are acute relapses treated?

An acute relapse normally will improve within 4 to 12 weeks. The patient is given methylprednisolone (Solu-Medrol) intravenously for 3 to 5 days, followed by corticosteroids in a tapering regimen for 3 days to reduce the symptoms and hasten improvement. Steroids have no effect on the course of the disease, and no evidence indicates that steroids alter disability.

45. What type of cognitive deficits do patients with MS experience?

About 65% of patients with MS have cognitive impairments, and the range of severity is from mild to global and severe. Brain atrophy is the most likely cause of cognitive impairments.
Generally, the impairments associated include
1. Memory (31%)
   - Verbal
   - Visual
   - Explicit (learning)
   - Forgetfulness
   - Delayed recall of recent events and conversation
2. Information processing/attention (25%)
   - Distractibility, slowed mental process
   - Unable to multitask
3. Executive function (19%)
   - Abstract/conceptual reasoning, decision making
   - Planning, correcting errors
   - Overcoming habitual responses
   - Problem solving, organizing
   - Difficulty with novel situations
4. Visuospatial, constructional, visual perceptual (16%)
   - Abnormal depth perception
   - Collisions and near misses while driving

- Impaired relation of self-position to environment
- Bumps into things
- Generally inattentive to this deficit
5. Language (9%): related to impairments in processing, attention and concentration, and memory

46. What are the areas of focus in rehabilitation for the patient with MS?

The rehabilitation nurse may see newly diagnosed patients, as well as patients experiencing relapses or progressive symptoms, receiving a wide variety of therapies. Each patient is assessed carefully, and an individualized plan is created collaboratively with the interdisciplinary rehabilitation team. Regardless of presenting symptoms, health teaching will always be first and foremost. Within the realm of teaching, the nurse will learn what alternative modalities the patient is using currently (30% use complementary medicines) so as to assess safety and effectiveness. The plan may include the following approaches for these problems:

1. Depression (25% to 55%)
   - Counseling
   - Referral to psychotherapy
   - Stress management
   - Monitoring for suicidal tendencies
   - Antidepressants
   - Biofeedback
   - Relaxation
   - Recreational therapy
2. Weakness
   - Strengthening exercises
   - Protective splints
3. Spasticity
   - Stretching, positioning
   - Cold baths
   - Antispasmodic medications
4. Pain
   - Increased activity
   - Improved posture
   - Muscle relaxation
   - Reduced pain behavior
   - Transcutaneous electrical nerve stimulation
   - Analgesics
5. Fatigue
   - Teaching of energy conservation
   - Increased rest periods
   - Stress management
   - Improved endurance
6. Memory/cognitive impairment (65%)
   - Teaching of compensatory strategies
   - Modification of home environment

7. Impaired balance/tremor/incoordination
   - Balance exercises
   - Gait training
   - Walking aids
   - Compensatory strategies
   - Splints
8. Impaired sensation: visual compensatory strategies
9. Constipation
   - Bowel program
   - High-fiber diet
   - Increase in activity
   - Sitting balance exercises
   - Transfer techniques
   - Hand function exercises
10. Reduced independence in activities of daily living
    - Transfers
    - Mobility
    - Hand function
    - Bed mobility
    - Hygiene skills
    - Trunk stability
    - Balance
    - Home equipment
11. Bladder dysfunction
    - Bladder program
    - Fluid regimen
    - Sitting balance
    - Transfers
    - Hand function
    - Anticholinergics
    - Self-catheterizations
12. Sexual dysfunction
    - Decrease in spasticity
    - Mobility
    - Balance
    - Hand function
    - Contractures release/prevention
    - Prosthesis
    - Education
    - Counseling
13. Dysarthria/impaired communication
    - Decrease in spasticity
    - Oral and breathing exercises
    - Communication boards
14. Dysphagia
    - Evaluation of nutrition
    - Diet
    - Swallowing exercises

- Education, monitoring, and training
- Tube feeding
15. Complications prevention: decubiti, contractures
  - Protective equipment
  - Mobility
  - Positioning
  - Evaluation
  - Exercises and increased activity
  - Skin assessment
  - Range of motion
  - Nutrition
  - Stretching

Key Points

- Fibromyalgia affects 5 million to 6 million persons in the United States, resulting in more unemployment and work absenteeism than rheumatoid arthritis and osteoarthritis combined. The need for rehabilitation measures to improve this syndrome or to assist the patients to adapt to it is profound.
- The nursing goals for patients with rheumatoid arthritis are prevention of functional loss and deformity, pain reduction, and optimal therapy compliance.
- Early recognition of HIV dementia is key to reduce the patient's risk for injury.
- Patients with Guillain-Barré syndrome must understand that the recovery process will occur in descending order, with the last symptoms clearing first.
- For patients with multiple sclerosis, health teaching is first and foremost, regardless of type and presenting symptoms. Development of an individualized plan collaboratively with an interdisciplinary team is key.

Internet Resources

National Fibromyalgia Association
http://www.fmaware.org/patient/coping/managingfm.htm

Arthritis Foundation
http://www.arthritis.org/default.asp

Center for HIV Information
http://hivinsite.ucsf.edu/

National Multiple Sclerosis Society
http://www.nmss.org/

Multiple Sclerosis Foundation
http://www.msfacts.org/

Bibliography

1. Aminoff MJ: Nervous system. In Tierney LM, McPhee SJ, Papadakis MA, editors: *Current medical diagnosis and treatment: adult ambulatory and inpatient management*, ed 41, New York, 2002, Lange/McGraw-Hill.

2. Barker E: The neurologic manifestations of HIV. In Barker E, editor: *Neuroscience nursing: a spectrum of care*, ed 2, St Louis, 2002, Mosby.

3. Brassell MP: Nursing management of the patient with rheumatoid arthritis. In Derstine JB: Hargrove SD, editors: *Comprehensive rehabilitation nursing*, Philadelphia, 2001, WB Saunders.

4. Bush M: Nursing management: arthritis and other rheumatic disorders. In Lewis SM, Heitkemper MM, Dirksen SR, editors: *Medical-surgical nursing: assessment and management of clinical problems*, ed 6, St Louis, 2000, Mosby.

5. Cooke JF, Orb A: The recovery phase in Guillain-Barré syndrome: moving from dependency to independence, *Rehabil Nurs* 28(4):105-108, 2003.

6. Del Bene M, Polak M: Neuromuscular and autoimmune disorders. In Barker E, editor: *Neuroscience nursing: a spectrum of care*, ed 2, St Louis, 2002, Mosby.

7. Frankel D: Multiple sclerosis. In Umphred DA, editor: *Neurological rehabilitation*, ed 4, St Louis, 2001, Mosby.

8. Freeman E, Winland-Brown JE: Hematologic and immune problems. In Dunphy LM, Winland-Brown JE, editors: *Primary care: the art and science of advanced practice nursing*, Philadelphia, 2001, FA Davis.

9. Hallum A: Neuromuscular diseases. In Umphred DA, editor: *Neurological rehabilitation*, ed 4, St Louis, 2001, Mosby.

10. Halper J, Kennedy P, Miller CM, and others: Rethinking cognitive function in multiple sclerosis: a nursing perspective, *J Neurosci Nurs* 35(2):70-81, 2003.

11. Hellmann DB, Stone JH: Arthritis and musculoskeletal disorders. In Tierney LM, McPhee SJ, Papadakis MA, editors: *Current medical diagnosis & treatment: adult ambulatory and inpatient management*, New York, 2002, Lange/McGraw-Hill.

12. Hickey JV: Peripheral neuropathies. In Hickey JV, editor: *The clinical practice of neurological and neurosurgical nursing*, ed 5, Philadelphia, 2003, Lippincott Williams & Wilkins.

13. Konkle-Parker DJ: The regulatory and immune systems and the patient with HIV. In Hoeman SP, editor: *Rehabilitation nursing: process, application, & outcomes*, ed 3, St Louis, 2002, Mosby.

14. Marek J: Management of persons with inflammatory and degenerative disorders of the musculoskeletal system. In Phipps WJ, Sands JK, Marek JF, editors: *Medical-surgical nursing: concepts and clinical practice*, ed 6, St Louis, 1999, Mosby.

15. Neal LJ: Neuromuscular disorders. In Hoeman SP, editor: *Rehabilitation nursing: process, application, & outcomes*, ed 3, St Louis, 2002, Mosby.

16. Oelke KR: Rheumatologic and autoimmune disorders. In Tierney LM, Saint S, Whooley MA, editors: *Essentials of diagnosis & treatment*, ed 2, New York, 2002, Lange/McGraw-Hill.

17. Terebelo S: Rheumatoid arthritis, *Clin Rev* 13(2):58-63, 2003.

Chapter 27

Degenerative Disorders Rehabilitation

Jeanne Flannery and Susan R. Bulecza

1. **What is the common link among degenerative, neuromuscular, and debilitating disorders that is important to the rehabilitation nurse?**

   Degenerative, neuromuscular, and debilitating disorders, which include things such as chronic pain syndromes, dementias, and progressive and debilitating disorders, are not curable and create a personal and societal burden. Dealing with multiple losses is overwhelming. The common link is the goals of rehabilitation for all of them, which include
   - Management of symptoms
   - Education of the patient and family
   - Maintenance of function
   - Slowing of progression or prevention of complications
   - Assisting the patient and family to cope
   - Support to help the patient accept the effects of the disorder realistically
   - Enhancing the patient's quality of life
   - Linking to resources

ALZHEIMER'S DISEASE

2. **What is the status of dementia in the United States today?**

   Dementia currently is viewed as approaching epidemic proportions in prevalence. About 78 million baby boomers are approaching old age, and Americans are living longer, with current research indicating the possibility of reaching age 129. Because Alzheimer's disease is responsible for more than 50% of all the dementias and its incidence increases with old age, Americans are facing a national tragedy. Because dementia is progressive and causes language deficits, personality disintegration, impaired visuospatial skills, psychiatric disturbances, and cognitive deficits ranging from memory impairment to confusion, disorientation, and stupor, the picture is that of the mind's dying; then after many years, the body follows. The health care system, particularly the long-term care facilities, truly is facing a crisis.

3. **What is Alzheimer's disease?**

   Alzheimer's disease is a syndrome, classified as a cortical dementia, and is the primary cause of dementias in the United States. The disease is compared to other classifications of dementia, such as the subcortical types, including Parkinson's disease and Huntington's disease, which are extrapyramidal syndromes, and to the dementias with cortical and subcortical dysfunction, such as human immunodeficiency virus dementia, which is an infection dementia. Alzheimer's disease is characterized by a slow loss of intellect that the patient is not aware of until the patient cannot accomplish routine tasks or impaired judgment creates problems. Prevalence in the United States is about 5 million and will increase to 15 million by 2050, unless prevention or a cure has been developed by then.

Dementia of the Alzheimer's disease type is manifested by slowly progressive deterioration in behavior and intellect, resulting in alterations in memory, intellect, judgment, personality, social behavior, and ability to perform normal tasks of daily living.

4. What is the incidence and epidemiology of Alzheimer's disease?

Although Alzheimer's disease can occur at any age, most all known cases are in persons more than 40 years old when first seen, and the greatest number are usually 65 or older. Projections for development of the disease vary. One approach is that 5% to 6% of the population will acquire Alzheimer's disease and that 11% are affected in the over-85 group.

Others suggest that the percentage is much higher, such as 15% in the over-65 group, and 47% in the over-85 group. Some say one in three over the age of 90 are at risk for Alzheimer's disease.

Those who have Down syndrome (trisomy of chromosone 21) have a high risk of developing Alzheimer's disease by the fourth decade. Mothers who delivered a Down syndrome child at age 35 or younger have a fivefold increased risk for Alzheimer's disease.

Additional risks include brain trauma (risk increased 80%), low intellectual capacity, low level of education with a lifelong job that requires little mental stimulation, small head (sixteenfold increased risk over large head size), and exposure to electromagnetic fields, such as a sewing machine (seamstresses have a higher risk).

5. What is the cause of Alzheimer's disease?

The cause of Alzheimer's disease is unknown. Several facts are known, and several theories may relate to the cause:
- Aluminum-toxicity theory: The aluminum concentration in the brain increases with age; its effects are unknown.
- Inflammatory process: Inflammation may cause the formation of amyloid precursor protein and buildup of plaque; a reactant has been found in cerebrospinal fluid; ultimate development of the radicals may cause cell destruction.

- Slow-virus theory: A virus with an incubation period of 2 to 30 years may have entered through a disruption of the blood-brain barrier, but no virus has been isolated.
- Genetic predisposition: 10% to 30% of patients with Alzheimer's disease have an inherited form. Persons with a first-degree relative have a fourfold risk of Alzheimer's disease. If a person inherits the gene from one parent, probability for Alzheimer's disease is a threefold increase, but if inherited from both parents, the risk is increased fivefold. Chromosome 19 may have four variants or alleles on one of its genes that controls apolipoprotein E, a plasma protein involved in transporting cholesterol. Most persons have the apoprotein E2 allele. If a person has apoprotein E4 proteins, the proteins cannot bind and protect microtubules, so they are degraded into neurofibrillary tangles. Persons with the apoprotein E4 allele develop Alzheimer's disease at least 10 years sooner than those with other alleles.

6. What is the pathophysiology of Alzheimer's disease?

The pathophysiology is determined usually on autopsy. No way exists to validate the presence of the disease through any current tests. Two major pathophysiological changes occur: senile neuritic plaques and neurofibrillary tangles. Each of these changes occurs in normal, aging brains, but the changes exist in greater numbers in patients with Alzheimer's disease.

Senile plaques are microscopic patches of tissue degeneration debris composed of granular deposits and remains of neuronal processes. The central core is amyloid β-peptide, which is a fragment of amyloid precursor protein. The protein is associated with the cytoskeleton of neuronal fibers and normally is degraded into extracellular fluid. In Alzheimer's disease the degrading process is modified, and intact amyloid β-peptide molecules are released, and they accumulate throughout the neocortex and in the hippocampus and amygdala. This process compromises the hippocampus function of information processing, creation of new memories, and retrieval of old memories.

The neurofibrillary tangles, which consist of fibrous proteins that are wound around each other, are found in the cytoplasm of abnormal neurons and persist after the neuron has died and disappeared. The tangles may be caused by the cdk5 enzyme. They are found in the same locations as senile plaques and interfere with cortical input and output by interrupting transmission of neurochemicals, so that the hippocampus essentially is "disconnected" and becomes functionless.

Neurochemically, a reduction occurs in choline acetyltransferase, which is necessary to synthesize acetylcholine, the excitatory neurotransmitter required for memory. This reduction correlates with the number of neuritic plaques and the degree of dementia.

On autopsy one finds gross atrophy of the cortex, especially in the parietal and temporal lobes and the anterior frontal region. The normal brain weighs about 1380 g, and an Alzheimer's disease brain may weigh less than 1000 g.

7. Describe the signs and symptoms of Alzheimer's disease.

Alzheimer's disease progresses through three stages that commonly occur over 7 years but may extend to 25 years. Although each patient progresses differently, the expected manifestations for each stage are as follows:

1. Stage I (1 to 3 years): Early stage
   - Is forgetful (attempts to cover through use of lists)
   - May lose job for poor performance
   - Has vague uncertainty in initiating actions
   - Has difficulty acquiring new information
   - Has poor word list generation
   - Has mild anemia
   - Is apathetic, irritable, depressed
2. Stage II (2 to 10 years): Confusional stage
   - Shows profound memory loss
   - Neglects personal hygiene
   - Demonstrates signs of global aphasia
   - Demonstrates apraxia (cannot perform previously learned tasks)
   - Demonstrates agnosia (cannot interpret sensory stimuli)
   - Has severe impairment in judgment
   - Lacks insight and abstract thinking
   - Loses social graces, which causes embarrassment to family, resulting in isolation
   - Has voracious appetite
   - Wanders from home, particularly at night
   - Sleep-wake cycle is reversed, and patient becomes active at night
   - Has sundown syndrome (darkness intensifies confusion)
   - Is paranoid about all lost belongings, believing someone took them
   - Has bouts of irritability and increased physical activity; repetitive behavior; otherwise, is apathetic
   - Is anxious and evasive
   - Overresponds to stimuli and becomes agitated, combative, and verbally abusive
   - Gets lost in familiar surroundings, including home
   - Slowing of electroencephalogram
   - Cannot be left alone
3. Stage III (may be short: 1 to 2 years, but can last 10 years): Late stage
   - Confined to bed, immobile
   - Incontinent of urine and feces
   - Totally dependent for all care
   - Becomes emaciated from lack of eating
   - Has flexed posture and limb rigidity and is unable to stand
   - Loses global cognitive functions
   - Is unable to communicate
   - Loses emotional responses
   - Does not recognize family
   - Electroencephalogram is diffusely slow
   - Is prone to seizures

- Computed tomography shows ventricular dilation (hydrocephalus) and sulcal enlargement
- Requires institutional care
- Death usually results from aspiration, pneumonia, or infection

8. What treatment is available for patients with Alzheimer's disease?

The following drugs have been approved for treatment of Alzheimer's disease:
- Tacrine (Cognex) 10 to 40 mg/day: inhibits cholinesterase to improve moderate dementia
- Donepezil (Aricept) 5 to 10 mg/day: inhibits cholinesterase to improve mild to moderate dementia
- Rivastigmine (Exelon) 1.5 to 12 mg/day: inhibits cholinesterase to improve mild to moderate dementia
- Galantamine (Reminyl) 16 to 24 mg/day: inhibits cholinesterase to improve mild to moderate dementia
- Risperidone (Risperdal) 0.5 to 2 mg/day: manages dementia-related psychosis
- Quetiapine (Seroquel) 5 to 10 mg/day: manages dementia-related psychosis
- Citalopram (Celexa) 20 to 40 mg/day: inhibits serotonin reuptake to improve depression

9. How is rehabilitation for the patient with Alzheimer's disease focused?

The rehabilitation nurse is a part of a collaborative interdisciplinary team to assist the patient and family cope with difficult symptoms that progressively worsen. The burden of caring for the patient with Alzheimer's disease is great; and education, support, and provision of resources are vital to maintain the patient in the home for as long as possible. The rehabilitation nurse assists the patient and family in the following ways:
- Teach the family about the disease process so they know what to expect.
- Refer the family to social services, legal, and financial counselors to prepare for determination of legal competence, writing of the will, power of attorney, medical directives, health care surrogacy, in-home care, and ultimate institutionalization.
- Assess the stage of Alzheimer's disease and provide assistance with the current manifestations.
- Determine safety in the home and help with modifications.
- Determine degree of independence the patient is safe to have (being alone, making decisions, driving).
- Recommend a structured plan of the day each day, with a routine that is followed; counsel to avoid new experiences and trips.
- Provide resources for the family as the need arises, such as respite care and in-home care.
- Teach family the degree of monitoring required to keep the patient safe: the patient will drink or eat anything perceived to be edible such as fruit-shaped soap or cleaning fluids. The patient will wander away and be lost or walk into moving traffic or fall into a pond. The patient will require the kind of attention given to a toddler.

- Teach the family to speak in short, direct, one-step sentences, such as "eat your food."
- Show how to involve the patient in activities to provide exercise such as raking, sweeping, and bouncing a ball.
- Remind the family to show caring; the tendency may be only to scold for the many accidents and crises created.
- Explain that the patient will sleep less and will be up during the night. The patient should have as active a day as possible with a brisk walk in early evening. Siderails and a bed alarm should be used. Locks should be placed at tops of doors to prevent the patient's exit from the home.
- Give small frequent feedings with only one or two foods. Stay with the patient and give brief directions, such as "chew your food." Use plastic bowls and cups.
- Prepare to spend a lengthy time each day with hygiene. Do not argue, just direct.
- Use clothing for the patient that is easy to slip on.
- Remind the family that toileting problems will emerge from misperceptions long before incontinence is present. A picture of a toilet can be placed on the bathroom door.
- Limit fluids after the evening meal.
- Take the patient to the bathroom every 2 to 3 hours.
- Give medications in a crushed or liquid form.
- Tell the family to report to the nurse when the patient is becoming unmanageable because of psychiatric behaviors. Medications may need adjusting.
- Encourage the family to join a support group. Provide contact information. Even some telephone support groups are available because families whose members have Alzheimer's disease often are confined to the home.
- Teach the family about the cognitive decline and how to use the short-term memory deficit to manage behavioral exacerbations. To reason or argue with the patient is fruitless; one must just redirect the patient to a different task or move to a different room. This ends the outbursts.
- Use music for calming.
- When it seems that getting the patient to take medication is impossible, sometimes just having another caregiver do it will work.
- Teach the family about facilities that are designed especially for patients with dementia. These facilities usually keep a waiting list, so the family should investigate well in advance of the time the facilities will be needed.
- Explain what hospice care is and provide contact information so that as the patient reaches the last stage the family can receive assistance and support.

PARKINSON'S DISEASE

10. What is Parkinson's disease?

Parkinson's disease is a chronic, progressive, degenerative central nervous system disorder of the substantia nigra in the basal ganglia.

11. What population is most affected by Parkinson's disease?

About 2% of persons over the age of 65 and more than 1 million persons in the United States have Parkinson's disease. Incidence increases with age, and one in three persons over age 85 has the disease. Although the mean age of onset is 58 to 62, the incidence is growing among persons in their twenties. Men have a slightly higher risk (3:2), and all races are affected.

12. What is the cause of Parkinson's disease?

The cause of primary Parkinson's disease is generally unknown (idiopathic). Secondary types have a known precipitating factor, such as mutations in the α-synuclein gene in the familial Parkinson's disease. From 15% to 20% of persons with Parkinson's disease have a relative with it. Drugs such as neuroleptics (e.g., Thorazine), antiemetics (e.g., Compazine), antihypertensives (e.g., Aldomet), and an illicit drug, MPTP (1-methyl-4-phenyl-1,2,3,6-tetrahydropyridine), can produce Parkinson's disease. The Parkinson's disease resulting from prescribed drugs is generally reversible with cessation of the drug; however, MPTP causes permanent cell destruction. Parkinson's disease also can result from cyanide, manganese, or carbon monoxide poisoning, encephalitis, and head trauma. Exposure to pesticides may be related to the dramatic increase in idiopathic Parkinson's disease that is expected to continue for decades. Evidence indicates that environment has some role as a trigger.

13. How is the pathophysiology of Parkinson's disease explained?

Genetic, environmental, and dietary factors or combinations of factors lead to oxidative stress in the substantia nigra compacta (nuclei in the midbrain) and production of oxygen free radical by-products of hydrogen peroxide, superoxide ions, and hydroxyl radicals. These chemicals interact with the cell membrane lipids of the neurons, leading to lipid peroxidation, which disrupts the membrane and causes dopamine-producing neuronal death in the substantia nigra and acetylcholine-producing neuronal death in the pedunculopontine nuclei, also in the midbrain.

The cells in the substantia nigra produce the neurotransmitter dopamine, which normally inhibits the motor pathway through the thalamus to contribute to normal voluntary muscle innervation. Dopamine also inhibits the motor pathway through the pedunculopontine nucleus to contribute to normal postural and girdle muscle function.

In Parkinson's disease about 80% of the dopamine-producing cells in the substantia nigra have degenerated before symptoms occur. An imbalance occurs between dopamine and acetylcholine in the extrapyramidal systems, which leads through a feedback pathway of disinhibition of basal ganglia control, resulting in less facilitation of voluntary muscles and too much facilitation of postural muscles. Resulting problems are hypokinesia (decreased active movement and lack of automatic movements, such as facial expression and arm swing during walking), rigidity, resting tremor, freezing during movement, and visuoperceptive impairments that block movement.

Lewy bodies, which are pigmented eosinophilic intraneural inclusion granules, are present in the remaining cells in the substantia nigra. Lewy bodies are related directly to the dementia aspect of Parkinson's disease; the loss of acetylcholine-producing neurons in the pedunculopontine nuclei also is thought to be directly related. Neurofibrillary tangles and amyloid plaques found in the brains of patients with Parkinson's disease on autopsy are characteristic of Alzheimer's disease. Dementia occurs in 30% to 50% of patients with Parkinson's disease.

14. How is Parkinson's disease diagnosed?

Diagnosis is clinically based and depends on the presence of one to four of the priority features on one side of the body, with the most common feature being tremor. The other features are rigidity, hypokinesia (bradykinesia/akinesia), and postural instability (flexed posture, shuffling gait, retropulsion, and festination).

15. How is the course of Parkinson's disease described?

The progressive disease advances through five stages as presented in Box 27-1.

Box 27-1.   The five stages of Parkinson's disease

- Stage I: unilateral symptoms
- Stage II: bilateral symptoms with posture and gait changes, but preservation of postural reflexes
- Stage III: moderate impairment, including postural instability (loss of postural reflexes); preserved ability to ambulate independently, but with hypokinesia
- Stage IV: considerable assistance required; severe disease, with added rigidity, festination, and retropulsion
- Stage V: confinement to wheelchair or bed; end-stage disease requiring total care

---

16. Describe the collective signs and symptoms of Parkinson's disease.

Table 27-1 presents the major manifestations of Parkinson's disease, and Table 27-2 presents the secondary manifestations. Box 27-2 presents other manifestations, most associated with autonomic dysfunction.

17. What are the treatment goals of Parkinson's disease?

Treatment goals of Parkinson's disease include treating symptoms and preventing complications, with the reminder that Parkinson's disease is progressive:
- Increasing movement, as well as range of motion
- Maintaining or increasing chest expansion
- Improving equilibrium
- Maintaining or restoring functional abilities

Table 27-1. Major manifestations of Parkinson's disease

Signs/dysfunctions	Manifestations
Tremor (75% early stage)	Pill-rolling tremor of fingers, exaggerated at rest and ceasing with purposeful movement
	Tremor in jaw, chin, tongue, hands, legs
	Resolution of tremor during sleep
Rigidity: increase in muscle tone; "lead pipe" resistance to passive motion	Cogwheel-ratchet–like movement, sudden jerks when passive extension or flexion is attempted
	Muscle stiffness, aching
Bradykinesia/akinesia (hypokinesia): poverty of movement precipitated by lack of coordination of antagonistic muscle groups	Inability to initiate movement
	Inability to change movement
	Slow movement
	"Freezing" during movement: motor block; difficulty turning in bed
	Lack of arm swing with walking
Postural instability: deficits in proprioception and kinesthetic processing; occurs in later stages	Flexed posture and shuffling gait; broad stance on turns
	Loss of balance; frequent falls (cannot catch self with hands)
	Retropulsion: movement backward is not checked, but accelerates until patient collides with a stationary object or falls
	Festination: upper body moves faster than lower, causing the patient to chase center of gravity at a trot with short steps, gradually gaining momentum, but patient remains off balance

Table 27-2. Secondary manifestations of Parkinson's disease

Signs/dysfunctions	Manifestations
Fine motor deficits	Micrographia; illegible handwriting
	Clumsiness; difficulty with activities of daily living
Impaired verbal communication	Voice tremors
	Monotone
	Slow speech
	Whisperlike muffled voice
	Slurring
	Dysarthria
Masked facies (hypomimia)	Expressionless
Infrequent blinking	Blank stare straight ahead

Continued

Table 27-2. Secondary manifestations of Parkinson's disease *continued*

Weakness and fatigue	Low initiation
	Impairment of rapidly alternating movements (dysdiadochokinesia)
	Muscle cramps of legs, neck, and trunk
Cognitive impairment/dementia (30%-50%)	Visuospatial and discrimination deficits
	Decreased psychomotor speed
	Decreased attention and concentration
	Difficulty shifting attention
	Decreased verbal fluency
	Impairment in procedural learning
	Mobility to use working memory
	Hallucinations
	Delusions
	Anxiety
	Apathy
	Mood swings
	Paranoia
	Cortical disinhibition
	Depression (50%)
	Predisposition to Alzheimer's disease

Box 27-2. Other manifestations of Parkinson's disease, most associated with autonomic dysfunction

- Drooling (sialorrhea); decreased swallowing; dysphagia
- Seborrhea: oily, greasy skin
- Excessive perspiration (diaphoresis)
- Complaints of pain, burning, coldness
- Orthostatic hypotension
- Urinary hesitation; frequency; incontinence
- Constipation; decreased peristalsis and stomach emptying; dysmotility
- Fragmented sleep; frequent awakenings; rapid eye movement sleep disorder
- Decreased libido; male impotence

18. **What pharmacological therapies can be used for Parkinson's disease?**

The following classes of drugs are useful in managing the symptoms of Parkinson's disease:
- Dopamine agonists (e.g., bromocriptine [Parlodel]): after initial treatment to delay start of levodopa
- Monoamine oxidase β inhibitors (e.g., selegiline [Eldepryl]): may slow progression of early Parkinson's disease
- Anticholinergics (e.g., trihexyphenidyl [Artane]): used early when tremor is the predominant symptom
- Precursor amino acid (e.g., carbidopa-levodopa [Sinemet]): crosses blood-brain barrier and is converted to dopamine
- Antiviral (e.g., amantadine [Symmetrel]): promotes release of dopamine; beneficial early in mild disease or to enhance effect of Sinemet
- Catechol O-methyltransferase inhibitors (e.g., tolcapone [Tasmar]): given only with Sinemet to prolong its effect
- Specific drugs to manage the related symptoms

19. **What other therapies can be used for Parkinson's disease?**

Other therapies for Parkinson's disease are
1. Stereotactic ablative surgery
   - Pallidotomy: relief of all symptoms
   - Thalamotomy: suppression of tremor
2. Deep brain stimulation in the medial globus pallidus and thalamus with an implanted electrode: suppression of tremor
3. Constructive surgery with fetal substantia nigra grafts: restore dopamine synthesis

20. **Describe the rehabilitation nursing management for the patient with Parkinson's disease.**

Because patients with Parkinson's disease are managed at home by the family until end-stage disease, when the physical burden is too much for the caregiver or when dementia makes home care impossible, the nurse often is the contact person for the collaborative interdisciplinary team that is needed. The nurse, as case manager, coordinates the care and refers the patient and family to the appropriate resources for care.

The most important aspect of care is the support and teaching for the patient and family. The nurse must recognize increasing caregiver burden and assist in modification of care to ease it. Unless the caregiver also can maintain an acceptable quality of life, the patient will need to be placed in a long-term facility. Such placement not only reduces satisfaction in the patient and family but also reduces independence, quality of life, and financial assets.

21. What is included in the rehabilitation nurse's teaching plan?

The teaching plan should include the following areas:

1. Disease progression: Provide explanation for expectations for each stage.
2. Medication therapy: Discuss all aspects of management:
   - Dosages
   - Indications
   - Side effects
   - Timing
   - Wearing-off effects
   - On/off effects
   - Drug holiday
   - Precautions for best absorption in relation to protein
3. Safety: Assist family in modifications of the home environment to prevent falls.
4. Nutrition: Discuss purpose of high-carbohydrate, low-protein diet for improved medication uptake.
   - Weekly weights (may overeat)
   - Adequate fluids and fiber
   - Modifications of food consistency with small bites when swallowing is impaired
   - Positioned upright to eat
   - Never leave patient alone while eating
5. Activities of daily living: Provide support to family to allow patient to do for himself or herself as long as possible.
   - Allow time to do task (may take a long time).
   - Teach importance of a daily complete bath.
   - Teach skin assessment to prevent breakdown.
   - Explain need for mouth care every 4 hours.
   - Determine if artificial tears are needed to protect the eyes.
6. Elimination: Help family to learn to do a bowel program to maintain regularity; help family to determine modifications if urinary incontinence develops (urinal, commode chair nearby).
7. Exercise/mobility: Explain importance of helping the patient to remain active.
   - Encourage deep breathing exercises.
   - Teach range of motion exercises to be done 4 times a day.
   - Recommend position change every 2 hours when patient is in bed.
8. Sleep/relaxation: Maintain activity during day.
   - Alternate exercise with rest periods.
   - Avoid afternoon naps.
   - Caution about sleep aids (little value).
   - Provide quiet, restful environment.
   - Teach relaxation techniques.
9. Orthostatic hypotension: Teach use of elastic stockings; remind to change position gradually.
10. Intolerance to heat/cold: Teach importance of climate control, especially in summer.
11. Communication: Suggest family sing together with patient.
    - Have patient read aloud.

- Have frequent engaging conversations with the patient.
- Teach family to wait for the patient to answer.
12. Depression: Teach family the signs to report; make referral to psychotherapist when needed.
13. Dementia: Teach family what behaviors to expect and how to respond.
    - Patient may experience personality changes.
    - Memory loss, confusion, irritability may cause concern and frustration.
    - Teach family how to use compensatory strategies with the patient.
    - Assist family with referral for neuropsychological evaluation of patient, if appropriate.
14. Institutional care: Assist the family through the decision-making process when home management is too difficult.
    - Help family through reframing so they are not overburdening themselves with guilt.
    - Discuss end-of-life issues and decisions that need to be made before a crisis occurs that requires resuscitation.
    - Refer to appropriate resource (elder law attorney).

HUNTINGTON'S DISEASE

22. What is Huntington's disease?

Huntington's disease is a hereditary degenerative disease of the basal ganglia and cerebral cortex. The defect is on chromosome 4 and is inherited as an autosomal dominant trait. Children of a parent with Huntington's disease have a 50% chance of having it. Although incidence is low (5 to 10 per 100,000), the disease is devastating and has no cure. Perhaps about 30,000 persons with Huntington's disease live in the United States, but more than 125,000 are at risk for inheriting it. In a small percentage (10%) of juvenile onset cases more rapid progression occurs, with death occurring in 5 to 10 years.

Huntington's disease is most prevalent among persons with western European lineage. Because of late onset, children already will be born before the affected parent is diagnosed. Generally, subtle personality changes and movement disorders manifest by age 35 years, and 90% of the patients have dementia by age 48. Death usually occurs 10 to 20 years after diagnosis from a complication, such as aspiration, infection, or heart failure. Progression of the disease is relentless, and many patients commit suicide.

23. Does a genetic test for Huntington's disease exist?

Persons who have a family member with Huntington's disease can be tested for the disease. An ethical issue arises, however, because there is no cure. Offspring of a person with Huntington's disease simply might elect to have no children, rather than learn early in life of such a horrifying future. The knowing can cause more deleterious responses than the not knowing. Those that choose not to be tested still can cling to hope of 50% chance, even though testing might confirm 100% clear. All offspring of a person with Huntington's disease should receive genetic counseling.

24. What is the pathophysiology of Huntington's disease?

Huntington's disease involves an excessive buildup of glutamine, used in protein synthesis, in neurons in the basal ganglia that leads to intranuclear inclusions that interfere with mitochondrial function.
- Cells in the caudate muscles and putamen die (striatum).
- Gliosis follows (scarring).
- Brain atrophy begins in the frontal, temporal, and parietal lobes.
- Degenerative changes become apparent in the neocortex and thalamus.
- Neurotransmitters acetylcholine and γ-aminobutyric acid are lost.
- An excess of dopamine occurs in relation to acetylcholine and γ-aminobutyric acid loss.

Because basal ganglia operate to create readiness to perform a task through preparatory adjustments, assist in the ability to initiate and carry out a pattern of movements smoothly and in proper sequence to accomplish a goal, and direct postural adjustments necessary before action can take place, such degeneration of neurons with the accompanying loss of their neurotransmitters causes some movements to be lost and others to go unopposed. Balance is lost. Dementia causes loss of perception to cues registered internally to direct actions, suppress response, or develop a habitual response, which causes inability to plan and execute complex tasks and loss of automatic movements.

25. What is the presentation of a person with Huntington's disease?

Depending on which of the four stages the patient is in, the symptoms vary widely over time. Table 27-3 presents the four stages.

Table 27-3. Stages of Huntington's disease	
Stage	**Symptoms**
Early	Fidgetiness, nervousness, anxiety
	Exaggerated facial expressions
	Forgetfulness
	Swaying, tilted gait
	Emotional volatility, irritable, violent
	May be enraged or suicidal
Middle	Swallowing slow and difficult, frequent aspiration, choking
	Complaints of trouble in closing mouth, chewing; mucus accumulation
	Greatly impaired gait, wide-based stance, lateral swaying
	Loss of balance
	Loss of automatic arm movements with walking
	Knee flexion
	Cognitive decline; lack of judgment, decrease in intelligence quotient, paranoia, anger

Table 27-3.	**Stages of Huntington's disease** *continued*
Late	Indistinct speech; deterioration in writing
	Weight loss
	Involuntary movements become severe
	Bed rest most of time
	Chorea: nonrhythmic, rapid, irregular, unpredictable, brief, jerky movements from one body part to another in a continuous, random order
	Unintelligible speech
	Episodes of extreme thirst or hunger
	Depression, agitation, panic, hallucinations
	Reversed sleep-wake cycles
	Akathisia: inner sense of restlessness; may prevent sleep
Final	Bed rest
	Somnolent
	Contractures
	Incontinent
	Retaining of fair comprehension

26. What treatment is being researched?

Early trials in the transplantation of fetal brain cells or stem cells into the striatum have shown the grafts to live and not become diseased. However, this is only one part of the brain; therefore such transplantation could not correct widespread degeneration. Other trials are using orally administered minocycline, which crosses the blood-brain barrier, to see whether it will block the enzymes that cause cell death.

27. What rehabilitation management is important for the patient with Huntington's disease?

The patient with Huntington's disease needs the help of the entire rehabilitation team to make the plan of care. The goals in the earlier stages involve maintaining function, reducing tone, and increasing stability. Later, the goals are more focused on preventing total immobility and assisting caregivers in transfers and use of adaptive equipment. Some strategies that are helpful for the patient with Huntington's disease are

1. Provide counseling and referral to appropriate resources for
   - Legal, financial, estate planning advice
   - Planning for unemployment and future health insurance
   - Helping in preparing instructions for care of the patient when dementia causes inability to make decisions
2. Refer the patient to a dentist quarterly for periodontal examinations.

3. Make a referral to speech pathologist early so that patient and family can learn interventions needed for
   - Swallowing
   - Prevention of aspiration
   - Methods to manage better food intake
4. Make a referral to dietitian early so that family can appreciate the importance of intake and can learn how to plan diet.
   - Daily caloric intake of 6000 kcal just to maintain weight, once chorea begins
   - Preparation of food: soft or blended; six servings per day
   - Small bites; food warmer or colder than mouth temperature
5. Teach family Heimlich maneuver.
6. Use relaxation exercises before dementia prevents their use to reduce extraneous movements.
7. Use slow rocking to reduce movements once dementia prevents relaxation exercises.
8. Obtain physical therapy to provide exercises to improve:
   - Strength
   - Flexibility
   - Balance
   - Coordination
   - Breathing
9. Use rhythmical auditory stimuli to improve cadence of gait; use metronome rather than music.
10. Help patient learn use of communication board before dementia so that patient may be able to communicate when speech is unintelligible.
11. Make a referral to psychologist to help patient and family manage progressive dementia.
12. Assist family to modify home to increase safety of patient and prevent falls:
    - Shower chairs
    - Handrails
    - Side rails that are padded
    - Helmet
    - Mattress on the floor
    - Sports padding on elbows, knees
    - Velcro fasteners on sneakers
    - Air splints
13. Teach range of motion, turning, hygiene, and skin care, and other measures to prevent hazards of immobility for the time when the patient is more in bed.
14. Teach family to maintain a consistent daily schedule to lessen patient's emotional outbursts.
15. Prepare family for development of urinary frequency and management of ultimate incontinence.
16. Teach family that, as patient becomes somnolent, the patient will require regular cognitive stimulation (the patient may still have fair comprehension).
17. Prepare family how to access and use hospice care when patient is in final stages.

Key Points

- The common link between all of the degenerative, neuromuscular, and debilitating disorders is the similar rehabilitation goals, which include management and education, maintaining function, assistance with coping, enhancing quality of life, and linking with resources.
- Five million Americans have Alzheimer's disease; and by 2050, 15 million Americans will have the disease if no prevention or cure is developed by then.
- The incidence of Parkinson's disease in persons in their twenties is growing. Currently more than 1 million Americans have Parkinson's disease, with 1 in 3 persons over 85 being diagnosed with it.
- Up to 50% of persons with Parkinson's disease have dementia.
- More than 125,000 Americans are at risk for inheriting the devastating, incurable, autosomal dominant Huntington's disease. Because Huntington's disease does not usually manifest until after 40, the patient already has had children. Possibly the person diagnosed with the disease already has grandchildren.

Internet Resources

Alzheimer's Association, Inc.
http://www.alz.org

Alzheimer's Disease Educational Referral Center
http://www.alzheimers.org

American Parkinson Disease Association
http://www.apdaparkinson.com

National Parkinson Foundations, Inc.
http://www.parkinson.org

The Parkinson's Disease Foundation
http://www.pdf.org

Huntington's Disease Society of America
http://www.hdsa.org

International Huntington Association
http://www.huntington-assoc.com

Bibliography

1. Barker E: Management of degenerative disorders. In Barker E, editor: *Neuroscience nursing: a spectrum of care,* ed 2, St Louis, 2002, Mosby.
2. Barker E: Management of movement disorders. In Barker E, editor: *Neuroscience nursing: a spectrum of care,* ed 2, St Louis, 2002, Mosby.

3. Edwards N, Ruethiger KM: The influence of caregiver burden on patients' management of Parkinson's disease: implications for rehabilitation nursing, *Rehabil Nurs* 27(5):182-186, 2002.
4. Flannery J: Degenerative neurologic disorders. In Burrell LO, Gerlach MJ, Pless BS, editors: *Adult nursing: acute and community care,* ed 2, Stamford, CT, 1997, Appleton & Lange.
5. Hickey JV: Neurodegenerative diseases. In Hickey JV, editor: *Neurological and neurosurgical nursing,* ed 5, Philadelphia, 2003, Lippincott Williams & Wilkins.
6. Melmick ME: Basal ganglia disorders: metabolic, hereditary, and genetic disorders in adults. In Umphred DA, editor: *Neurological rehabilitation,* ed 4, St Louis, 2001, Mosby.

Chapter 28

Neuromuscular and Debilitating Disorders Rehabilitation

Jeanne Flannery and Susan R. Bulecza

POSTPOLIO SYNDROME

1. **What is postpolio syndrome?**

   Postpolio syndrome occurs in some individuals who have a history of poliomyelitis. The syndrome can affect previously affected and nonaffected muscles. The average time of development is about 35 years after infection. Although the cause of postpolio syndrome is unknown, research has shown a correlation between the initial impairments and physical activity level in the years before onset. Postpolio syndrome can cause neuromuscular, musculoskeletal, and psychosocial problems (Box 28-1).

Box 28-1. Common symptoms of postpolio syndrome

- Fatigue
- Deep muscle pain
- Joint pain
- Weakness in previously affected or unaffected muscles
- Cold intolerance
- Atrophy
- Problems with activities of daily living

---

2. **Because the cause of postpolio syndrome is unknown, what has been suggested as possible causes?**

   Several theories have been put forth as possible explanations for postpolio syndrome. One theory is that the normal loss of neurons through aging further reduces the number of functional neurons in already damaged areas, resulting in decreased strength and function. Another theory suggests that neurons that may have shown recovery histologically may not have returned physiologically to a normal state, resulting in premature aging and failure. Regardless of the cause, evidence is lacking to support a reactivation of the poliovirus or autoimmune involvement.

3. **How is postpolio syndrome diagnosed?**

   Postpolio syndrome is diagnosed by the following criteria:
   - Confirmed paralytic polio history
   - Partial or complete recovery of muscle strength and function
   - 15-year, or greater, period of stability
   - Development of two or more of the previously mentioned symptoms
   - Absence of any other medical condition that would be indicated by these symptoms

   An important note is that many individuals who may have been diagnosed with a nonparalytic polio because they only had a mild weakness and fully recovered in fact may have had paralysis. These individuals may develop severe cases of postpolio syndrome. Therefore comprehensive assessment is critical when determining diagnosis.

4. **What are important goals for the patient in order to manage postpolio syndrome?**

   The important goals are to
   - Gain an understanding of the syndrome and its relationship to the prior acute polio infection
   - Effectively manage and prevent pain
   - Reduce muscle workload to compensate for decreased capacity
   - Use adaptive devices to reduce postural and gait deviations
   - Optimize function, safety, and quality of life

5. **Because pain is a major problem with postpolio syndrome, what are some interventions to consider for pain reduction?**

   Typically, pain associated with postpolio syndrome is categorized as muscle or joint pain. Muscle pain can be due to multiple causes and is of different types. This pain can affect already weakened muscles or muscles that were considered to be normal and often is diffuse and unrelieved by medication. The pain is exacerbated by activity and decreases with rest. A unique characteristic is that pain occurs 1 to 2 days after physical activity (Box 28-2).

Box 28-2. Management to prevent pain in postpolio syndrome

- Activity pacing with frequent rest periods
- Techniques to conserve energy, such as using an elevator instead of stairs
- Use of nonfatiguing activities, such as using rolling carts instead of carrying items

Patients need to be educated that recovery is prolonged and depends on compliance with treatment plans in addition to the severity and duration of the pain. Research has shown that improvement and resolution of pain depends greatly on the patient's compliance.

Joint pain is considered not to be a direct symptom of postpolio syndrome. Such pain usually results from long-term damage to joints from abnormal gait and posture as a result of the initial polio infection. Osteoarthritis has a higher incidence rate in individuals with postpolio syndrome and can be a complicating factor in joint pain. Treatment for joint pain is similar to sports injury management. Identification and elimination of the cause of the pain is important (Box 28-3).

Box 28-3.   Treatment for pain in postpolio syndrome

- Rest
- Mechanical postural correction
- Cold therapy
- Nonsteroidal antiinflammatory drugs
- Orthotics
- Range of motion

---

6. How is postpolio syndrome fatigue different from general fatigue?

Postpolio fatigue is different from general fatigue in that no relationship exists between occurrence of fatigue and activity, and fatigue does not resolve with a usual amount of rest. Postpolio syndrome fatigue has been described as a progressive loss of strength during activity, muscle heaviness sensation, and a progressive weakness. These descriptions are different from those usually associated with general fatigue. Treatment is similar to that described for muscle pain. Recovery may be prolonged to as much as 12 months from onset.

7. Why do patients with postpolio syndrome have cold intolerance?

The cold intolerance is due to decreased vasoconstriction from abnormal sympathetic nerve cell response, resulting in heat loss. Most patients will not want to use local application of cold pack to affect joints because they feel they will not be able to tolerate it. However, patients have been found to be able to tolerate the cold, which is often more effective than heat, which can increase edema and pain.

8. Do individuals with postpolio syndrome have sleep disturbances?

Yes, sleep disturbances have been reported by more than half of the individuals who have postpolio syndrome. Pain has been identified as a common cause. Therefore, nurses must thoroughly assess sleep status and pain in their patients.

9. **What are some techniques for helping patients conserve energy?**

Some energy-conservation techniques are to
- Combine several activities into one trip rather than two or three trips in a day
- Identify different, less strenuous ways of doing tasks (e.g., sitting rather than standing and using a rolling cart to carry items)
- Identify assistive devices and technology that can be used (e.g., motorized carts or chairs at stores)
- Break up long or large activities or tasks into parts with rest periods
- Identify whether others can assume responsibility for the more physical components of a task

10. **Why may a patient resist orthotics or other assistive devices?**

Many individuals with postpolio syndrome have been able to reduce the need for orthotics such as braces or crutches over time, or may have never needed them at all, after their initial illness. Therefore these individuals resist the use of assistive devices now with postpolio syndrome because such use is a disturbance of their body image and will be seen as a visible sign of disability. Giving the patient a specific rationale for why the orthotic is needed is critical, such as the orthotic will help prevent a fall or fracture, reduce pain, or enhance posture.

11. **Does exercise help patients with postpolio syndrome?**

Exercise, in general, can be detrimental to the patient with postpolio syndrome because it increases muscle workload, pain, fatigue, and muscle weakness. In later phases of recovery, gentle stretching and joint exercises may be tried, but only under close monitoring and evaluation. The reduction of exercise is a difficult concept for the patient with postpolio syndrome to understand because many were encouraged to do strenuous exercises during recovery at the time of their initial illness.

12. **What psychosocial issues do patients with postpolio syndrome frequently have?**

Patients with postpolio syndrome may have a number of psychosocial issues. They may distrust the medical treatment plan because it is counter to their prior experience during the initial illness. Because these individuals are usually in their fifties and sixties, they may be at the peak of their career and suddenly not be able to work any longer because of the effects of the syndrome. They may suffer from anxiety and depression because of role change in the family or community. These individuals have, throughout their lives, worked hard to appear normal and blend in. As a result of postpolio syndrome, they may no longer view themselves as normal or fitting in, and self-esteem decreases. Because of these emotions, many patients will have difficulty complying with treatment plans. Therefore for the nurse to provide support, be patient, and allow the patient time to process information and make decisions is important.

MYASTHENIA GRAVIS

13. What is myasthenia gravis?

Myasthenia gravis is an incurable autoimmune disease that affects the neuromuscular junction through destruction of the acetylcholine receptor sites. The cause of the autoimmune response is unknown. Although the disease can affect either gender, women more often are affected than men by a ratio of 3:2. Myasthenia gravis can affect all ages; however, women are affected more often in their twenties and thirties, whereas men are often not affected until their fifties and sixties. Onset is gradual.

14. What are characteristics of myasthenia gravis?

Characteristics of myasthenia gravis are fatigue and fluctuating muscle weakness that increases with exercise and improves with rest. Muscles most often affected are extraocular and those involved with mastication, swallowing, speech, and facial movement. The severity of myasthenia gravis depends on how many acetylcholine receptors are destroyed.

15. What are signs and symptoms of myasthenia gravis?

The signs and symptoms of myasthenia gravis correlate with the severity of the disease. Muscle weakness may be localized, affecting only the eye muscles, or it may be generalized, involving respiratory muscles. Generally, ocular muscles are always involved regardless of other muscle involvement. Presenting symptoms may include the following:
- Ptosis: may be asymmetrical
- Diplopia
- Difficulty chewing or swallowing
- Respiratory problems
- Limb weakness

Symptoms may vary in intensity throughout the day. Disruption of sensation, coordination, and reflexes does not occur.

16. How is myasthenia gravis diagnosed?

The following tests help to diagnose myasthenia gravis:
- Anticholinesterase testing: Edrophonium (Tensilon) is administered in a weakened muscle; if weakness improves, the test is positive for myasthenia gravis. This is considered a confirmatory test.
- Antibody titer for acetylcholine receptors: The titer usually is elevated in 80% to 90% of individuals with myasthenia gravis.
- Repetitive muscle stimulation: If amplitude decreases rapidly, the test result is considered positive for myasthenia gravis.
- Single fiber electromyography: Electromyography detects delay or absence of neuromuscular transmission in muscle fiber pairs. The test is 99% sensitive in confirming myasthenia gravis.

- Mediastinal magnetic resonance imaging: An enlarged thymus is present in many with myasthenia gravis because of a thymoma.

17. How is myasthenia gravis classified?

Table 28-1 presents myasthenia gravis classifications.

Table 28-1. **Myasthenia gravis classifications**	
Class	**Signs/symptoms**
Class 1	No disability: Minor complaints and signs
Class 2	Slight disability: Signs present after exertion May have daily activity restrictions
Class 3	Moderate disability: Signs present always Restricted activity Needs assistance with activities of daily living
Class 4	Severe disability: Requires continuous support with activities of daily living Respiratory function impaired
Class 5	Severe disability: Assisted respiratory function required

18. How is myasthenia gravis treated?

Treatment of myasthenia gravis focuses on reducing symptoms. The medication of choice for initial treatment is pyridostigmine (Mestinon), an anti-cholinesterase. The nurse must ensure that the patient takes medication on time, for symptoms will increase if medication is delayed, potentially resulting in the patient's being unable to swallow the pills. A thymectomy also may be done for symptom relief and possible remission if the patient is less than 60 years old. Plasmapheresis and/or immunoglobulin G therapy may be used in patients who have not responded well to conventional therapy.

19. What rehabilitation considerations are important for the patient with myasthenia gravis?

Important rehabilitation considerations are
- Patient education: For patients to understand what myasthenia gravis is and its effects and the importance of complying with the medication regimen is critical.

- Functional assessment: An initial assessment is key to determining how much assistance with daily activities will be needed and for determining any need for assistive devices or activity restrictions. Ongoing functional assessment is critical to ascertain medication effectiveness and compliance.
- The nurse should plan medication administration so that the effect is maximized during meal time to facilitate chewing and swallowing. Meals may need to be six smaller meals to minimize fatigue.
- The nurse should teach patient energy conservation techniques to manage activity and work.
- Patients with severe disability will need comprehensive assistance and environment modifications so that they can be managed at home.

AMYOTROPHIC LATERAL SCLEROSIS

20. What is amyotrophic lateral sclerosis (ALS)?

Amyotrophic lateral sclerosis, also known as Lou Gehrig disease, is an incurable, terminal, degenerative motor neuron disease that affects upper and lower motor neurons.
- *Amyotrophic* means progressive muscle wasting, the primary lower motor neuron component of the disease.
- *Lateral sclerosis* means demyelination of the corticospinal tracts of the lateral column of the spinal cord, resulting in scarring, which lowers symptoms indicative of upper motor neuron damage.

Characteristics of ALS include voluntary muscle weakness and atrophy, with the ability to speak, swallow, and breathe also affected. Currently, the cause of ALS is unknown. However, several proposed theories have been proposed, with the leading theory being that a defect in glutamate metabolism, transport, and storage allows an excess of glutamate to occur, which results in a toxic effect on motor neurons.

21. Are there different types of ALS?

Yes, the three types of ALS are
- Progressive muscular atrophy: primarily lower motor neuron loss affecting the limbs
- Primary lateral sclerosis: only involving upper motor neurons; prolonged illness course with survival as long as decades
- Progressive bulbar palsy: may be upper or lower motor neuron loss or a combination of both

22. Is one gender affected more frequently?

Yes, males are affected more often, with a ratio of 3:2. Incidence is about 1 to 2 cases per 100,000 population. The disease is about 3 times more common than myasthenia gravis and is less common than multiple sclerosis. Onset is generally around 30 years of age, but can occur earlier or later. Average survival is about 4 years after diagnosis with a range of 2 to 5 years.

23. What are signs and symptoms of ALS?

Disease onset is insidious; so by the time a patient complains of weakness, about 80% of the motor neurons have been lost in affected areas. Inability to perform functional activities such as dressing or tying shoes causes a patient to seek care. Physical examination by the health care provider usually identifies a greater degree of weakness and atrophy than reported by the patient.
Other signs and symptoms may include
• Fatigue
• Spasticity and hyperreflexia
• Fasciculations
• Dysarthria
• Dysphagia
• Dyspnea
• Babinski's and Hoffman's reflexes

A definitive characteristic of ALS is an asymmetrical pattern of progression with areas of normal muscle fibers in atrophied muscles. Confirmatory diagnosis is based on physical assessment, clinical presentation, and exclusion of other diseases with similar symptoms. No diagnostic or laboratory test is specific for ALS.

24. What are the rehabilitation goals for patients with ALS?

The rehabilitation goals are
• Maintain function and independence as long as possible
• Reduce and prevent complications caused by muscle weakness and atrophy
• Ensure patient and family understanding of the disease and its progression
• Ensure that the plan of care is patient-centered and allows the patient a degree of control

25. Is the patient's cognition and intellect affected by ALS?

No, the patient's cognition and intellect are not affected; therefore the patient must be involved in planning care. Also, alternative communication plans need to be developed so that the patient will still be able to communicate after losing the ability to speak.

26. How are ALS patients managed?

Because little in the way of medication is available, only one drug, riluzole, is used in the care of patients with ALS; management must be multidisciplinary and focus on symptom and progression management. Table 28-2 provides a brief example.

27. Because dysphagia is a major problem for patients with ALS, what are some ways to manage it?

Some ways to manage dysphagia follow:
• Changes in eating position (upright), head position (flexed), food temperature, and food viscosity can enhance eating ability and reduce aspiration risks.

Table 28-2.   **Management plan for amyotrophic lateral sclerosis**

Identified need	Goal	Action
Physical therapy	Optimize independence	Range of motion exercise Supportive and adaptive devices (e.g., braces and canes)
Occupational therapy	Facilitate ability to perform activities of daily living	Adaptive and electronic equipment (e.g., special utensils)
Speech therapy	Maximize communication ability	Vocal projection techniques or voice synthesizers
Nutrition assessment	Ensure adequate intake and reduce risk of aspiration	Caloric assessment Swallowing evaluation Gastrostomy tube
Respiratory assessment	Ensure adequate ventilation and function	Pulmonary function studies Incentive spirometry Respiratory therapy Respiratory support (e.g., ventilator)
Psychosocial	Enable patient/family to develop appropriate coping mechanisms	Counseling Patient/family education
Home care	Ensure support/resources are available for home care management	Referrals to community services and home health agencies Home assessment for equipment/ modification needs
Medical	Minimize complications	Medication management for symptoms
End-of-life planning	Ensure advance directives, financial, and personal needs are addressed	Health care surrogate appointed Advance directives written Legal referral

- Assistance with feeding can increase intake.
- Medications or supplements such as papaya tablets can assist in management of excessive secretions.
- Maintain adequate hydration to reduce secretion viscosity.
- Place a feeding tube to maintaining adequate nutrition.

28. **Respiratory function is another area of concern with patients with ALS. How can function be optimized?**

Respiratory function can be optimized by
- Postural drainage with cough facilitation and suctioning
- Breathing exercises and incentive spirometry
- Sleep position assessment
- Noninvasive assistive devices (e.g., BiPAP)
- Long-term ventilation: The nurse should discuss the pros and cons thoroughly and early with the patient and family. If the patient chooses ventilator support,

a home assessment is critical to environmental compatibility and identification of any needed modifications.

29. What two factors must one consider and prevent regarding exercise?

Two factors one must consider and prevent are
* Disuse atrophy: Disuse accelerates functional loss and mobility.
* Overuse injury: Ongoing assessment of patient's exercise program is critical to prevent further damage from excessive overuse and fatigue.

30. What are the abilities of patients with ALS as the disease progresses?

Table 28-3 presents the progression of the disease.

Table 28-3. Stages of amyotrophic lateral sclerosis		
Stage	**Functional status**	**Characteristics**
Stage 1	Independent	Mild weakness Able to ambulate No assistance needed with activities of daily living (ADL)
Stage 2	Independent	Local areas of moderate weakness Needs assistance with some ADL Able to ambulate
Stage 3	Independent	Severe weakness in hands, wrists, and ankles Moderate assistance needed with ADL Ambulatory but easily fatigued Changes in respiratory effort
Stage 4	Partially independent	Increased upper extremity weakness with decreased function and severe lower extremity weakness Wheelchair dependent Can do some ADL but fatigues easily
Stage 5	Partially independent	Moderate to severe extremity weakness Greater dependence with ADL Wheelchair dependent
Stage 5	Dependent	Bedridden Total care required Severely impaired or no speech

31. What is a major psychosocial concern for patients with ALS?

Coping ability for the patient and family is one of the major concerns. For the nurse to assist the patient and family to identify appropriate coping mechanisms to manage the emotional, social, and physical stress of the disease and its progression is critical. Collaboration with and referral to counselors, pastoral services, social workers, and hospice agencies can identify interventions for and provide services to the patient and family.

MUSCULAR DYSTROPHY

32. Is muscular dystrophy one disease or a category of diseases?

Muscular dystrophy is a category of diseases. These diseases are hereditary and are characterized by progressive muscle weakness, atrophy, and scarring. These diseases differ from others in this chapter in that there is not an associated nerve dysfunction. These diseases have variable degrees of severity, mortality, and age of onset. Several types affect primarily male individuals, whereas others are not gender specific. Additionally, some types have cardiac-related complications that are of more concern than the affected skeletal muscles. Mental retardation is common in the early-onset types.

33. What are the different types of muscular dystrophy?

Table 28-4 lists all the types of muscular dystrophy.

Table 28-4. Types of muscular dystrophy

Type	Onset	Progression
Duchenne's muscular dystrophy	2-6 years old, males only	Slow, survival into twenties
Becker's muscular dystrophy	Adolescence or adulthood, males only	Slow, survival into middle to late adulthood
Emery-Dreifuss muscular dystrophy	5-13 years old, males only	Slow, cardiac complications
Limb-girdle muscular dystrophy	10-40 years old	Slow, late onset, cardiac complications
Facioscapula-humeral muscular dystrophy	Before age 30	Slow, survival up to decades after diagnosis
Myotonic dystrophy	30-40 years old	Slow, survival to 50-60 years of age
Oculopharyngeal muscular dystrophy	20-40 years old, specific to ethnic groups: Jewish Americans, French Canadians, Hispanic Americans from New Mexico and Colorado	Slow, swallowing difficulty common
Distal muscular dystrophy	40-60 years old	Slow, non–life threatening
Congenital muscular dystrophy	Birth	Slow

34. How are muscular dystrophy diseases diagnosed?

Diagnosis varies for each disease, but common diagnostics include physical assessment, muscle biopsy, electromyography, and laboratory studies, such as creatine kinase.

35. How are muscular dystrophy diseases treated?

Because no cure exists for any of the muscular dystrophy diseases, treatment focuses on management of symptoms and prevention of complications.

36. What are rehabilitation goals for muscular dystrophy diseases?

Rehabilitation goals are
- Prevent contractures.
- Prolong strength and functional ability.
- Optimize mobility and independence through use of assistive devices and equipment.
- Maintain optimal respiratory and cardiac function.
- Promote realistic expectations.
- Ensure appropriate home and community integration and adaptation.
- Assist in patient and family development of positive psychosocial behaviors and strategies.
- Ensure the patient and family understand the disease and progression.

37. Why is maintenance of appropriate exercise important?

Appropriate exercise
- Helps maintain mobility
- Reduces the development of contractures
- Assists in maintaining optimal respiratory function
- Reduces obesity risk

Studies have shown that with appropriate exercise activities, walking ability was prolonged. Even for patients who could no longer walk, periodic standing helped prolong muscle strength. Long periods of bed rest should be avoided because it hastens weakness. Use of orthotics, such as ankle braces, are also of great value for prolonging mobility and exercise ability. The patient and family must understand that overuse and excessive fatigue can be detrimental for the patient. Therefore the patient should follow only the prescribed exercise program, and the nurse should provide reevaluation periodically to ensure appropriateness and need for modification.

38. What are some of the psychosocial issues?

Critically important is that a psychosocial assessment with appropriate referrals be done. Whether a child or an adult is affected by these diseases, the progressive consequences of these diseases are often profound and life-altering for the patients and their families.

For the parents of an affected child, the issues range from inability to achieve developmental milestones, overprotection, unrealistic expectations, and fear of having other affected children to anticipatory grieving. For an adult, the issues range from loss of independence and productivity, financial difficulties, depression, and fear of uncertain outcome to end-of-life decisions.

Key Points

- Generally, ocular muscle weakness, leading to ptosis and diplopia, always occurs, regardless of the severity of myasthenia gravis.
- Amyotrophic lateral sclerosis affects persons around 30 years of age, more frequently men; and because it is currently incurable and degenerative, survival is about 4 years after diagnosis in the more common progressive type.
- Because respiratory failure is an ultimate expectation, decisions about ventilatory support must be made early in the disease course of ALS.
- Muscular dystrophy, a hereditary category of diseases, affects persons across the life span, depending on the type, with slow progression of disability.

Internet Resources

Postpolio Syndrome Resources
http://www.ppsr.com

Myasthenia Gravis Foundation of America, Inc.
http://www.myasthenia.org

Amyotrophic Lateral Sclerosis Association
http://www.alsa.org

Muscular Dystrophy Association
http://www.mdausa.org

Facioscapulohumeral Dystrophy Society
http://www.fshsociety.org

Muscular Dystrophy Family Foundation
http://www.mdff.org

International Myotonic Dystrophy Organization
http://www.myotonicdystrophy.org

The National Institute of Neurological Disorders and Stroke
http://www.ninds.nih.gov

Bibliography

1. Barker E: Management of degenerative disorders. In Barker E, editor: *Neuroscience nursing: a spectrum of care,* ed 2, St Louis, 2002, Mosby.

2. Barker E: Management of movement disorders. In Barker E, editor: *Neuroscience nursing: a spectrum of care,* ed 2, St Louis, 2002, Mosby.

3. Del Benne M, Polak M: Neuromuscular autoimmune disorders. In Barker E, editor: *Neuroscience nursing: a spectrum of care,* ed 2, St Louis, 2002, Mosby.

4. Flannery J: Degenerative neurologic disorders. In Burrell LO, Gerlach MJ, Pless BS, editor: *Adult nursing: acute and community care,* ed 2, Stamford, CT, 1997, Appleton & Lange.

5. Hallum A: Neuromuscular diseases. In Umphred DA, editor: *Neurological rehabilitation,* ed 4, St Louis, 2001, Mosby.

6. Hickey JV: Neurodegenerative diseases. In Hickey JV, editor: *Neurological and neurosurgical nursing,* ed 5, Philadelphia, 2003, Lippincott Williams & Wilkins.

7. Mandler RN: Muscular dystrophy. In Biller J, editor: *Practical neurology,* ed 2, Philadelphia, 2002, Lippincott.

Chapter 29

Chronic Pain Rehabilitation

Jeanne Flannery

CHRONIC PAIN

1. **Why is chronic pain of interest to the rehabilitation nurse?**

   Chronic pain influences the patient's relationship with family, friends, co-workers, and health care providers. Chronic pain disturbs the patient's ability to meet role responsibilities, work, and social activities.

   Generally, patients who have chronic pain have endured it for years and have sought assistance from a variety of care providers. They often have disability, depression, fear, and pain behavior. About 45% of Americans seek medical care for chronic pain, most commonly back pain. The majority receive inadequate care.

2. **What is pain behavior?**

   Pain behavior is a set of behaviors linked to the pain but serving no purpose in relieving the pain, such as exaggerating the description of the pain to get stronger narcotics.

3. **What is chronic pain?**

   Chronic pain is not of malignant origin and persists past the time the disorder needed to heal. Chronic pain therefore does not respond well to interventions directed at correcting the disorder. The pain must have been present for at least 3 months. Chronic pain does not serve the protective purpose that acute pain provides. The pain is poorly localized, is continuous, or recurs at intervals, with poorly defined time of onset, lasting for months or years.

4. **What are the results of inadequately treated chronic pain?**

   Psychological changes, such as depression and feelings of hopelessness and helplessness, lead to withdrawal from work and normal activities. Physical activity is decreased; strength and endurance is decreased; appetite is reduced; sleep patterns are disturbed; and constipation develops. Chronic pain becomes a syndrome that not only deteriorates the patient's quality of life but also affects the patient's whole sphere of acquaintances. Table 29-1 provides further details on the physiological effects.

Table 29-1.   Physiological effects of inadequately treated pain

System	Effects
Musculoskeletal	Spasms
	Decreased mobility
Immunological	Decreased cellular immunity
	Impaired cellular immunity
	Impaired wound healing
	Increased risk for infection
Central nervous system	Fatigue
	Sympathetic stimulation
Gastrointestinal	Nausea/vomiting
	Decreased mobility
	Decreased secretions
	Paralytic ileus
Cardiovascular	Vasoconstriction
	Venous stasis
	Deep vein thrombosis
	Pulmonary embolism
	Hypertension
	Tachycardia
	Increased myocardial oxygen demand
Pulmonary	Hypoxia
	Decreased vital capacity
	Pneumonia
	Atalectasis
Endocrine	Increased metabolic rate
	Vagal inhibition
	Increased catecholamine release
Renal	Increased water retention
	Decreased urinary output

5. **What is the pathophysiology of pain?**

Nociceptors connect to A delta fibers (myelinated, fast-conducting) that transmit sharp, stabbing localized pain and also connect to C fibers (unmyelinated, slow-conducting) that transmit aching, burning, or itching diffuse pain. Histamine, bradykinin, serotonin, substance P, and prostaglandins are sensitizing chemical substrates that are released from damaged tissue. The pain message travels to the dorsal horn of the spinal cord where it synapses with second-order neurons that do three things:
- Most deliver the pain message to the thalamus through ascending tracts
- Some connect to motor neurons causing reflex movement
- Some connect to autonomic nervous system to create sweating, increased blood pressure and heart rate, local vasodilation, and piloerection.

Awareness of pain occurs at the thalamus. From the thalamus the impulse is relayed to the frontal lobes and limbic system for pain interpretation. Projections to the temporal lobes create pain memory and those to the hypothalamus create the autonomic response to pain.

6. How is pain physiologically modulated?

Systems of modulators act on ascending and descending pathways. First, in the ascending gating control, blocking mechanisms come from the substantia gyrus that are stimulated to close the gate to permit pain transmission. The A beta fibers that carry messages from pressoreceptors and mechanoreceptors close the gate, blocking pain transmission.

Additionally, the descending pathways have endogenous opioid peptides in the amygdala, hypothalamus, midbrain, medulla, and dorsal horns:
- Enkephalins
- β-Endorphins
- Dynorphin

These chemicals block the release of substance P. Neurotransmitters such as serotonin and L-dopa inhibit discharge of nociceptive neurons, and γ-aminobutyric acid inhibits in the dorsal horns.

7. How is pain classified, based on pathophysiology?

Pain is classified as
1. Nociceptive (somatic, visceral): arises from bone, muscle, skin, or viscera
2. Neuropathic (neural): generated from a central or peripheral nervous system structure; may be called neurogenic pain
   - May be the result of abnormally processed pain
   - May result from chronic diseases such as diabetes or peripheral vascular disease
   - May result when neurons continue to transmit pain messages in the absence of a stimulus

8. What is allodynia?

Allodynia is pain sensation occurring from a nonpainful stimulus.

9. What are the primary pain syndromes?

The primary pain syndromes include
1. Trigeminal neuralgia: paroxysmal, unilateral severe pain lasting seconds to minutes in the distribution of the trigeminal nerve
   - Triggered by talking, brushing teeth, chewing, or a cool breeze on the cheek
   - Does not extend
   - No structural course

2. Chronic regional pain syndrome
   a. Type I (formerly known as reflex sympathetic dystrophy): follows mild trauma without nerve injury
      • Begins within a month of the injury
      • A disproportionate response
      • Not limited to a single peripheral nerve
      • Constant burning pain that increases with movement
      • Impaired motor function
      • Allodynia (hyperalgia, edema, abnormal sweating, abnormal blood flow, and trophic changes in area of pain)
   b. Type II (formerly known as causalgia): follows trauma with nerve injury
      • Intense burning pain
      • Usually in hand or foot
      • May be a greatly delayed onset
      • Pain exacerbated by light touch, temperature change, movement, visual/auditory stimuli, stress
      • Symptoms spread proximally
      • Impaired motor function
      • Allodynia (hyperalgia, edema, abnormal sweating, abnormal blood flow, and trophic changes in area of pain)
3. Central pain
   a. Diffuse, poorly localized, continuous severe pain; sometimes worsens
   b. Results from damage to central nervous system; pain is burning, gnawing, aching, crushing
   c. May be paroxysmal with new pain on top of continuous pain
   d. Touch, cold, or heat produce allodynia that lasts beyond stimulus
   e. Pain occurs weeks to years after original injury

10. What is involved in the assessment of a patient in pain?

Assessment of a patient in pain requires
1. A complete neurological assessment
2. A pain assessment including
   a. Observation during movement (also including outside of treatment room when the patient is unaware of the observation)
   b. Origin/onset
      • When did the pain start?
      • What was happening at that moment?
      • Was there an injury?
   c. Position: Have patient *show* where the pain is.
   d. Pattern
      • Is the pain constant or periodic?
      • Does the pain radiate or travel?
      • What time of day does the pain occur? What activities are affected by pain?
      • Has the pain changed?
      • Is the pain worsening, the same, or improving?

  e. Quality
   • What adjectives describe the pain?
   • Is the pain mechanical (pressing, stabbing)?
   • Is the pain chemical (burning)?
   • Is the pain neural (numb, pins and needles)?
   • Is the pain vascular (throbbing)?
  f. Duration (How long does the pain last?)
  g. Quantity
   • What is the intensity of the pain?
   • Has the intensity changed?
  h. Radiation
   • Describe the radiation.
   • Can the radiation be reversed?
   • How?
  i. Signs/symptoms
   • Does the pain cause any functional limitations?
   • Are any changes in lifestyle necessary?
   • Does the pain cause any problems with work?
   • Can leisure time still be enjoyed?
   • How is the patient's personality?
   • Has the personality changed with the pain?
   • Are there any benefits from the pain?
  j. Treatment
   • What has been tried? How effective was the treatment?
   • What are the expectations from treatment?
  k. Visceral symptoms (If physical symptoms have visceral origin and link to pain, referral should be made to the physician.)

11. What is the focus in the physical examination of a patient with chronic pain?

The examination should include
1. Observation of gait and movement; use of assistive devices
2. Assessment of body type; any anomalies
3. Assessment of posture: sitting, standing; note any automatic adjustment; position of head, trunk, extremities
4. Inspection of the skin: scars, elasticity, trophic changes
5. Palpation of soft tissues: temperature, edema, tenderness
6. Palpation of anatomical structures: discomfort with movement
   • Empty: no resistance
   • Spasm: muscular resistance
   • Capsular feel: rubbery
   • Bone: hard, smooth movement
   • Soft tissue: no resistance on movement
7. Range of motion measurement: resistance, less than full range of motion, pain, weakness
8. Muscle strength measured (scale of 1 to 5)
   • Strong and painful
   • Weak and painful

- Weak but pain does not increase
- All movements painful
- Strong and painless (normal is l5)

9. Neurological assessment: bilateral
   - Reflexes (2+ is normal)
   - Sensation: touch, sharp, vibration (first to be lost), contralateral symptoms
   - Allodynia, hyperalgia, chronic regional pain syndrome
   - Coordination
   - Stretch and pressure tests to nerve trunks

10. Neurovascular assessment: headache, temporal arteries, diabetic neuropathy

The patient may not be able to tolerate all these activities at once and may need this examination to be done in several sessions, in spite of managed care. If pressed, the patient may be so stressed that the diagnosis is not accurate.

12. **In assessing the pharmacological therapy of a patient who has chronic pain, how should the rehabilitation nurse evaluate?**

The World Health Organization recommends a three-step approach in treatment. Therefore the nurse should use this model as a guide. Table 29-2 presents the pattern.

Table 29-2. World Health Organization analgesic protocol

Steps	Pain level	Type of drug	Action
Step 1	Mild	Nonopioids: Aspirin Acetaminophen NSAIDs* (ibuprofen, naproxen, indomethacin)	Provide concurrent treatment for cause. Use adjuvants as needed: Tricyclic antidepressants Antiseizure drugs Anxiolytics Antihistamines Benzodiazepines Caffeine Dextroamphetamine Corticosteroids
Step 2	Mild to moderate	Opioids: Codeine Oxycodone	Continue step 1 drugs. Add step 2 drugs. Use adjuvants as needed.
Step 3	Moderate to severe	Opioids: Morphine Hydromorphone (Dilaudid) Methadone (Dolophine) Fentanyl	Continue step 1 drugs. Replace step 2 drugs with step 3 drugs. Use adjuvants as needed.

*NSAID, nonsteroidal antiinflammatory drug.

13. When should the rehabilitation nurse expect to use adjuvant drugs?

Adjuvant drugs commonly are used with neuropathic pain. They have analgesic properties or they increase the effects of other analgesics synergistically. Table 29-3 presents some of the adjuvant drugs.

Table 29-3. Adjuvant drugs

Drug	Class	Action
Clonidine (Catapres)	Antihypertensive	α_2-Adrenergic agonist Affects pain receptors at central and peripheral levels.
Dextromethorphan	Over-the-counter cough suppressant	NMDA* receptor antagonist is used concurrently with morphine.
Carbamazapine (Tegretol) Phenytoin (Dilantin)	Anticonvulsant	Stabilizes neuronal membranes and suppresses spontaneous firing (trigeminal neuralgic).
Gabapentin (Neurontin)		Action is not understood.
Amitriptyline (Elavil) Nortriptyline (Pamelor) Desipramine (Norpramine) Paroxetine (Paxil) Fluoxetine (Prozac)	Antidepressant • Tricyclic • Selective serotonin reuptake inhibitor	Is effective in neuropathic pain. Single dose at bedtime blocks reuptake of serotonin.
Baclofen (Lioresal) Metaxalone (Skelaxin) Tizanidine (Zanaflex)	Muscle relaxant/antispasmodic	Relieves pain of muscle spasms.
Botulinum toxin (Botox)		Relieves severe spasticity and dystonia.
Alprazolam (Xanax) Lorazepam (Ativan)	Anxiolytic/(benzodiazepine)	Has no analgesic properties, but with sedation, use of analgesics may be reduced when muscle tension is reduced.
Lidocaine (usually intrathecal or epidural) Mexiletine (oral) Lidocaine (transdermal; Lidoderm)	Local anesthetic	Blocks sodium channels in pathways for pain transmission.

*NMDA, N-methyl-D-aspartate.

14. What invasive procedures can be used to treat chronic pain?

Table 29-4 presents some invasive procedures for treating chronic pain.

Table 29-4. **Procedures to relieve chronic pain**

Procedure	Effect
Invasive procedures	

Epidural steroid injection	Most common procedure for
	   Herniated disk
	   Spinal stenosis
	May require 2-3 injections 2 weeks apart.
	May provide temporary to permanent relief.

Nerve blocks	Peripheral nerve block
	Intravertebral facet nerve block: for pain from degenerative change in facets
	Sympathetic nerve block
	   Stellate ganglion: for arms, hands, face pain
	   Celiac plexus: for visceral, abdominal pain
	Ablation with alcohol or phenol for permanent block

Acupuncture	Needles stimulate large fiber (C) input, which inhibits small fiber (A) input; endorphins are released; autonomic system is influenced.
Surgical procedures	
Dorsal column stimulation (radiofrequency patient-controlled transmitter)	Treats chronic back pain that has failed to respond to all else; also treats phantom pain. Electrodes are implanted to increase β-endorphins release, which activates serotonin inhibitor system.
Peripheral nerve stimulation	For localized pain: posttraumatic neuralgia Electrode is implanted around nerve.
Deep brain stimulation	For unremitting central pain, such as thalamic stroke Stimulates periventricular and periaquaductal gray matter in upper midbrain.
Ablative procedures:	
• Dorsal rhizotomy	Surgically destroy the sensory nerve root via thermal lesions, cryotherapy lesions, or open surgery. Must cover several unilateral spinal levels to be effective.
• Radiofrequency lesioning	For lumbosacral vertebral facet joints or postherpetic pain of trunk
• Percutaneous trigeminal rhizotomy	For trigeminal neuralgia (may be permanent) or radiofrequency (lasts 6 months)
• Sympathectomy	To control causalgia and visceral pain of upper abdomen Ipsilateral lesion of lumbar sympathetic chain controls pain in foot (may produce impotence). Cervical chain lesion, for pain in upper extremity, may produce Horner's syndrome.
Surgical decompression	Relieves pain and parasthesia from pressure on nerve root. Causes scarring, which may produce pain.
Intradiscal electrothermaplasty	Wire is inserted percutaneously into herniated disk and heated. Relief is gained by 6 months as disk deteriorates.

Table 29-4. Procedures to relieve chronic pain *continued*

Cordotomy	Percutaneous needle and radiofrequency current destroy sensory tract over affected dermatomes ipsilaterally. Relieves central pain from spinal cord injuries and brachial plexus avulsion.
Implantable pump	Dispenses morphine, hydromorphone, fentanyl, or clonidine with morphine into intrathecal space. Controls pain that is intractable. Use of baclofen controls spasticity.

15. **What physical interventions are available to the patient with chronic pain?**

Table 29-5 presents physical interventions for the patient with chronic pain.

Table 29-5. Physical interventions for chronic pain

Types	Description
Dermal cutaneous stimulation	Includes massage, vibration, application of heat and cold/ice, mentholated substances, or acupressure, which soothes, numbs, or serves as a counterirritant to ice and mentholated substances.
Transcutaneous electrical nerve stimulation	Stimulates large fibers (A), which inhibit pain transmission. Produces endogenous opiates.
Ultrasound	Heats deep tissue via sound waves. Stimulates C fibers and relieves pain distal to application. Stimulates large fibers (A) and relieves spasm. Treats neuropathies, herpes zoster, and muscle spasm.
Phonophoresis	Chemicals are delivered via ultrasound up to 2 inches deep: Lidocaine ointment Hydrocortisone cream Salicylate cream
Cryotherapy	Cooling is by ice packs, ice massage, immersion, or evaporation of vapocoolant spray. Treats tendonitis, rheumatoid arthritis, and pathological conditions of the disk.
Iontophoresis	Chemical ions are driven through skin by electrical current: Lidocaine ointment: before ROM,* stretching, joint mobilization Hydrocortisone: for arthritis, bursitis, inflammation Epsom salts (magnesium): for muscle spasm or localized ischemia

*ROM, range of motion.

Continued

Table 29-5. Physical interventions for chronic pain *continued*

	Iodine: for pain from adhesions (softens fibrotic tissue)
	Salicylate: for joint inflammation, myalgia
	Acetic acid: dissolves calcium deposits
	Lithium: breaks down gouty tophi
Massage	Indirectly stimulates A delta and A beta fibers, producing gating mechanism.
	Provides reflex relaxation of muscle tissue.
	Relieves ischemic pain.
Myofascial release	Releases imbalances and restrictions within the fascia and normalizes through pressure and stretching.
	Treats headaches and chronic pain.
Joint mobilization	Passive oscillations allow collagen fibers to loosen, enhancing accessory movements and free ROM without pain; also repetitions relieve pain through the spinal gating mechanism.
Therapeutic touch	Energy is transferred from the healer and then a repatterning of the patient's energy state occurs.
	Relieves headache, anxiety, and tension.
	Provides heat to affected area.
Point stimulation (acupressure)	Uses same mechanism as acupuncture.
	Deep pressure is applied in circular motion up to 5 minutes on meridian points.
Exercise	ROM stretching, aerobic exercises
	Relieves pain through gating mechanism and release of endorphins.
	Reconditions and strengthens muscles.

16. **What cognitive strategies can be used to relieve the patient's chronic pain?**

    Box 29-1 presents the cognitive strategies effective in relieving pain.

Box 29-1. Cognitive strategies for pain relief

Relaxation techniques: Establish a self-induced state incompatible with pain.
- Visualization
- Guided imagery
- Meditation

> **Box 29-1. Cognitive strategies for pain relief**   *continued*
>
> - Progressive muscle relaxation
> - Body scanning: separating self from the pain and the reaction to the pain
> - Hypnosis: more vivid images, deeper focus; altered state; subconscious mind is open to suggestion, bypassing the critical conscious mind; allows pain to be perceived differently
>
> **Attention diversion:** An active process of concentrating on stimuli in environment, which blocks awareness of the pain.
>
> **Humor:** As little as 10 minutes of belly laughter a day can produce 2 hours of pain-free sleep.
> - Releases energy and tension; creates muscle relaxation
> - Distraction
>
> **Operant conditioning:** Conditioning addresses the learned aspects of pain and separates the behavior and the response. (One can condition the body to tolerate higher levels of activity before pain.)
>
> **Biofeedback:** The patient is trained to change selectively certain physiological processes, such as muscle tension, skin temperature, blood pressure, and heart rate and to gain control over them (effective for headaches, muscle spasms, and chronic pain).

17. **What goals should the rehabilitation nurse have in caring for the patient with chronic pain?**

The nurse focuses on teaching the patient about the cause, prevention, and relief measures related to the pain so that the patient can be empowered and in control of the pain. The nurse must address medications extensively so that the patient understands limits and interactions. Safety is a basic foundation for all the education.

The nurse also must relieve the patient's fear about addiction, so that the patient will take the medications as prescribed. The nurse should mention all alternative modalities to learn which ones the patient would be comfortable trying. The nurse then can teach alternative modalities the patient accepts so as to enhance the effects of medication. The nurse accepts and validates the patient's pain but reminds the patient that the patient can remain in control, rather than be controlled by the pain to the point of no longer being functional. The nurse assists the patient to regain functionality and achieve a better quality of life. The nurse makes certain the patient has a list of the medications in his or her wallet. The nurse provides reinforcement regarding side effects and untoward reactions so that the patient understands when to call the physician or 911 in emergencies. If the nurse can influence the patient/family to participate in a support group, then the nurse can get them in contact with the group.

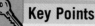

Key Points

* Chronic pain does not respond well to intervention directed at correcting the disorder that produced it, for this pain persists past the time the disorder needed to heal. Chronic pain does not serve a protective purpose and is poorly defined.

* The three chronic pain syndromes are trigeminal neuralgia, chronic regional pain syndrome, and central pain.

* The World Health Organization provides a guide for treatment of patients with chronic pain in a three-step approach, depending on the level of pain, recommending the drugs to use.

Internet Resources

American Chronic Pain Association
http://www.theacpa.org

American Council for Headache Education
http://www.achenet.org

American Pain Society
http://www.ampainsoc.org

Bibliography

1. Faria SH, Flannery JC: Reflex sympathetic dystrophy syndrome: an update, *J Vasc Nurs* 16(2):25-30, 1998.

2. Hickey JV, Brown R: Management of chronic pain: a neuroscience prospective. In Hickey JV, editor: *The clinical practice of neurological and neurosurgical nursing,* ed 5, Philadelphia, 2003, Lippincott Williams & Wilkins.

3. Karapas ET, Barker E: Management of the neuroscience patient with pain & headache. In Barker E, editor: *Neuroscience nursing: a spectrum of care,* ed 2, St Louis, 2002, Mosby.

4. Mayberry BG: Chronic pain. In Biller J, editor: *Practical neurology,* ed 2, Philadelphia, 2002, Lippincott Williams & Wilkins.

5. Misabelli-Susens L: Pain management. In Umphred D, editor: *Neurological rehabilitation,* ed 4, St Louis, 2001, Mosby.

Chapter 30

Nursing Management for Wounds

Sharon A. Aronovitch

1. **Why do some wounds develop necrotic tissue along the surgical incision?**

   Necrotic tissue that develops along a surgical incision is called a reperfusion injury. This injury occurs when blood supply is restored to ischemic tissues. The renewed availability of oxygen to tissues produces a large amount of free radicals. Research has shown that free oxygen radicals cause damage to epithelium because of lipid peroxidation. Neutrophils then cause occlusion of capillaries in the reperfused tissue. As proteins are upregulated during reperfusion injury, an increase in capillary permeability results in leakage of proteins and fluid into tissue, which causes tissue necrosis.

2. **What are oxygen free radicals?**

   An oxygen free radical is an oxidant or unstable O_2 compound that is produced by the body during normal body processes. The radical is produced more abundantly during exposure to environmental agents such as pollution, smoking, and alcohol consumption. Oxygen free radicals may cause cellular damage resulting in the inability of the cell to function normally. The chain reaction of free radicals can be halted when two free radicals interact. Neutrophils use free radicals to attack bacteria because lipids are susceptible to free radical injury (lipid peroxidation).

   Carbohydrates are damaged readily by free radicals. An enzyme system is present in all tissues that will disarm free radicals and is located in the cytoplasm of the cell (superoxide dismutase, catalase, glutathione peroxidase). This system converts free radicals to harmless compounds.

3. **How can the rehabilitation nurse assist patients to strengthen their systems against free radicals?**

   Giving patients antioxidants to combat the destruction caused by free radicals when they have an injury is advisable. The most common antioxidants recommended are β-carotene (vitamin A, converted as needed), vitamin C, and vitamin E. Each of these antioxidants gives up electrons to free radicals, thereby stopping the domino effect of cellular destruction.

4. **Is 1 L per shift (8 hours) of an intravenous solution of D$_5$W adequate hydration and nutrition for a patient recovering from a wound if the patient does not feel like eating?**

No, an intravenous solution typically used to provide hydration is not an adequate nutrition source for the patient. A well-known fact is that hospitalized patients can lose anywhere from 4% to 25% of their total body weight. Patients recovering from a spinal cord injury can expect a weight loss ranging from 15% to 25% of their preinjury weight.

Many health care providers presume that because patients are well nourished when they are admitted to a health care facility, that a few days of intravenous solutions will not change the patients' nutritional status. However, that is an erroneous assumption to make when providing care to any patient who is recovering from an injury, whether the injury is traumatic or surgical, particularly if intravenous solution is the only means of providing hydration and nutrition.

An intravenous solution of 1000 ml D$_5$W given every 8 hours provides the patient with only about 500 Kcal per day. Each 5% dextrose solution of 100 ml is equivalent to 5 g of dextrose, and a gram of dextrose is about 3.3 Kcal. Aside from the caloric intake being grossly inadequate, no protein or vitamins needed for wound healing are being provided.

5. **What is the difference between inflammation, a localized infection, and wound sepsis?**

Inflammation to the wound site involves erythema, minimal edema, localized heat, and pain as a result of the tissue injury. Inflammation is the first step of the healing process and is required in order for wound closure to occur.

A *local infection* at the site of injury also has redness. The granulation tissue, if present, in the wound bed will be friable. The periwound, or area surrounding the wound, will have cellulitis rather than mild to minimal edema, as in inflammation. An infected wound produces heat and pain. Also, a noticeable increase in wound size occurs; drainage increases (usually purulent); and the drainage has a foul odor.

A systemic infection, or *sepsis*, that results from a wound or injury is evidenced by an elevated white blood cell count, fever, tachycardia, tachypnea, confusion, and fatigue. The body temperature may become extremely elevated. If the process is not treated quickly, *septic shock* may develop, threatening the patient's life.

6. **Is there a special way to perform a wound culture?**

Wound cultures are to be obtained only from a wound after thoroughly cleansing the wound with normal saline. The culture is taken from the pink, healthy tissue present in the wound environment. If the wound has no healthy pink tissue from which to obtain a culture, then to obtain a culture just because it has been ordered is a waste of the nurse's time and the patient's money.

Culturing necrotic or hard black eschar results in a false positive for the micro-organisms that are causing the wound infection. If the nurse cultures nonhealthy wound tissue, the health care provider then will be writing antibiotic orders based on wound debris. The most accurate wound culture is from a tissue culture obtained from a punch biopsy or tissue biopsy that can be performed only by a physician or other qualified health care provider.

The easiest wound culture is obtained using a swab system; however, this type of culture is only viable for 30 minutes outside of a refrigerated environment. One must remember that wounds are "dirty" and contain a multitude of micro-organisms, meaning that all wounds will culture bacteria. Wounds should be cultured only if there are signs of clinical infection, such as fever or purulent drainage, or the patient is immunocompromised even if the patient has no signs and symptoms of an infection.

7. How does a major wound affect a patient's quality of life?

To promote the healing process of a wound, the nurse must realize that all injuries to the skin, no matter the size or location, affect the patient's quality of life and psychological well-being. The impact on the patient's quality of life is related to the patient's degree of mobility, nutrition, self-esteem, and possible iatrogenic illness. Immobility can be devastating to a patient who must be resting in bed, in a prone position, to treat a sacral pressure ulcer when the only means of ambulation is by wheelchair.

Such immobilization eliminates the possibility of ambulation for the duration of treatment, which could be months. Self-esteem can be affected when the patient's wound has a large amount of foul-smelling drainage or when the dressing contin-uously falls off. The psychological impact of wounds can be from financial stressors and result in self-esteem issues and severe emotional stress. Other psychological stressors related to tissue and or bone injury include loss of independence, fear associated with possible death or amputation, and diminished social contact because of hospitalization that may cause isolation and depression.

8. What is the difference between grafts and flaps?

Grafts are described as the following types:
- Full-thickness tissue grafts are used to cover nonextensive repairs of the face, neck, and hands. A full-thickness tissue graft is a segment of epidermis and dermis that is detached totally from the original site. The usual donor sites are those where the skin is thin, such as the prepuce, scrotum, labia minora, upper eyelid, and supraclavicular region. The problem with using these sites is that unwanted hair growth can occur at the grafted location.

- Split-thickness grafts contain the epidermis and a portion of the dermis and are used to cover extensive defects or as a biological dressing to control or eliminate infection. The usual donor sites are from "hidden areas" such as the abdomen, thigh, and buttocks.
- Other sources of tissue grafts come from cadavers (allograft); animals, usually the pig (xenograft); or placental membrane (amnion). There are not many types of biosynthetic wound dressings used as skin grafts. A few of the most common products are Biobrane (a strong flexible nylon fabric; Bertek Pharmaceutical Inc., Research Triangle Park, North Carolina) and Apligraf (bovine collagen and human epidermal keratinocytes that are from neonate foreskin; Norvartis Pharmaceutical Corp., East Hanover, New Jersey).

Flaps are used typically to repair large cavernous wounds. The most common types of tissue flaps are
- Skin flap (section of skin with all layers and subcutaneous tissue moved from one location to another while maintaining vascular attachment to its original location)
- Myocutaneous flap (contains muscle and its blood supply with an attached paddle of skin and is a relatively hidden donor site that may leave a functional deformity)
- Free flap (contains various tissue types that are disconnected from the donor site with blood supply reestablished directly in the recipient site and has a hidden donor site with no functional deformity)

These tissue flaps also are referred to by terms related to positioning of the flaps, such as
- Random: The specific blood supply is not known, and the blood supply to the flap is derived from nonspecific dermal and dermal vessels in the wound environment.
- Rotation: The base of the flap is immediately adjacent to the defect to be filled.
- Advancement: The defect lies beyond the tip or distal portion of the flap that is raised, undermined, and pulled/pushed into the defect.
- Transposition: The tissues are moved over or under intervening normal tissue to fill the defect.

9. **Is nursing care provided to a wound that has been grafted different from that for a wound that has been flapped?**

Graft failure occurs because of decreased vascularity in the wound bed, infection, hematoma, technical error, movement of the tissue graft, and poor storage of grafts. Survival of a tissue graft therefore depends on the production of adequate capillary blood flow (a process that takes 3 to 4 days), the proximity of graft to the recipient area (meaning that the closer the donor site is to the injury to be repaired, the more likely the take of the tissue graft will heal optimally), and immobilization of the tissue graft. Box 30-1 presents nursing responsibilities following a tissue graft.

Box 30-1. Nursing responsibilities following tissue graft

1. Assessing for adequacy of blood flow by using a cotton swab on periphery of graft
   - Color
   - Temperature
   - Capillary refill no greater than 1 second
2. Observation for hematoma
3. Observation for the presence of infection

   Flap failure occurs as a result of
   1. Poor design of the flap immediately before surgical removal
   2. Surgical, technical, or mechanical complication
   3. Patient-related factors such as
      - Advanced age
      - Cachexia
      - Elevated hematocrit
      - Polycythemia vera
      - Smoking

Box 30-2 presents nursing responsibilities following a surgical flap placement.

Box 30-2. Nursing responsibilities following surgical flap placement

1. Assessing for adequacy of blood flow by checking the flap site:
   - Color
   - Temperature
   - Capillary refill within 1 second
2. Observation for hematoma and the presence of infection
3. Observation for infection

---

10. How does the rehabilitation nurse decide which type of dressing product to use on a patient's wound?

The decision in choosing a wound dressing is based on the functions of the dressing and the type of wound needing care. Products differ based on their
- Hydrating ability of the wound environment
- Adhesiveness
- Absorbency
- Conformability
- Ability to eliminate dead space
- Ability to immobilize tissue and thereby minimize scarring

Using a dressing product that contains wound fluid (occlusive dressing) in the wound bed provides a natural antibacterial solution and polymorphonuclear neutrophils. Occlusive dressings, those that protect the wound environment from the outside environment, stimulate growth factors and generate an electrical potential within the wound bed. Dressing products are classified into the categories found in Table 30-1.

Table 30-1.   Categories of dressing products

Type of product	Action	Examples of products
Hydrocolloids	Fluid impermeable; mold to body; absorb wound exudate; safe, easy way to débride necrotic tissue	DuoDerm Restore ComFeel RepliCare Tegasorb Cutinova hydro ULTEC
Semipermeable membrane dressing	Similar in appearance to plastic wrap, but with an adhesive backing	ACU-Derm BIOCLUSIVE BlisterFilm OpSite POLYSKIN II Tegaderm
Barriers	Usually require a secondary dressing; can be protective ointment	Carrington ILEX ProShield Lantiseptic No-sting Skin Protectant Barrier Cream
Hydrogels	Absorb wound exudate; mold to body; cool burned or excoriated tissue; fluid impermeable (sheets only); safe, easy way to debride necrotic tissue; 80%-90% water/normal saline; most now contain glycerin to increase the viscosity of the product	AQUASORB Biolex Carrasyn Clearsite Elasto-Gel NORMLGEL Nu-Gel Royal-DERM Wound Hydrogel Vigilon SoloSite
Collagen	Absorbs wound exudate; molds to wound environment; safe, easy to use	Multidex (only recommended for use on patients who have diabetes) Kollagen Dermagran

Table 30-1. Categories of dressing products *continued*

Alginate	Easy to use; absorbs wound exudate; hemostatic and antibacterial (helps to decrease odor naturally) properties; safe, easy way to remove slough tissue	AlgiDERM CURASORB KALTOSTAT Sorbasan Bard Absorptive
Absorptives	Absorbs more than 20 times weight of product; many forms (paste, beads, flakes, unit dose); fill dead space of wound; safe, easy way to débride soft, necrotic tissue	Bard Absorptive Dressing HYDRON Triad Wound Paste Iodasorb (a cadexomer iodine that is safe to the wound environment) MESALT
Foam dressing	Easy to use; not traumatic to wound bed; absorbs wound exudate; fluid impermeable	LYOFOAM Allevyn Flexzan MITRAFLEX Hydrasorb NU-DERM
Composite dressing	Easy to use; semiocclusive dressing combining features of moisture-retentive dressing; not traumatic to wound bed; absorbs wound exudate; fluid impermeable	LYOFOAM "A" Polymem Transorb VENTEX Viasorb Alldress Fibrocol
Enzymes	Only use to débride necrotic tissue and should not be used on healthy wound bed; antiseptics containing iodine, hexachlorophene, benzalkonium chloride will inactivate the enzymes	Elase Collaganase/Santyl Panafil Accuzyme

11. Describe sponge dressings.

Sponge dressings include the following types:
1. Dry (Woven sponges are made of 100% cotton and are a coarse or fine mesh.)
2. Impregnated with a solution or substance that maintains a moist environment but is not occlusive:
   - Adaptic (Johnson & Johnson, Somerville, New Jersey)
   - Aquaphor (Smith & Nephew, Largo, Florida)

- CarraGauze (Carrington Laboratories, Inc., Irving, Texas)
- Dermagran Wet Dressing (Derma Sciences, Inc., Princeton, New Jersey)
- Scarlett Red (Kendall, Mansfield, Massachussetts)
- Vaseline Gauze (Kendall)
- Xeroflo (Kendall)
- Xeroform (Kendall)

3. Synthetic (i.e., polyester or rayon) and nonwoven (This type of sponge product feels softer than a sponge made of 100% cotton fibers.)

12. When is a sponge dressing appropriate to use?

The following sponge types are listed with their appropriate use:
- Dry dressing should be used only on dry, closed wounds.
- Coarse gauze sponges are used for débriding (e.g., wet to moist or moist to dry dressing).
- Fine mesh gauze is used when débriding is needed, but healthy tissue is present.
- Nonwoven sponges were manufactured to wick drainage from the wound environment. These sponges can and should be used as the secondary or outermost dressing layer over a moist dressing.

Sponges are not an occlusive dressing and should not be used when an occlusive environment is more appropriate for a healthier healing process.

To place a dry dressing over a moist wound is never appropriate; this only results in desiccation of the wound bed and pain to the patient when the dressing is removed.

13. How does the rehabilitation nurse know which dressing to choose for a dermal wound?

Figure 30-1 presents a simplistic model of which dressing to choose for a dermal wound.

14. Why are only pressure ulcers staged?

The National Pressure Ulcer Advisory Panel developed a staging system that is used nationally and internationally. The staging system was developed specifically to categorize pressure ulcers based on the depth of tissue injury.

15. Describe the staging system for pressure ulcers.

Box 30-3 presents the staging for pressure ulcers.

16. What is the difference between arterial and venous ulcers?

Wounds that are located on the lower extremities can be arterial (ischemic) ulcers or venous ulcers. *Arterial ulcers* have a primary cause of peripheral vascular disease that includes risk factors of smoking, hyperlipidemia, diabetes, and hypertension.

Arterial ulcers typically are located on the foot (between and on toes, metatarsal heads, pharyngeal heads), lateral malleolus, and pretibial region. Wound appearance of an arterial ulcer includes well-defined margins; black or necrotic tissue; and a deep, pale wound bed that does not bleed freely.

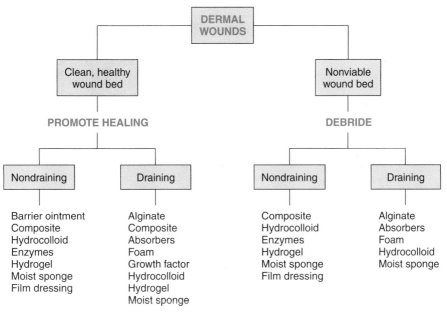

Figure 30-1. Dressings for dermal wounds.

Box 30-3. Stages of pressure ulcers

Stage I is an observable pressure-related alteration of intact skin for which indicators, compared with an adjacent or opposite area on the body, may include changes in one or more of the following:
- Skin temperature (warmth or coolness)
- Tissue consistency (firm or boggy feel)
- Sensation (pain, itching)

The ulcer appears as a defined area of persistent redness in lightly pigmented skin; whereas in darker skin tones the ulcer may appear with persistent red, blue, or purple hues.

Stage II is a partial-thickness wound and could be an intact blister.

Stage III is a full-thickness wound.

Stage IV is also a full-thickness wound that invades the muscle, tendon, and bone.

Stage III and Stage IV pressure ulcers can have necrotic and/or slough tissue and exudate. If all that can be visualized of a pressure ulcer is solid black eschar, that wound cannot be staged until the depth of the wound is visualized. Patients possibly can develop pressure ulcers during a surgical procedure. This type of pressure ulcer initially appears as a burnlike lesion or mottled skin.

Venous ulcers are located in the area of the ankles and medial malleolus. Skin changes of the lower extremity include nonpitting edema; reddish-brown discoloration (hemosiderin); evidence of healed ulcers; dilated, tortuous superficial veins; and increased warmth and edema with a history of deep vein thrombosis. The ulcer has uneven wound margins, ruddy granulation, and a superficial wound bed that bleeds easily. The primary cause is vein dysfunction related to an increase in venous pressure that leads to edema and eventually ulceration. Venous ulcers typically are seen in patients with congestive heart failure, incompetent valves in the venous system of the lower extremity, obesity, pregnancy, and muscle weakness caused by paralysis or arthritis. The primary treatment includes an absorptive dressing and compression of at least 40 to 50 mm Hg.

17. What is the VAC?

The acronym VAC stands for vacuum-assisted closure and is a product available from Kinetic Concepts Incorporated (San Antonio, Texas). The VAC is a negative pressure therapy system used to accelerate wound healing. This product is used to facilitate removal of excess wound fluid, stimulate granulation tissue production, and reduce the bacterial count. The product consists of a foam sponge that is placed in the wound bed and is sealed in place using an adhesive drape. A tube attached to a pump and placed within the dressing provides subatmospheric pressure. The use of negative pressure increases circulation to the wound environment, thereby increasing nutrition and oxygenation of the wound bed. This product is not recommended for use on wounds associated with cancer, fistula, necrotic tissue, or osteomyelitis.

18. What type of solution should the rehabilitation nurse use in a wound?

The safest solution to place in a wound is that which is safest to place in an eye: normal saline.

Dakin's fluid, acetic acid, povidone iodine (Betadine), and hydrogen peroxide should be used only for specific purposes and for short durations of time. Dakin's fluid and Betadine have a higher bactericidal effectiveness and lower cytotoxicity than acetic acid.
• Dakin's fluid (sodium hypochlorite) is diluted bleach in a 5:10 solution using distilled water that produces a 0.25% solution. Dakin's fluid is useful to dissolve necrotic tissue, control odor, and is bactericidal to staphylococci, streptococci, methacillin-resistant *Staphylococcus aureus, Klebsiella pneumoniae, Enterobacter cloacae, Serratia marcescens, Proteus mirabilis, Pseudomonas, Escherichia coli,* and *Bacteroides fragilis*. However, the fluid is cytotoxic at 0.25% to fibroblasts; therefore prolonged use of this solution inhibits wound healing. A noncytotoxic solution of Dakin's fluid is 0.005% (1:200), but the solution will not inhibit bacterial colonization or infection.
• Acetic acid is diluted vinegar and has been purported to be useful in managing *Pseudomonas* and gram-positive bacteria; however, recent data show a weak bactericidal effect. Acetic acid changes the color of exudates and destroys fibroblasts.
• Povidone-iodine solution contains 10% polyvinylpyrrolidone iodine that is water-soluble iodine bound to polyvinylpyrrolidone and a synthetic polymer.

Betadine is effective against *Staphylococcus aureus* and should never be used with débriding agents. As with the other chemical solutions, Betadine destroys fibroblasts, dries the wound bed, discolors the wound bed and surrounding tissue, and is a chemical irritant.

- Hydrogen peroxide usually is used to manage anaerobic bacteria; however, its cytotoxicity outweighs its bactericidal effect. Hydrogen peroxide always should be flushed out of a wound bed because it is an irritant to granulation tissue. Incidents also have been reported of pulmonary emboli caused by hydrogen peroxide used to irrigate a wound, forcing the effervesent bubbles into the vascular system.

Key Points

- Free oxygen radicals cause damage to the epithelium, so patients should be given antioxidants to combat the destruction.
- To differentiate between inflammation in a wound and a local infection of the site is important.
- The nurse should culture wounds only when pink healthy tissue is present in the wound environment and after cleansing with saline.
- Choosing a wound dressing is based on the functions of the dressing and the type of wound needing care.
- The staging system for pressure ulcers categorizes the ulcer based on the depth of the tissue damage.
- Vacuum-assisted closure is a negative pressure therapy system used to accelerate wound healing.
- The safest solution to place in a wound is normal saline.

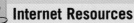

Internet Resources

Wound, Ostomy and Continence Nurses Society
http://www.wocn.org

American Academy of Wound Management
http://www.aawm.org

Association for the Advancement of Wound Care
http://www.aawc1.com/

National Pressure Ulcer Advisory Panel
http://www.npuap.org

Wound Care Society
http://www.woundcaresociety.org

Bibliography

1. Aronovitch SA: Dressing sponges: how do you decide which one to use, *Nursing 95* 25(7):52-54, 1995.
2. Doughty D: A rational approach to the use of topical antiseptics, *J Wound Ostomy Continence Nurs* 21(6):224-231, 1994.
3. Smith C: Oxygen, oxygen free radicals and reperfusion injury, *Wounds* 8(1):9-15, 1996.
4. Stotts NA: Nutritional assessment and support. In Bryant R, editor: *Acute and chronic wounds: nursing management,* St Louis, 2000, Mosby-Year Book.
5. Wysocli AB: Anatomy and physiology of skin and soft tissue. In Bryant R, editor: *Acute and chronic wounds: nursing management,* St Louis, 2000, Mosby-Year Book.

Chapter 31

Palliative Care and End-of-Life Issues

Denise A. Tucker

1. **The patient has an advance directive and was diagnosed with pneumonia and a stroke. The physician wrote a do-not-resuscitate (DNR) order on the patient's chart. Why is this patient, at the end of life, receiving rehabilitation if the patient will not be getting well?**

   Patients at the end of their lives may need rehabilitation too. One should remember that the focus of their care is not necessarily the same as for relatively healthy, younger patients. The focus of care for patients nearing the end of their lives is comfort measures and palliative care. Returning to a higher level of functioning may assist these patients in becoming more comfortable. The health care providers, working in concert with the family and an interdisciplinary team, support these patients to help them achieve their highest level of functioning. One should remember that prognostic predictions are uncertain; no one ever has achieved 100% accuracy at predicting when death will occur. Even when patients have been diagnosed with terminal illnesses and their deaths have been predicted within 6 months, they may survive weeks, months, or even years longer than the original predictions. These patients deserve to live life to the fullest extent possible while they are able to do so.

   Therefore one should not think it unusual at all to see patients with DNR orders and advance directives who are in rehabilitation facilities or are receiving aggressive therapy. These patients greatly benefit from rehabilitation principles and techniques, and this enhances their quality of life. The patients may even go home when the acute crisis is resolved, at which time the DNR order is no longer active.

2. **How is the best quality of life for the patient determined?**

   Quality of life is individual and unique for each person; it may not be assumed or ascribed to another person without knowing the frame of reference from which the person comes. Quality of life is one of the highest considerations when providing care for patients. Only through holistic assessment and discussion with the patient and/or family can a patient goal be set.

3. **The patient is on "comfort measures only," receiving 3 to 5 mg morphine sulfate intravenously as needed for shortness of breath or pain. The patient**

has needed progressively higher doses over the past few days. Is morphine the best choice for pain relief for this patient?

Patients at the end of their lives frequently require opioid medications for pain and symptom management. Morphine is an excellent choice for this type of patient because morphine
  • Increases venous pooling, thus decreasing preload and the workload on the heart
  • Decreases the work of breathing, relieving respiratory symptoms
  • Decreases anxiety, allowing for relaxation

4. **Patients are afraid to use the morphine because they think they might become addicted. How can the nurse assure them?**

Studies have shown repeatedly that patients receiving medication for actual pain rarely become addicted to the medication. Actually, patients tend to receive less medication for pain than is therapeutic. If patients receive pain medication at an adequate level for their pain, and when they actually need it, addiction is not an issue.

5. **What is physical dependence on a drug?**

Patients may become physically dependent on opioid medications. Physical dependence means that if the drug were withdrawn after having been given over a period of time, during which the body has become physiologically accustomed to receiving the medication, the patient would suffer withdrawal symptoms such as nausea or feelings of malaise. If such a drug is to be withdrawn, typically the patient is weaned gradually from the drug to decrease the probability of withdrawal symptoms.

6. **Is drug tolerance the same as addiction?**

Tolerance to the drug occurs when the body becomes accustomed to maintaining certain levels of medication in the bloodstream; the body becomes adept at clearing the drug from the system, taking shorter and shorter times to do so; and higher doses are required to achieve the same effect. Tolerance is not the same as addiction; addiction is more of a psychological desire for the medication, whereas tolerance is a physiological occurrence in any person receiving doses of the drug over time. Patients who have developed addictions repeatedly report the desire to use the drug, even if they are physically harmed from its use; they have developed cravings for the drug; and they cannot control their compulsive use of the drug. This is to be expected with morphine, an opioid medication. Because morphine has no dose ceiling, higher doses may be prescribed if the patient continues to be monitored.

7. **What is the likelihood of the patient receiving such a high dose of morphine that respiratory depression is occurs?**

Patients who have been receiving continuous doses of morphine or other opioid agents become physiologically accustomed to the medication. Therefore the likelihood that the patient will suffer respiratory depression is minimized if the dose has been increased gradually, while the patient is monitored continuously for respiratory difficulties. Respiratory depression is most likely to occur when opioid medications are first administered in the beginning stages of treatment with the medication.

8. **The patient has a DNR order and is in intense pain. The nurse has been giving the patient high doses of morphine. The nurse asks the rehabilitation advanced practice nurse, "What if, after I give the patient this dose of pain medication, the patient dies right then?"**

If the patient is nearing the end of life and the morphine will relieve the pain, why should the medication not be given, even if it hastens the patient's death? The patient already has a DNR order written by the physician and has requested pain medication. The intent of the medication is not to hasten death but to ease pain.

Because giving morphine or other pain medication actually may hasten the patient's death, however, some nurses are uncomfortable filling such a request. The "principle of double effect," or the "last dose syndrome," occurs when the following three principles are true:
- The actual act is not intrinsically wrong in itself.
- The good effect occurs directly because of the action.
- The good effect is desirable enough that the risk of the bad effect occurring is acceptable.

Thus even though morphine may depress respirations and lower the blood pressure, the relief of pain as a result of the morphine injection generally compensates for its administration.

Some nurses may feel uncomfortable giving medications near the end of life for fear of affecting the timing or cause of the patient's death. The nurse must remember that the person is dying from the disease process; the medication is intended to relieve pain. Nurses may ask another nurse to administer the medication when uncomfortable doing so, if that is an option under the circumstances.

9. **The patient's daughter is afraid that if she requests a "DNR" status in the hospital, the nurses and physicians will not provide care for her mother in the same manner as other patients. Does a DNR order also mean the patient will not be cared for?**

No, DNR does not mean *do not care*. A DNR order is a physician's order stating that the person will not be resuscitated in the event of a cardiac or respiratory arrest.

Priorities have shifted from curative treatment—which often includes aggressive therapies such as cardiopulmonary resuscitation, endotracheal intubation and placement on mechanical ventilation, defibrillation or cardioversion, and vasopressive medications to increase blood pressure and regulate the heart beat—to carative treatment, including aggressive pain management and symptom control. Carative therapy provides comfort to the patient and also is identified as palliative care or "comfort measures only." Patients, at the end of their lives, require palliative care to increase their comfort and assist them in the dying process. Aggressive treatment aimed at prolonging an inevitable death may greatly increase the patient's/family's suffering during its administration.

10. **What is palliative care?**

Palliative care has at its goal the control of uncomfortable symptoms and pain management. The aim is to comfort the patient (and family members) and relieve pain and suffering. Health care providers who administer palliative care must view the patient holistically and take into account all aspects of the patient's care. An interdisciplinary team—made up of nurses, physicians, aides, physical therapists, respiratory therapists, spiritual advisors, music therapists, and others—works with the patients and their families as a unit. The team's focus is that death is accepted as the normal progression of life, and care is based on the symptoms presented by the patient. Care is individualized because this process is subjective and differs for each patient.

11. **The patient has pain medication that is combined with acetaminophen. What concerns should the rehabilitation nurse have when giving these types of medications?**

The nurse should be cautious when administering pain medications with acetaminophen. Acetaminophen has a dose ceiling of 4 g per 24 hours; if more acetaminophen is given, liver damage might occur and the patient could present with distressing gastrointestinal signs and symptoms. Hydrocodone/acetaminophen (Lortab) and oxycodone/acetaminophen (Percocet) are examples of medications combined with acetaminophen.

If the patient is in a unit with self-administration of medications, or if the patient is at home and family are responsible for medications, the nurse should teach the patient to limit acetaminophen use to 4 g or less daily. If the pain is not controlled with the appropriate dose, another type of analgesic agent may be necessary. The rehabilitation nurse should reassess the patient for changes in physical condition before the medication is changed.

12. **What medications, other than narcotics, might be given for patients with chronic pain?**

The nurse may anticipate epidural or intrathecal administration of opioids or local anesthetic agents. Additionally, nonopioid analgesic agents may be administered. Such agents might include nonsteroidal antiinflammatory drugs, steroids, tricyclic antidepressants, anticonvulsants, muscle relaxants, or benzodiazepines. Topical analgesics and anesthetic agents also may be applied directly to the affected area. These medications are considered adjuvant therapy for patients with chronic pain and are prescribed often for patients with chronic pain, especially at the end of life.

13. Can anything else be done for patients with chronic pain?

Direct peripheral nerve and spinal cord stimulation may be administered in an attempt to decrease the sensation of pain. Surgery is required to implant the stimulation device, however. Nerve blocks and trigger point injections also may be administered to decrease the sensation of pain. Transcutaneous electrical nerve stimulation is a treatment that has been shown to be effective for pain relief in a variety of conditions. Electrodes are placed on the skin and electrical current applied at different pulse rates (frequencies) and intensities stimulates these areas so as to provide pain relief.

Nonpharmacological therapies also may be administered for patients whose pain is unrelieved. Cognitive-behavioral therapies, such as support groups, guided imagery, relaxation techniques, distraction, spiritual counseling, prayer, and cognitive reframing may be useful. Physical measures such as turning and repositioning the patient, applying heat or cold to affected areas, and massage also may be useful to decrease painful stimuli.

14. The home care rehabilitation nurse needs to switch the patient from an oral analgesic to an equivalent intravenous dose. Should the nurse give the same dose of the medication?

The nurse should check an equianalgesic table (Table 31-1) to ensure that the correct dosage is given to the patient. Typically, smaller doses are needed when the medication is given intravenously or intramuscularly; larger doses are needed for the oral route. If too much medication is given to the patient, an unintended overdose might occur.

15. The terminally ill patient has signs and symptoms of discomfort other than the documented pain. What do these include?

Signs and symptoms of discomfort may include
- Respiratory symptoms, such as dyspnea and cough
- Gastrointestinal symptoms, such as anorexia, constipation or diarrhea, and nausea
- General and systemic problems of fatigue and weakness
- Psychological symptoms, such as depression and anxiety.

16. How should the nurse address the problems of discomfort?

A thorough assessment of all body systems is important to do first. Diagnostic testing may be undertaken to determine the cause of the problem, but the risk-benefit ratio, as well as patient prognosis and current condition, must be kept in mind before any testing is implemented. If an acute, treatable crisis has occurred that can be determined by testing, then testing is warranted. Symptomatic con-

Table 31-1. **Equianalgesic dosing information**

Medication	Parenteral dose	Oral dose
Buprenorphine	0.3-0.4 mg q 6-8 hours	—
Butorphanol	2 mg q 3-4 hours	—
Codeine	75 mg q 3-4 hours	130 mg q 3-4 hours
Hydrocodone	—	30 mg q 3-4 hours
Hydromorphone	1.5 mg q 3-4 hours	7.5 mg q 3-4 hours
Levorphanol	2 mg q 6-8 hours	4 mg q 6-8 hours
Meperidine	100 mg q 3 hours	300 mg q 3-4 hours
Methadone	10 mg q 6-8 hours	20 mg q 6-8 hours
Morphine	10 mg q 3-4 hours	30 mg q 3-4 hours
Nalbuphine	10 mg q 3-4 hours	—
Oxycodone	—	30 mg q 3-4 hours
Oxymorphone	1 mg q 3-4 hours	—
Pentazocine	60 mg q 3-4 hours	150 mg q 3-4 hours

Please note that the advanced practice rehabilitation nurse must review each patient's clinical response to specific medications and dosages. Although the given dosages are approximately equal, there may be individual variations with differing medications and dosages.

One must use caution when changing medications from one type to another (for example, from meperidine to morphine): the possibility exists that the patient may not be able to tolerate a different medication at that equianalgesic dose. Therefore the advanced practice nurse may need to begin the second medication at a lower dose and reevaluate patient response.

trol is necessary even when the patient's disease is incurable.

17. **What can be done for respiratory complaints?**

The rehabilitation nurse teaches the patient/family strategies in energy conservation for the patient. Respiratory symptoms of dyspnea may be relieved by
- Repositioning the patient, elevating the head of bed
- Oxygen administration
- Pursed-lip breathing
- Indirect room fans that can increase the circulation of air
- Chest physiotherapy
- Caffeinated beverages that may improve ventilation (dilation of bronchi)
- Relaxation and guided imagery that may relieve anxiety that exacerbates dyspnea

18. **What can be done to relieve the gastrointestinal problems?**

Gastrointestinal symptoms may be treated by medications specific to the cause, such as appetite stimulants for anorexia and antiemetics for nausea. Dietary modifications specific to constipation, such as increased fluids and fiber, or clear liquids for patients with diarrhea, may be instituted.

19. Will any care help fatigue and weakness?

Physical and occupational therapy may be helpful for severe fatigue. Gentle range-of-motion exercises can help alleviate weakness. Maintaining a regular wake-sleep schedule that mimics the patient's usual circadian rhythm as much as possible can help alleviate fatigue.

20. What should be done for depression and anxiety?

Medications may be indicated specifically for anxiety and depression, along with counseling. Many emotional issues stem from fears and emotions that are difficult to discuss or confront. Much can be achieved through active listening and guided discussion. If these concerns become problematic, further counseling may be indicated.

Many medications specific to typical symptoms that occur at the end of life are available today. The hospice nurse is a valuable resource for the rehabilitation nurse when exploring options and should be consulted.

Key Points

- Patients receiving analgesics for actual pain rarely become addicted.
- The likelihood that a patient will develop respiratory depression from gradual increments of opioids is unlikely because the body becomes physiologically accustomed to the medication, even in high doses.
- Palliative care aims to control discomfort in all categories and considers holistic needs of the patient at any point in the patient's life, not just as end-of-life care.

Internet Resources

Center to Advance Palliative Care
http://www.capc.org

National Hospice and Palliative Care Organization
http://www.nhpco.org

Pain Medicine and Palliative Care
http://www.stoppain.org

International Association for Hospice and Palliative Care
http://www.hospicecare.com

Palliative Care
http://www.growthhouse.org/palliat.html

Bibliography

1. Coyle N, Layman-Goldstein M: Pain assessment and management in palliative care. In Matzo ML, Sherman DW, editors: *Palliative care nursing: quality care to the end of life,* New York, 2001, Springer.

2. Eagan KA, Labyak MJ: Hospice care: a model for quality end-of-life care. In Ferrell BR, Coyle N, editors: *Textbook of palliative nursing,* New York, 2001, Oxford University Press.

3. End-of-Life Nursing Education Consortium: ELNEC training program (revised), Robert Wood Johnson Foundation, January 2003.

4. Fink R, Gates R: Pain assessment. In Ferrell BR, Coyle N, editors: *Textbook of palliative nursing,* New York, 2001, Oxford University Press.

5. Kazanowski MK: Symptom management in palliative care. In Matzo ML, Sherman DW, editors: *Palliative care nursing: quality care to the end of life,* New York, 2001, Springer.

6. Kuebler KK, Berry PH: End-of-life care. In Kuebler KK, Berry PH, Heidrich DE, editors: *End-of-life care: clinical practice guidelines,* Philadelphia, 2002, WB Saunders.

7. McCaffery M, Pasero C: *Pain clinical manual,* ed 2, St Louis, 1999, Mosby.

8. Mickle J: Cancer pain management. In St Marie B: *Core curriculum for pain management nursing,* Philadelphia, 2002, WB Saunders.

9. Paice JA, Fine PG: Pain at the end-of-life. In Ferrell BR, Coyle N, editors: *Textbook of palliative nursing,* New York, 2002, Oxford University Press.

10. Super A: The context of palliative care in progressive illness. In Ferrell BR, Coyle N, editors: *Textbook of palliative nursing,* New York, 2001, Oxford University Press.

11. Vasco MR, Guiterrez K: Opioid analgesics. In Guiterrez K, Queener SG, editors: *Pharmacology for nursing practice,* St Louis, 2003, Mosby.

Chapter 32

Pediatric Rehabilitation

Susan R. Bulecza

1. **When planning care for children with disabilities, are there any main differences between children and adults that need to be considered?**

   The three main differences to consider for children with disabilities are presented in Box 32-1.

Box 32-1. **Special considerations for children with disabilities**

- First, child development is dynamic, and different developmental stages alter the child's needs and outcomes. Illness and disability can delay or arrest normal development.
- Second, the epidemiology of childhood disabilities differs from adults in that there are many rare or low-incidence conditions and few common ones; whereas adult disabilities often consist of few rare conditions and several common ones.
- Third, children's health and development largely depend on their families' health and socioeconomic status.

---

2. **What impact do differences between children and adults have on rehabilitation nursing care?**

   The differences between care for children and adults can have significant negative impact if the rehabilitation nurse does not understand them as they influence timing of services, goals, interventions, and outcomes, follow-up frequency, and role of caregiver. For example, a 3-year-old child predominantly uses diaphragmatic abdominal breathing. Therefore placement of braces or casts that restrict abdominal movement will restrict breathing.

   Physiological differences occur in all body systems and processes. Functional differences exist in the areas of mobility, self-care, skin care, bowel and bladder care, spasticity, social interaction and behaviors, and cognitive function and learning.

3. **How important are screening and assessment tools for pediatric rehabilitation nursing?**

A number of tools are designed specifically for assessing a child's abilities and limitations. By using these tools, the nurse and collaborative partners can collect a wealth of information for use in care planning, resulting in more individualized goals, interventions, and outcomes. Additionally, these tools can be used to evaluate interventions by providing a standardized measure of progress.

Table 32-1 presents some of the more frequently used tools and the appropriate use age range. This list is not an exhaustive list of all tools available.

Table 32-1. Age-appropriate assessment tools

Tool	Age
Pediatric Evaluation of Disability Inventory	6 months to 7 years
Functional Independence Measure for Children (WeeFIM)	6 months to 7 years
Bayley Scales for Infant Development II (Psychomotor Scale)	Birth to 36 months
Vineland Adaptive Behavior Scales	Birth to adult
Peabody Pictures Vocabulary Test—Revised	1-18 years
Peabody Developmental Motor Scales and Activity Cards	Birth to 6.11 years
Test of Early Language Development	2-8 years
Uzgiris-Hunt Ordinal Scales of Development	Birth to 24 months
Denver Developmental Screening II	1 week to 6 years
Miller Assessment for Preschoolers	2 years 9 months to 6 years 2 months
Hawaii Early Learning Profile	Birth to 36 months and 3-6 years
Home Observation for Measurement of the Environment	Birth to elementary age
Gesell Developmental Schedules	Birth to 6 years
Bruininks-Oseretsky Test of Motor Proficiency	4.6-14.6 years
McCarthy Scales of Children's Abilities	2.6-8.6 years
AAMR Adaptive Behavior Scale	3-16 years
Bender Gestalt Test	<3 years and 5-10 years
Minnesota Developmental Inventories	Infant to 15 months and 6 months to 6 years
Early Intervention Developmental Profile	Birth to 36 months
Sequenced Inventory of Communication Development—Revised	4-48 months
Infant and Toddler Temperament Questionnaires	4-8 months and 12-36 months
Gross Motor Function Measure	5 months to 16 years
Leiter International Performance Scale	2 years to adult
Test of Visual Motor Skills	2-13 years
Toddler and Infant Motor Evaluation	Birth to 42 months
Brigance Inventory of Early Development—Revised	Birth to 7 years
Milani-Comparetti Motor Development Screening Test	Birth to 3 years

4. **Why is beginning childhood-to-adult transition planning early important for children with disabilities?**

Frequently young persons with disabilities find themselves entering adulthood ill prepared to navigate the adult health care system or able to meet their self-care needs. To address the issues of self-care, education, employment, and independent living early in the rehabilitation process is important for maximum independence to be achieved. Families must be engaged and educated on the importance of addressing these issues early and understanding how successful transition through early developmental stages sets the pace for later transition. Social isolation and low expectations are major barriers to successful adulthood transition. Suggested activities with approximate ages for consideration in enhancing transition are found in Table 32-2.

Table 32-2.   Age-specific activities to enhance transition from childhood to adulthood

Age	Activities
Birth to 10 years	Encourage doing for self.
	Allow child to assist with family chores.
	Encourage interaction/participation in different activities and settings.
	Assist the child in taking responsibility for health care needs including talking with providers.
	Encourage children to talk about what they might like to be when they become adults.
10-14 years	Discuss career interest and how level of ability would affect various careers.
	With the child, identify school and community resources that provide employment opportunities, aptitude assessment, and vocational rehabilitation programs.
	Encourage and develop the child's ability to provide own self-care or to direct personal care attendants and to take responsibility for taking own medications.
	Encourage children to become their own advocates to meet their needs.
	Begin adult transition planning process, which includes school needs/resources, health care needs/resources, community resources, and independent living requirements.
14-20 years	Discuss with child how level of ability affects future health, including sexuality and expected body changes, vocation choice, marriage, and children.
	With child, identify and apply for appropriate financial and health care insurance resources such as supplemental security income, Medicaid, or private insurance.
	Assist child with finding an adult health care provider and transition from the pediatric provider.

5. **What federal guidelines exist for ensuring that children with disabilities receive appropriate accommodations in an educational setting?**

The federal law titled Individuals with Disabilities Education Act provides legal directives for ensuring that children with disabilities receive free, appropriate education. The law sets forth requirements, including nursing service standards for schools to develop an individualized education plan detailing accommodations necessary to create an environment appropriate for the child to succeed. School guidance counselors and the school district's office of exceptional student education are excellent resources for information and assistance.

6. **Are there nursing standards for pediatric rehabilitation practice?**

Several nursing standards for pediatric rehabilitation practice are available. The Association of Rehabilitation Nurses has published the "Pediatric Rehabilitation Nursing Role Description." Additionally, the "National Standards of Nursing Practice for Early Intervention Services" and "Care of Children and Adolescents with Special Health and Developmental Needs" have been developed.

7. **Is case management important in pediatric rehabilitation?**

Case management services are a critical service component for children with disabilities. In many cases pediatric rehabilitation nurses function in the role of case manager. Specific skills in the following areas are necessary to function in this role: assessment, care planning, evaluation, leadership, service delivery, quality assurance, and resource identification and utilization. These services need to be family centered and community based.

8. **What factors can affect nutrition?**

Children with disabilities are at high risk for alterations in feeding and nutrition because of anatomical, developmental, sensory, neuromotor, and psychosocial environmental conditions. Ongoing assessment is critical to ensure the child and family are able to compensate successfully and adapt to meet the child's nutritional needs. The more significant the disability or condition, the more potentially complex feeding and meeting nutritional needs become.

9. **Is obesity a risk for children with disabilities?**

Obesity is a risk factor for children with disabilities for several reasons:
- First, the child may not be able to indicate satiation to the care provider because of disability or developmental delay.
- Second, nutritional needs may be less than the volume of parenteral feeding being administered, resulting in overfeeding.
- Third, the child receives the standard number of calories for age without consideration for level of ability and activity or condition.
- Additionally, a child who is obese also may be receiving inadequate nutrition.

Consultation with a registered dietitian with experience and knowledge in nutritional management of children with disabilities or chronic conditions is important to meet nutritional needs.

10. What are some special considerations related to children with disabilities or chronic conditions regarding elimination patterns?

Bowel and bladder control and establishment of elimination patterns in "normal" children often can be frustrating and problematic for care providers but resolve as the child matures. However, a child with disabilities or chronic conditions may have unique challenges related to elimination and require establishment of a pattern that differs from conventional norms, which can be difficult for family and caregivers. Management requires team collaboration to establish the new "normal" and help anticipate needs related to the disability. Conditions that affect cognitive, sensory, and motor functioning and medications that alter bowel or bladder function can affect the child's and family's ability to manage elimination significantly. The pediatric rehabilitation nurse may need to be more involved for a longer period of time and provide more education for successful elimination patterns to be achieved. One must remember that the child needs to be involved in the performance of the bowel and bladder program as early as possible and to the maximum level of ability. Special consideration should be given to adapting procedures so that the child can perform activities as independently as possible.

11. What is the most common skin integrity problem in pediatric rehabilitation?

Pressure ulcers are the most common problem. Pressure ulcers most often occur with children who have insensate skin or are immobile. Most often breakdown occurs over bony prominences. However, very young children who are becoming more mobile but have lower extremity immobility, causing dragging of the lower limbs can have breakdown on toes, knees, and abdomen. Casts and braces are also frequent contributors to skin breakdown.

12. How does disability affect development of motor skills?

Obviously, a disability that is physically limiting affects normal motor skill development. However, the nurse needs to understand that learning through movement is a major developmental aspect and needs to be considered when a child is learning alternative methods of mobility. Young children are focused on motor movement and do not have the cognitive ability to assess the situation for danger. For instance, a young child learning to use an electrical wheelchair for the first time will be focused totally on the newfound mobility and will be unable to attend to obstacles in the way. Therefore the caregiver must ensure the path is clear.

13. Statistics show that injury is the leading cause of death for children under 19 years old. Are children with disabilities at higher risk?

Children with disabilities are at higher risk for injury because of several factors. Ambulatory children with cognitive disability may go outside safe environments into areas posing harm, such as streets and woods. Therefore to ensure safety measures are in place, such as door locks and fences, is important to lessen the risk. Likewise, children who use equipment for mobility and their caregivers need to be given instruction on proper safety equipment such as seat belts and proper use. Good communication between the child's caregiver and health care providers is key to ensuring that the child is given optimal opportunity for motor development without restriction from unfounded fear of injury.

14. **What are some of the sexuality issues relating to children with disabilities?**

Often children with disabilities are not provided with information on sexuality and how their disability affects sexual/reproductive potential. The nurse should discuss developmental patterns and stages pertaining to sexuality, such as gender identity, puberty, and sexual identity, with the child's caregivers at the appropriate intervals to develop compensation strategies specific to the child's disability, ensuring healthy sexual development. Special consideration needs to be given to children with obvious physical disabilities, for these may present barriers that increase isolation and limit social skill development.

As the child reaches adolescence and young adulthood, addressing sexual ability and issues such as pregnancy, birth control, sexually transmitted diseases, fertility, and genetic risk is essential. This is important for children with cognitive, as well as physical, disabilities.

15. **Do spiritual and religious beliefs positively influence children's and families' coping ability during rehabilitation?**

In general, families often report increased levels of spiritual support and more frequent engagement in religious activities when coping with illness/disability and subsequent rehabilitation. These families also report a greater level of adjustment. Additionally, when families attribute blame to fate or God's will for their children's situation, they are more likely to be better adjusted than families who blame themselves or the environment.

16. **Is a resource available for information on transporting children with special needs?**

The American Academy of Pediatrics published a document titled "Car Seat Shopping Guide for Children with Special Needs." The document can be found online at www.aap.org.

17. **Can car safety seats be obtained for short-term use?**

Often local and state resources are available that loan or rent specialty car seats. Each state, within its health or human services departments, has an office whose activities are devoted to children with special health care needs. This office can assist in identifying available resources.

18. **Before a child can be discharged home, what must be considered?**

Two main areas that must be considered are home environment and physical challenges of everyday life. An assessment of the home needs to be conducted before discharge to determine what modifications are needed and what special equipment will be necessary to accommodate the child's needs. If the child attends school and will be returning to the school environment, an assessment of the school needs to be conducted, as well as discussions with school personnel regarding necessary accommodations for an optimal learning environment. These accommodations may include an adjusted school day schedule; provision of a nurse or aid, and development of emergency plans, as well as school fire and evacuation plans specific to the child's health needs. Transportation issues need to be addressed as well. One comprehensive resource available to assist in planning is the "Children and Youth Assisted by Medical Technology in Educational Settings: Guidelines for Care" by Porter, Haynie, Bierle, and others. This document can provide guidance from entrance planning to staff skills checklists. A rehabilitation nurse or rehabilitation counselor, in collaboration with the facility's interdisciplinary team, should conduct this planning.

19. **What are the most common congenital central nervous system anomalies?**

Neural tube defects are the most common congenital anomalies that result when the neural tube fails to close. Spina bifida results when the spinal column fails to close. Box 32-2 presents the three types of spina bifida.

Box 32-2. Types of spina bifida

- Myelomenigocele (open spinal column with external sac containing neural tissue, spinal fluid, and possibly nerve fibers)
- Meningocele (open spinal column with external sac containing meninges)
- Myeloschisis (flattened spinal cord without meninges and often without skin covering)

Myelomeningocele is the most common, and myeloschisis is one of the most severe. All of these forms result in varying degrees of central nervous system, neuromuscular, and skeletal dysfunction and deformity. Physical and functional limitation depend on location and extent of lesion, primarily affecting lower extremity and bowel/bladder function. Cognitive function may be affected as well.

20. **What are the more common needs or problems for children with spina bifida?**

Latex allergy is a common problem for children with spina bifida, and potential development should be assessed continually. Ongoing surgical needs such as ventriculoperitoneal shunt revision and orthopedic correction are necessary as the child grows. These surgeries often require a degree of rehabilitation management in the postoperative phase. Additionally, frequent monitoring of the genitourinary system is required to minimize infection and enhance function. A comprehensive bowel and bladder program developed with extensive education provided to the child's caregivers is critical to ensure compliance. This plan needs to be reviewed periodically to ensure understanding, knowledge and ability to perform required skills, nutritional needs, how to handle social issues, and helping the child to gain independence with care.

21. What is cerebral palsy?

Cerebral palsy is a nonprogressive disorder that occurs before birth or during the birth process as a result of injury to the areas in the brain that affect purposeful movement and coordination. Even though this disorder is nonprogressive, periodic evaluation is needed to assess the child's growth and for any complications that can occur because of abnormal muscle tone. Additionally, these children are at risk for developmental delay and vision problems.

22. Are there different types of cerebral palsy?

Yes, Box 32-3 presents the four main types of cerebral palsy.

Box 32-3. Types of cerebral palsy

- Spastic: Characterized by abnormal reflexes and muscle tone with motor weakness and spasm; hemiplegia is the most frequent type
- Athetoid: Characterized by abnormal involuntary movement involving all extremities and facial muscles that disappear during sleep
- Ataxic: Characterized by hypotonia with coordination impairment; least common type
- Mixed: Combination of any of the above types; severe cognitive delay is frequently present

---

23. What are the major management issues with cerebral palsy?

Major management issues are nutritional, surgical, and functional ability. Nutritional assessment should be ongoing because energy requirements are increased so as to accomplish daily activities, but intake may be inadequate because of eating difficulties. Surgical intervention may be necessary at different intervals to improve function and reduce complications. Rehabilitation may be required postoperatively to optimize function. Ongoing assessment is required to determine functional abilities as the child moves through developmental stages so as to determine the need for more or different assistive devices and equipment. Bowel/bladder function and management should be a part of the assessment, for bowel/bladder dysfunction is common. Management of spasticity should be a high priority to maximize functional ability. Medications frequently are used for control and may require trials of different types before finding the most effective. For the rehabilitation nurse to conduct the assessment is important so that the nurse knows the child's method of communication to assess correctly developmental level and behaviors.

24. What are the most common craniofacial anomalies and their management issues?

The most common craniofacial anomalies are cleft lip with or without cleft palate and cleft palate alone. The degree, location, and severity of the cleft determines the level of feeding difficulty, middle ear disease risk, dental problems, and speech/hearing difficulty. Because initial repair is done early in life, maintenance of adequate nutrition is important to ensure optimal surgical weight.

25. Can an infant with a cleft be breast-fed?

Yes, the degree and location of the cleft determines whether the child can attach to the breast or whether the mother needs to pump the milk and deliver it via another method.

26. What are the main considerations the pediatric rehabilitation nurse should know regarding limb deficiencies in children?

Periodic assessment is needed to ensure proper fit of the prosthesis as the child grows and that the stump skin remains intact. The nurse should educate the child and caregiver on proper stump care and prosthetic maintenance to minimize skin breakdown and trauma to the site. The nurse also should provide information regarding phantom pain and potential occurrence. Provision of psychosocial support and counseling to children with limb deficiencies is important, especially those with traumatic or disease-related surgical amputation, so that they develop a positive self-esteem.

27. What is the most common neuromuscular disease in children?

Duchenne's muscular dystrophy is the most common neuromuscular disease in children, primarily affecting males, with only rare occurrence in females. Because this is a progressively debilitating disease that leads to death, the goal of care should be to maintain functional ability as long as possible. Periodic assessment is necessary to ensure that appropriate assistive devices are provided based on level of functional ability. Respiratory muscles often are affected late in the disease process; and the child or young adult becomes ventilator dependent, increasing the risk for pneumonia.

28. What is osteogenesis imperfecta?

Osteogenesis imperfecta is a group of inherited connective tissue disorders. These disorders result in brittle bones, increasing susceptibility to fracture,

short stature, and deformity. The four different types, I to IV, occur based on genetic variation.
- Type I: considered mild
- Type II: most severe
- Type III: moderately severe
- Type IV: considered mild

In addition to skeletal abnormality, other characteristic features are blue sclera, teeth abnormalities, and deafness (with some types). Some frequent complications are respiratory failure, quadriplegia, brainstem compression, and hydrocephalus in adolescence or adulthood. An important note is that the majority of these children have normal cognitive function and intelligence.

29. **What are key rehabilitation nursing actions regarding a child with osteogenesis imperfecta?**

The following are key rehabilitation nursing actions for children with osteogenesis imperfecta:
- Education of caregivers about the disease is critical to reduce the injury risk for the child. Content should focus on what osteogenesis imperfecta is, reducing fracture risk, proper positioning, treatment options, and use of supportive devices.
- Emotional support is another area of emphasis so the family is able to handle the complexity of care and deal with the psychosocial aspects of a child with a significantly disabling condition.
- Ongoing physical and developmental assessments are essential so that fractures are identified quickly and potential developmental delay is identified for appropriate intervention and guidance.
- Repetitive surgical management of fractures and for preventive support is a frequent therapy for these children, who require postoperative nursing interventions focused on maintaining function, pain management, and reducing complications.

30. **Is osteogenesis imperfecta sometimes mistaken for child abuse?**

Yes, therefore careful evaluation and history taking are important for differentiation. Misdiagnosis of osteogenesis imperfecta as child abuse can result in severe consequences for the child and family.

31. **What is important to know about congenital heart disease?**

A variety of anomalies are categorized under congenital heart disease. The severity of symptoms, ability to repair the anomaly, and residual limitations affect function and developmental outcomes. Education regarding care needs, limitations, and technological support are key for caregivers to feel competent to care for the child. Sensitive and appropriate psychosocial care for the family is also important to reduce high levels of fear and anxiety that are often present even with the simplest heart condition.

32. Does Guillain-Barré Syndrome occur in children and adolescents?

Yes, however, the syndrome is not so common. Management of the syndrome is similar to management in adults, except special consideration needs to be given to school issues and minimizing disruption of education.

33. What are the special considerations for a child with diabetes mellitus?

Although insulin-dependent diabetes mellitus (type 1) is the most common in children, the incidence of type 2 in children has been increasing. Manifestation and medical management of both types is similar to that for adults. Differences occur in education regarding blood glucose monitoring and insulin administration because a parent or other caregiver, as well as the child, will need to be given instruction. Additionally, collaboration with the school nurse and other school staff is essential to ensure understanding of the disease, accommodations needed in the school environment, and emergency management. Training of school personnel in blood glucose testing may be needed as well.

34. What is cystic fibrosis?

Cystic fibrosis is an inherited genetic disease. Both parents must be carriers in order for the child to develop the disease. Cystic fibrosis can affect multiple systems but mainly affects respiration and digestion. This disease affects the exocrine glands, causing them to produce thick, sticky secretions. These secretions clog the bronchi, small intestine, and pancreas, resulting in difficult breathing, poor gas exchange, and impaired absorption of fats and protein. Although advances in medical care have resulted in longer life expectancies and usually about half of affected persons will live to 30 years old, still no cure is available. Treatment focuses on managing symptoms and preventing complications because affected children frequently have recurring respiratory infections and poor weight gain.

35. What are the important care aspects for a child with cystic fibrosis?

Important care aspects for children with cystic fibrosis are
- Respiratory: maintaining airway patency and optimizing lung function through postural drainage, chest physiotherapy, and inhalation therapy
- Nutrition: assessing weight and growth, supplement use and knowledge, and elimination patterns
- Psychosocial: This disease has significant impact on the child and family. They need assistance in dealing with emotions related to the disease and its incurability, promoting optimal development, and achieving a balance between protection and independence.

36. What are the goals of nursing care when caring for a child with burns?

The goals of caring for a child with burns are helping the child to be as independent as possible, enabling skill return, and achieving optimal functioning.

Achievement of these goals requires interdisciplinary collaboration and coordination of therapies so that the child receives the maximum benefit of each therapeutic intervention.

37. **What behavior does a child with burns frequently exhibit?**

The child with burns commonly exhibits procrastination or avoidance before burn care time. The nurse should provide interventions to reduce fear, anxiety, and pain. Involving the child as much as possible also helps the child feel more in control. The nurse should anticipate common diversionary tactics such as needing to go to the bathroom or needing food or drink and incorporate them into the care routine. Additionally, the nurse should provide diversions such as music or videos during burn care to distract the child.

38. **What are children with spinal cord injury more at risk for than adults with spinal cord injury?**

Children and adolescents with spinal cord injury are more at risk for developing scoliosis because their skeletons are still growing. Braces may be necessary for prevention.

39. **What are some psychosocial concerns for children with spinal cord injury?**

How a child reacts to spinal cord injury depends on the level of physical, emotional, and cognitive development. Anger, depression, and noncompliance are frequent reactions that require interventions to facilitate healthy expression of feelings and concerns. Although these reactions are similar to adults, one must realize that normal developmental stages during childhood and adolescence are about gaining independence and self-identity. Therefore when a child or adolescent suffers a spinal cord injury, the significant impact to psychosocial development causes these reactions to be more pronounced and prolonged. Ongoing assessment and monitoring is critical for early intervention.

40. **In addition to traditional therapies, what is of major concern for a child with traumatic brain injury?**

Academic concerns should be addressed early in the child's rehabilitation. Educational and cognitive assessments should be comprehensive and include the following:
- Ability to take standardized tests
- Curriculum-based learning ability
- Strengths and weaknesses of learning style

Use of data from neuropsychological testing and functional analysis is essential to develop compensatory strategies. Giving these children appropriate and comprehensive accommodations and support is critical for them to be successful in the school environment. Coordination with school personnel early is critical. Additionally, all children with traumatic brain injury, regardless of severity of injury or residual deficits, should be evaluated and have collaborative education plans developed. Families also require education as to the child's rights related to school setting and to resources available in the community.

41. **Does gender affect outcome following moderate to severe traumatic brain injury in children?**

Research suggests that boys have statistically significant poorer outcomes than girls related to memory for new information, particularly during the first year following injury. Therefore taking this factor into consideration is important for long-range rehabilitation planning and reentry into the school environment.

42. **How does social support affect the caregivers of children with traumatic brain injury?**

Social support has been found to be a key diffuser of distress in caregivers. Although social support cannot completely mitigate the distress, it can substantially reduce the effect.

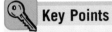

Key Points

- The three main differences between care for children and adults to consider when planning care for children are child development, epidemiology of childhood disabilities, and the relationship of the child's health and development to the family's health and socioeconomic status.
- Childhood-to-adult transition planning should begin early so as to maximize independence.
- Case management services are a critical service component for children with disabilities.
- The more significant a child's disability or condition is, the more potentially complex feeding and meeting nutritional needs become.
- The pediatric rehabilitation nurse may need to be more involved for a longer period of time, and provide more education, for successful bowel/bladder elimination patterns to be achieved.
- Children with disabilities are at higher risk for injury.
- Provision of information on sexuality and how the child's disability affects sexual/reproductive potential is important.
- Home environment and physical challenges of everyday life must be considered before a child can be discharged home.
- Children with spina bifida should be assessed for latex allergy continually.
- Major management issues for children with cerebral palsy are nutrition, surgery, and functional ability.
- Children with spinal cord injury have an increased risk for developing scoliosis.
- Educational planning always should be a part of case management for a child with disabilities.

Internet Resources

American Academy of Pediatrics
http://www.aap.org

Federation for Children with Special Needs
http://www.fcsn.org

Spina Bifida Information from the National Institutes of Health
http://www.ninds.nih.gov/health_and_medical/disorders/spina_bifida.htm

Shriners Hospital for Children, Spinal Cord Injury Rehabilitation
http://www.shrinershq.org/hospitals/sci.html

Muscular Dystrophy Association
http://www.mdausa.org

Cystic Fibrosis Research, Inc.
http://www.cfri.org

Bibliography

1. American Academy of Pediatrics: Managed care and children with special health care needs: a subject review (RE9814), *Pediatrics* 102(3):657-660, 1998.

2. American Academy of Pediatrics: Transporting children with special health care needs (RE9852), *Pediatrics* 104(4):988-992, 1999.

3. Aronovitch SA, Scardillo J: Latex allergy and the WOC nurse: a review of the literature, *J Wound Ostomy Continence Nurs* 25(2):93-101, 1998.

4. Donders J, Woodward HR: Gender as a moderator of memory after traumatic brain injury in children, *J Head Trauma Rehabil* 18(2):106-115, 2003.

5. Edwards PA, Herzberg DL, Hays SR, and others: *Pediatric rehabilitation nursing,* Philadelphia, 1999, WB Saunders.

6. Ergb MA, Rapport LJ, Coleman RD, and others: Predictors of caregiver and family functioning following traumatic brain injury: social support moderates caregiver distress, *J Head Trauma Rehabil* 17(2):155-174, 2002.

7. Jacobs JM: Management options for the child with spastic cerebral palsy, *Orthop Nurs* 20(3):53-60, 2001.

8. Luther B: Age-specific activities that support successful transition to adulthood for children with disabilities, *Orthop Nurs* 20(1):23-29, 2001.

9. McDaniel L, Cooper TJ, McDaniel R, and others: Postacute rehabilitation for pediatric brain injury, *Case Manager* 2(2):55-57, 2003.

10. Nierenberg B, Sheldon A: Psychospirituality and pediatric rehabilitation, *J Rehabil* 67(1):15-19, 2001.

Chapter 33

Gerontological Rehabilitation

Sandra H. Faria

1. **Why is awareness of rehabilitation for the gerontological patient important?**

   The number of aged persons in American society is growing and will continue to grow in future years as the baby boomers reach retirement age. Elderly ethnic minority groups are the fastest-growing subgroup of the elderly population. These minority elders have been shown to be at increased risk for morbidity and mortality because of socioeconomic, as well as health status, factors. These groups may use health services less often than those in a white majority group; therefore, they use folk cures or folk medicine along with health care services. This has implications for nurses who need to be knowledgeable about cultural and ethnic variations in health beliefs and practices. Additionally, nurses may need to take rehabilitation into the community rather than relying on individuals to come to a traditional health care setting.

2. **What is a gerontological rehabilitation nurse?**

   Gerontological rehabilitation nursing is a specialty area that requires knowledge of gerontology and of rehabilitation nursing. The nurse may work in a variety of settings. Working within long-term care facilities, skilled, intermediate, or residential care may be required. The role of the nurse may include caregiver, teacher, leader, mediator, consultant, and researcher. The nurse needs to know the physiological changes of aging and how these changes affect rehabilitation. The amount of time devoted to each of these roles depends on the patient's condition and the job description of the nurse.

3. **What are some settings in which a gerontological rehabilitation nurse may work?**

   The nurse may work in a variety of settings, including acute care hospitals, rehabilitation units, subacute care facilities, nursing homes, extended care facilities, and homes or community-based facilities. A long-term care facility may have different levels of care, including skilled, intermediate, and residential. These represent increasing levels of independence of the patient.

4. **Does everyone age alike?**

Everyone ages differently. Factors such as heredity, culture, socioeconomic factors, education, and social support may influence how a person ages. Life expectancy differs in genders and race. Many life changes occur with aging, including changes in living arrangements, income, and marital status.

Aging persons have been divided into three groups: the young-old, aged 65 to 74; middle-old, aged 75 to 84; and old-old, aged 85 and over. The old-old group often is called "frail elderly." The groups vary in their independence, in their functional abilities, and in their limitations.

5. **Are there cultural health-related differences among elderly individuals that may be important to nurses?**

Native Americans, Puerto Ricans, and Mexican Americans have a higher incidence of diabetes mellitus. Native Americans have a much higher incidence of poverty in their elders. Elderly African Americans tend to have more loss of functional abilities, and the incidence of hypertension is much greater. Heart disease, stroke, and cancer remain the primary causes of death in older Americans in all cultural groups.

6. **What are some changes to the integumentary system with aging, and how do those changes affect rehabilitation?**

The skin becomes dry and loses elasticity. The skin excretes less perspiration and has less subcutaneous tissue. The fatty tissue redistributes to the trunk of the body. These changes make the skin more prone to breakdown because of the dryness and less padding to bony prominences. The body temperature is altered because of decreased perspiration.

7. **What are the changes to the musculoskeletal system with aging, and how do those changes affect rehabilitation?**

The elder experiences joint stiffness, decreased muscle tone, and demineralization of the bones. These changes cause the person to be more prone to bone fractures, have pain in the joints, and experience altered mobility. The person has decreased muscle strength, as well, which modifies the way an elder rises from a sitting position or climbs stairs. Handles, railings, and bars for assistance may be required.

8. **What are the changes to the neurological system with aging, and how do those changes affect rehabilitation?**

The elder experiences slower reflexes and has a decreased ability to react to multiple stimuli within the environment. These changes result in the elder's taking more time to respond to stimuli. In addition, elders need to concentrate on one task at a time, rather than having multiple tasks to accomplish simultaneously.

9. **What are the changes to the genitourinary system with aging, and how do those changes affect rehabilitation?**

The elderly have an increase in incidence of incontinence, especially stress incontinence. They also may experience frequency and nocturia. Incontinence is a major reason for the elder to be institutionalized. Men may have benign prostatic hypertrophy, which causes urinary frequency and nocturia. The bladder tends to lose tone in men and women, therefore causing frequency. The person has an increase in risk for urinary tract infection because of these bladder changes.

10. **What are the changes to the gastrointestinal system with aging, and how do those changes affect rehabilitation?**

Peristalsis decreases with age; therefore gastric motility also decreases. A decrease in the amount of gastric juices/digestive enzymes affects digestion. Many elders wear dentures, which affects how they chew their food and affects what kinds of food they may eat. They may have more difficulty swallowing, which places them at high risk for aspiration. Because peristalsis is slower, constipation becomes a major problem. If dentures do not fit well, the elders tend not to eat well and therefore may lose weight.

11. **What are the changes to the circulatory system with aging, and how do those changes affect rehabilitation?**

With aging, the heart pumps less effectively. Hypertension incidence increases because of hardening, or stenosis, of the arteries. If the elder takes medication for hypertension, the incidence of orthostatic hypotension increases, which increases the risk of falls. The incidence of cardiac arrhythmias is greater. The person has less cardiac reserve; therefore the heart is less able to meet the demands placed on it.

12. **What are the changes to the respiratory system with aging, and how do those changes affect rehabilitation?**

The respiratory muscles stiffen, and resistance to airflow in the airways increases. This results in a decreased amount of inhaled oxygen with each breath. Therefore elders experience more shortness of breath with exertion and may require supplemental oxygen in the presence of lung disease.

13. **What is geriatric abuse, and why is it important to the gerontological rehabilitation nurse?**

Geriatric abuse can be of several types: physical, psychological/emotional, neglect, and financial. This abuse may occur in any culture and any socioeconomic level and may occur anywhere. Dependent and functionally impaired elders are especially at risk. All health care workers should be aware of this and keep eyes and ears open for vulnerable elders. Box 33-1 lists signs of abuse.

Box 33-1. Signs of elder abuse

- Poor hygiene
- Bruises
- Broken bones
- Malnutrition
- Dehydration
- Being left alone
- Being threatened
- Not being turned
- Being frightened
- Having savings and belongings stolen
- Being scammed
- Being defrauded out of home

---

14. **What are some nursing interventions when the nurse suspects abuse in the home?**

    Most states require that suspected abuse be reported, so the nurse should make accurate and thorough observations and do thorough documentation. Prevention is the best approach for the family. The nurse should make sure family members are aware of respite and community facilities that may assist them in caregiving.

15. **Why is patient safety of such grave concern to health care professionals?**

    Falls are the leading causes of accidental death in persons age 75 and older. Therefore safety measures are important to prevent such falls. The nurse may use specific fall risk tools to assess the patient's abilities, limitations, and needs.

16. **An important objective for the gerontological rehabilitation nurse is to promote wellness and self-care in the patient. What are the key areas involved in this endeavor?**

    Box 33-2 lists the key areas for promotion of wellness and self-care in elders.

Box 33-2. Key areas to promote wellness and self-care in elders

- Improving nutritional status, which is important for the patient (A thorough nutritional assessment should be done, and plans should be outlined to provide nutritionally sound meals.)
- Assessing skin integrity and providing skin care as appropriate
- Promoting mobility and functional independence
- Assessing bowel and bladder patterns and planning interventions as needed
- Taking measures to enhance cognition, communication, sensory perception, and learning

---

17. **What assessments should the nurse perform on an elderly patient to provide a good database for care?**

Box 33-3 presents important assessments necessary for older patients.

Box 33-3.   Important assessments for care of elders

- A functional assessment should be done to determine the patient's functional status.
- An environmental assessment should be done for the safety and well-being of the older adult with disabilities.
- A medication history provides good information to determine drug interactions in the older adult with chronic illness.
- A physical examination is necessary to determine how one factor affecting an older adult's health may exacerbate or aggravate another problem.
- A fall risk assessment determines whether impaired mobility puts the patient's safety at risk.

---

18. **Is alcohol abuse a problem with the elderly that may affect rehabilitation of these patients?**

Misuse of alcohol is often an overlooked problem with the elderly. Women are more likely to have late-onset alcohol problems. Alcohol is a depressant and affects judgment, coordination, alertness, and reaction time. When the person takes drugs with alcohol, the alcohol potentiates the drug effects. The gerontological rehabilitation nurse must ask, rather than avoid, questions regarding alcohol use. Oversedation, produced by the synergistic effect of alcohol and tranquilizers, pain medication, or sleep aids may reduce the patient's level of independence and increase the risk of falls or other injuries.

19. **Is interrupted sleep pattern a problem with the elderly?**

Although many Americans report sleep problems, the elderly are the most deprived of sleep. Sleep-related complaints are the second most common reason for elderly visits to physicians. Psychosocial changes, as well as chronic illness, are factors. For example, sleep disturbances among those with Parkinson's disease and their spouses were predicted best by their depression ratings. Sleep pathologies include sleep apnea, neurological diseases, diabetes, circulatory diseases, chronic pain, hiatal hernias, and Alzheimer's disease.

20. **What are conditions that may affect the cognitive perceptual pattern in the elderly?**

Three main conditions affect the cognitive perceptual pattern in elders (Box 33-4).

> **Box 33-4. Conditions affecting the cognitive perceptual patterns in elders**
>
> - *Pain* is not always considered relevant in the care of elders. Many older adults are reluctant to report pain because they believe that analgesia is addicting and they do not want to become dependent. Frequent intense pain is associated with depression and affects a patient's independence and self-care abilities. Careful interviews are important because many elders experience chronic transient pain but may describe it as an ache or discomfort, thus avoiding the verbalization of the nature of the pain.
> - *Acute confusion* is defined as an abrupt onset of changes and disturbances in attention, cognition, psychomotor activity, level of consciousness, and the sleep/wake cycle. Acute confusion, or delirium, is common on admission to an acute care facility and increases in incidence after admission. Acute confusion is characterized by fluctuations in mental function and is treatable; but if left undiagnosed, it may progress to chronic confusion.
> - *Chronic confusion,* or dementia, may be caused by many different conditions. The patient experiences a progressive decline in mental functioning, which in turn affects the patient's ability to perform activities of daily living. Therefore this may affect the patient's outcome directly in relation to rehabilitation.

21. Is depression a problem with the elderly?

Depression is one of the most common and treatable disorders in older adults. Depression can be difficult to distinguish from dementia because many of the symptoms of depression (memory loss and disorientation) are similar. If depression is unrecognized and untreated, it may become life threatening. Depression may have a direct influence on the patient's ability to perform activities in a rehabilitation program. Therefore for the gerontological rehabilitation nurse to be aware of the signs and symptoms and to evaluate the patient at all times is imperative.

22. What is the focus of rehabilitation after a stroke?

Stroke is the leading cause of disability in older adults and one of the leading causes of death in the United States. The focus of stroke rehabilitation includes training for mobility, activities of daily living, communication, nutrition, behavior, continence, social support, and sexual function. The goal is to regain or maintain as much independence as possible.

23. What are areas of concern in rehabilitation of the patient after a stroke?

Some areas of major consideration for these patients include cardiac care, skin care, respiratory toilet, and management of blood pressure. These are areas in which the gerontological rehabilitation nurse is well qualified to assess and implement measures to promote well-being for the patient. Support is strong for the need to regain or maintain activity and mobility after a stroke.

24. What are rehabilitation nursing interventions after a stroke?

The nurse should encourage use of the affected side to reduce neglect. When the patient is alone, the nurse should place as many objects (telephone and so on) as possible on the affected side so that the patient is stimulated continually to use compensatory strategies. The nurse should use a variety of teaching strategies for patient/family teaching and should keep sessions short to promote learning. The nurse should use terms such as "weak/strong" rather than "good/bad," should plan activities to allow frequent rest periods, and should foster a calm, unrushed environment by moving and speaking slowly and using simple sentences. The nurse should break any task into simple steps to enhance the patient's understanding and should work to build the patient's endurance slowly. The nurse should include the patient and the family in planning the care and should connect the family to a stroke support group or club. Depending on comorbidities, the elder patient may not have the endurance to tolerate 3 hours of therapy a day; therefore the patient may not qualify for acute rehabilitation. The family will need to share in the responsibility of providing therapy.

25. **What are areas of concern for all health workers in the patient with spinal cord injury?**

The health care team should be aware of the areas particularly affected by the combination of aging and spinal cord injury (Table 33-1). Important areas for concern in the elder with spinal cord injury is recognition of the level of the injury and maintaining spinal stability. These involve excellent communication between the rehabilitation nurse/team and the facility from which the patient was transferred.

Table 33-1. Effects of the combination of aging and spinal cord injury

Area of concern	Effects
Skin integrity	Decreased subcutaneous fat, decreased perspiration, and immobility lead to pressure sores.
Control of temperature	Peripheral vascular disease and spinal cord injury (SCI) lead to intolerance to temperature change.
Joint range of motion	Stiff joints and SCI lead to compromised extremities.
Muscle and bone mass	Osteoarthritis and no weight bearing lead to muscle atrophy and bone loss.
Gastric motility	Age and SCI lead to decreased motility.
Bowel/bladder	Age and SCI lead to incontinence.
Cardiopulmonary	Decreased function (age) and SCI lead to venous stasis, decreased cardiac output, decreased blood pressure, decreased tidal volume, and ineffective cough.
Nutrition	Slower gastric motility with age and inactivity lead to a need for increased protein, fiber, fluids, and vitamin intake.
Renal function	Function decreases with age and combined with immobility leads to decreased glomerular filtration rate and risk for neurogenic bladder.
Self-esteem	Poor bladder control in elders and SCI lead to feelings of helplessness and depression.

26. What are the areas in which nursing interventions are focused for the patient with spinal cord injury?

Areas in which the nursing interventions are focused are
- Promoting adequate respiration
- Preventing hazards of immobility and the effect on cardiac function (especially deep vein thrombosis and orthostatic hypotension)
- Establishing appropriate bowel and bladder programs
- Promoting adequate nutrition
- Preserving skin integrity
- Managing pain

Psychosocial issues include social support, quality of life, and caregiver burden. Table 33-1 provides detailed effects of these areas of concern.

27. How does Parkinson's disease affect rehabilitation of the patient?

Parkinson's disease is one of the most common neurological diseases and has been described as "shaking palsy." The course is variable and the progression is slow. Symptoms (Box 33-5) progress at a different rate in individuals. Some patients never portray the severe symptoms. Chapter 27 gives more information on Parkinson's disease.

Box 33-5. Parkinson's disease signs and symptoms

- Altered sleep pattern
- Bradykinesia
- Deficits in discrimination
- Deficits in visual/spatial perception
- Dementia
- Depression
- Difficulty swallowing, chewing
- Drooling
- Fatigue
- Festination
- "Freezing" movements
- Impaired judgment
- Inability to access working memory
- Inability to shift attention
- Learning deficits
- Listlessness
- "Pill-rolling" movements of fingers
- Rigid, masklike expression
- Rigidity

Box 33-5. **Parkinson's disease signs and symptoms** *continued*

- Stiff, shuffling gait
- Tremor
- Unexpected falls
- Unstable posture
- Voice tone changes

28. Nursing care of the patient with Parkinson's disease should aim primarily at what aspect of care?

Nursing care of the patient with Parkinson's disease is aimed at support/education. Areas include
1. Medication therapy:
   - Anticholinergics to reduce tremor and rigidity
   - Levodopa to alleviate akinesia and tremors
   - Dopamine agonists to prevent end-of-dose failure
   - Monoamine oxidase B inhibitors allow longer responsiveness induced by levodopa
2. Prevention of falls caused by the effect of the disease on balance and muscle tone
3. Disease progression: slow and variable
4. Nutritional needs: fluids, fiber, adequate calories
5. Risk for aspiration: swallowing is altered; patient drools; nurse must sit patient upright and assist to self-feed
6. Promotion of self-care: muscle rigidity and tremors affect movements
7. Promotion of sleep and relaxation: quiet environment, promote daytime activities, limit afternoon naps
8. Communication: problems caused by dysarthria and changes in voice quality

29. Many elders have joint replacement surgery because of arthritis or other conditions common in elders. What is the importance for the rehabilitation nurse?

Total hip arthroplasty is a common surgical procedure in elders. The patient response varies because of many factors (e.g., age and comorbidities). Nursing implications include two general areas to assess: injury factors and patient factors. Injury factors include
1. Bone and soft tissue quality (e.g., bruising)
2. Circulation and sensation assessment
3. Surgical site assessment:
   - Swelling
   - Signs of infection
   - Bleeding
4. Pulses assessment for adequate circulation to the extremity

Patient factors include
1. Psychological issues
2. Other unrelated diseases (e.g., diabetes)

Assessment of the patient's mental status should be ongoing, and nursing interventions should include those for other disease states as well.

The nurse should address concern for the fact that the elder may be intolerant of the typical physical rehabilitation regimen necessary for joint replacement and should make necessary modifications.

30. Why is rehabilitation so important to an elderly person?

Chronic diseases are prevalent in the elderly population. The elder experiences normal changes of aging and in addition may experience changes caused by chronic disease states. The gerontological rehabilitation nurse can intervene to assess the patients as a whole and offer nursing interventions that will increase their mobility and functioning, therefore increasing their quality of life.

31. Is pain considered a problem in the elderly?

Pain is often a problem in the elderly because of mobility changes compared with when they were younger. Decreased production and liberation of enkephalins (a natural analgesic) may be a secondary effect of aging. A tendency toward decreased activity results in tightness of muscle groups that may cause pain. Environmental influences such as poor nutrition, disease, or injury may lead to posture changes that can cause discomfort in the patient. Many diseases (arthritis, stroke, fractured bones) may cause pain in the elderly; therefore the nurse's objective is to provide comfort measures to relieve pain and to teach the patient to cope with chronic pain.

32. What pain-relief measures are effective?

A variety of treatment measures may be used for pain:
1. Hot and cold compresses often are used in physical therapy departments to relieve pain.
2. Transcutaneous electrical nerve stimulator is a device that "distracts" the pain transmission, thereby decreasing painful sensations through electrical impulses.
3. Palliative pain relief measures often are used in patients with long-term or chronic pain. These measures may decrease the need for pain medication and include
   - Relaxation therapy
   - Touch
   - Music therapy
   - Subdued lighting
   - Massage therapy

Other pain-relieving measures may include positioning and turning schedules so that patients have no pressure points that may become sore and irritated. The nurse should give pain medications as appropriate and should use pain-rating scales. The nurse may give narcotic or nonnarcotic drugs and should give pain medication 30 minutes before each physical therapy session. Nurses should not hesitate to administer pain medications to the patient as they are needed.

33. What if the elder is fearful of becoming addicted to pain medication?

Nurses should not hesitate to administer pain medications to the patient as they are needed. An important point for the nurse and patient/family to remember is that active participation in the rehabilitation program cannot occur if the patient is in too much pain or is too uncomfortable. The nurse should stress this to the patient and family members because many are fearful that the patient will become addicted to pain medication. Addiction is not a consideration as long as the medication is needed to relieve pain.

34. Why do some elders get osteoporosis?

Osteoporosis is a common disease in elders that is preventable. The effects are devastating. Women are affected more often than men because of the lack of the protective effect of estrogen after menopause. Women in northern climates are thought to be more at risk because of decreased hours of sunlight exposure. Men, however, are not immune to this disease. Many elderly men experience hip fractures as a result of osteoporosis.

35. What are risk factors for osteoporosis?

Osteoporosis has many risk factors; some are controllable and some are uncontrollable. Controllable risk factors include
* Inactivity
* Inadequate calcium and vitamin D intake
* Cigarette smoking, alcohol consumption, and excessive caffeine intake
* Lack of exposure to sunlight.
Uncontrollable risk factors include
* Menopause
* Advanced age
* Thin, small-boned frame
* European or Asian descent
* Fair-skinned blonde appearance
* History of anorexia or bulimia
* Surgical removal of reproductive organs
* History of endocrine disease

36. **What are the components of a teaching program for prevention of osteoporosis?**

The nurse should stress the importance of a nutritional diet to the patient, especially the importance of calcium and vitamin D intake. Calcium supplements ensure that the patient has an adequate calcium intake. The patient should modify controllable risk factors. Weight-bearing activity is important to maintain healthy bones and joints. Fall prevention in the home is an important teaching objective. Bone density imaging (Dexascan) and physical examination by the physician should be done routinely (usually every 2 years).

37. **What is polypharmacy, and why is it a problem for the elderly?**

Polypharmacy is the use of many medications by the elderly. Polypharmacy is a problem because many times elders go to several different physicians and fail to tell the physicians what drugs they are taking already. Of course, the question should be posed in the office. Even when the question is asked, elderly patients may not remember all the drugs to report. Therefore they are taking many drugs prescribed by many different physicians and filled at different pharmacies. The rehabilitation nurse case manager is a valuable resource for addressing this overwhelming problem among the elderly, for often the problem is not discovered until the patient is brought to the emergency department in a toxic state from an overdose of a medication that has been prescribed by different physicians under different trade names.

38. **What can the nurse do to help the patient if polypharmacy is a problem?**

Communication between health care professionals is of utmost importance. The nurse can assist with this by getting an accurate picture of the patient's medication regimen on admission to the rehabilitation facility. The nurse should request a written list of medications, including over-the-counter medications, from the family. The nurse can ask a family member to bring in all the medications the patient is taking at home. The nurse should compare the written list with the medications in the bag. This should give a good picture of the patient's medication history. Including over-the-counter medications is important because many persons forget about them and do not consider them "real medications." Many over-the-counter drugs may affect the action of prescription drugs; therefore to know which ones the patient may be taking is essential. Additionally, all herbal preparations should be listed. The next step is to communicate the medication list with all physicians who are consulting with the patient. The nurse should encourage the patient to use one pharmacy so that the pharmacist can get to know the patient. The pharmacist can be invaluable in recognizing drug interactions in the patient's medical regimen.

The rehabilitation nurse then needs to sit with the patient and family and teach about each medication, the reason it was prescribed, side effects, time of dosage in relation to other drugs and food, and precautions. Additionally, the nurse increases the patient's awareness of the possibility of different trade names for the same medication, so that any time a new physician orders medication, all the patient's medications are discussed.

39. What is Alzheimer's disease?

Alzheimer's disease is a severe form of dementia resulting from degeneration of the limbic system, which affects many elders in American society. About half of the elders above the age of 85 have Alzheimer's disease. The signs and symptoms that the patient portrays are a result of deterioration of the brain that affects the patient's ability to think, remember, and perform activities of daily living. Alzheimer's disease is characterized by progressive forgetfulness.

40. What are the warning signs of Alzheimer's disease?

The disease involves progressive forgetfulness and gradual increase in symptoms. Chapter 27 gives more information on Alzheimer's disease. The warning signs and progressive symptoms are
- Recent memory loss that may affect job skills
- Depression and anxiety
- Increasing difficulty performing tasks
- Problems with language
- Emotional outbursts; combativeness
- Disorientation
- Inability to recognize familiar objects
- Decreased judgment
- Difficulty with abstract thinking
- Misplacing things
- Changes in behavior
- Personality changes
- Loss of initiative
- Distractibility, nonattentiveness
- Noncommunicative; little social interaction
- Severe short-term memory loss

41. What can the nurse do to help the patient and family as Alzheimer's disease progresses?

As the patient progresses through the stages of Alzheimer's disease, the patient becomes more dependent on others for care. Patients lose the ability to recognize their friends and family, become unable to manage their bodily functions and activities of daily living, wander and become lost, and are not aware of happenings in their environment. Most perceptions of their environment create fear, agitation, paranoia, and depression. Many persons require institutionalization because the family becomes unable to care for them at home because of behavioral changes. As the patient progresses in this disease, it becomes important to provide support for the caregiver because the stress of providing constant care for these patients may be overwhelming, especially when the caregiver is also an elder.

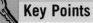

Key Points

- Promoting wellness in the elderly patient includes improving nutritional status, assessing skin care, assessing bowel and bladder function, promoting mobility and functional independence, and enhancing cognitive functioning, learning, communication, and sensory perception.
- Elderly patients have the greatest amount of sleep disturbance of all ages.
- Depression is one of the most common and treatable disorders in older adults.
- Pain is often a problem in the elderly because of reduced mobility, posture changes, and many diseases such as arthritis and because of fractures, which cause pain.
- Nurse case managers need to address polypharmacy to prevent toxicity and nontherapeutic effects.

Internet Resources

Gerontological Nursing Interventions Research Center
http://www.nursing.uiowa.edu/gnirc

National Gerontological Nursing Association
http://www.ngna.org

The Gerontological Society of America
http://www.geron.org

Hartford Gerontological Nursing Initiative
http://www.gerontologicalnursing.info

American Society on Aging
http://www.asaging.org

Bibliography

1. Durnbaugh T, Kramer JF, Speechley M, and others: Comparison of clinic- and home-based rehabilitation programs after total knee arthroplasty, *Clin Orthop* 410:225-234, May 2003.
2. Easton K: *Gerontological rehabilitation nursing,* Philadelphia, 1999, WB Saunders.
3. Lewis SM, Heitkemper MM, Dirksen SR: *Medical-surgical nursing: assessment and management of clinical problems,* ed 5, St Louis, 2000, Mosby.
4. Radwanski HB: Gerontological rehabilitation nursing. In Hoeman S, editor: *Rehabilitation nursing: process, application, & outcome,* ed 3, St Louis, 2002, Mosby.
5. Rovach CR, Wilson SA: Dementia in older adults. In Stanley M, Beare P, editors: *Gerontological nursing,* ed 2, Philadelphia, 1999, FA Davis.
6. Salisbury SA: Cognitive assessment of the older client. In Chenitz WC, Stone JT, Salisbury SA, editors: *Clinical gerontological nursing,* Philadelphia, 1991, WB Saunders.
7. Sehy YA, Williams MP: Functional assessment. In Chenitz WC, Stone JT, Salisbury SA, editors: *Clinical gerontological nursing,* Philadelphia, 1991, WB Saunders.
8. Stanley M: Acute confusion. In Stanley M, Beare P, editors: *Gerontological nursing,* ed 2, Philadelphia, 1999, FA Davis.

Levels of Cognitive Functioning Assessment Scale (LOCFAS): Using Levels 1-5 from the Rancho Los Amigos Scale

Jeanne Flannery

DIRECTIONS

1. After familiarizing yourself with the clustered behaviors in each level described on LOCFAS, begin to observe the patient without disturbing him/her for a few minutes (3-5). From this brief observation of his/her random interaction with uncontrolled environmental stimuli, you will have a general idea of what level to anticipate (Level I as opposed to Level V).
2. Proceed to observe and elicit responses. Continue upward on the scale assessing for observable behaviors for each level. Cease assessment at the point that no expected behaviors for a whole level can be observed. The cognitive level is designated as the *highest* level at which the *preponderance* of matching behavioral responses occurs. There is always a scatter of responses above and below this level. The next higher level in which two or more behaviors are checked is also recorded. The patient is assessed for his best effort since these behaviors indicate the patient's capacity to move up to a higher level. A certain amount of overlap between levels is expected since human behavior is not precise. Variation downward during the day, particularly in relation to distractions, fatigue, and stress, is expected to occur.
3. The assessment may take approximately 15 minutes. It can be incorporated within other aspects of routine care and, therefore, no exact time frame is set. Observations begin with the caregiver's first encounter with the patient and may extend through whatever activities in which the patient and caregiver normally engage until adequate assessment data are gathered.
4. Note the expected behavior for each of the 10 categories is stated in capital letters (A-J) for each level.

LEVEL I. NO RESPONSE

A. **Attention to the Environment:**   NONE
   1. Appears unaware of environment; eyes usually closed
B. **Response to Stimuli:**   NONE
   2. Completely unresponsive to tactile stimuli and position changes
   3. Completely unresponsive to auditory stimuli

4. Completely unresponsive to visual stimuli
   (This is not to be confused with pupillary response to light, which is reflexive.)
5. Completely unresponsive to painful stimuli
6. Completely unresponsive to gustatory stimuli

C. Behavior Status: **REFLEXIVE**

7. May have primitive responses such as chewing, rooting, blinking, eye opening, which are unrelated to specific stimuli

D. Ability to Process Information: NONE
E. Ability to Follow Commands: NONE
F. Awareness of Person (Self):   NONE
G. Awareness of Time (Present):   NONE
H. Ability to Perform Self-Care: NONE
I. Ability to Converse: NONE
J. Ability to Learn New Information: NONE

LEVEL II. GENERALIZED RESPONSE

A. Attention to the Environment: NONE
B. Response to Stimuli: NONSPECIFIC, INCONSISTENT

8. May respond to external stimuli, such as position changes, with physiologic changes such as increased BP, P, or R,* or increased perspiration
9. Responds to painful stimuli with generalized reflex action (nonpurposeful gross body movement, as decerebration or decortication)
10. Repetitive stimuli produce a change in the level of response, either dampening or heightening it (e.g., stroking may reduce physiological changes or intensify response, which occurred initially)
11. Demonstrates nonpurposeful variations in responses to the same stimulus; delayed, limited response

C. Behavior Status: **AWAKE**

12. May be awake but unaware of environment unless directly stimulated
13. Demonstrates inconsistent, infrequent visual fixation; may have roving eye movements, but is incapable of visual tracking
14. Behavioral response may be the same regardless of stimulus (e.g., eye opening; startle; gross body movement; decerebration upon tactile, painful, or auditory stimulus)

D. Ability to Process Information: NONE
E. Ability to Follow Commands: NONE
F. Awareness of Person (Self):   STIMULI TO BODY PRODUCE
                                                             GENERAL RESPONSE
G. Awareness of Time (Present):   NONE
H. Ability to Perform Self-Care: NONE
I. Ability to Converse: NONE
J. Ability to Learn New Information: NONE

LEVEL III. LOCALIZED RESPONSE

A. Attention to the Environment: NONE
B. Response to Stimuli: SPECIFIC, INCONSISTENT

15. Tracks briefly a moving object in visual field (when awake) only if stimulus intensity gains attention; inconsistent response

16. Demonstrates withdrawal responses or facial grimacing to tactile stimuli (pressure, temperature, texture) but inconsistently
17. Responds specifically to the stimulus (e.g., resists restraints, swallows food, relaxes to stroking, pulls at NGT*), but inconsistently
18. Responds inconsistently to same stimulus (e.g., turns toward or away from a sound)

C. **Behavior Status:**   **BEGINNING AWARENESS**
19. Awakens to stimuli; has sleep/wake cycles; awakens spontaneously
20. Demonstrates purposeful visual orientation and fixation
21. Moves body parts purposefully, if able

D. **Ability to Process Information:**   **NONE**
E. **Ability to Follow Commands:**   **INCONSISTENT, DELAYED**
22. Response to commands is delayed
23. Responds more consistently with some persons than with others (e.g., may look at regular caregiver when called, but may not do it with others)
24. Demonstrates inconsistent attention and language comprehension; but when there is a response, it is unequivocally meaningful (e.g., may not respond to command "touch your nose" when it has been followed before)

F. **Awareness of Person (Self):**   **VAGUE, NOT MEASURABLE**
G. **Awareness of Time (Present):**   **VAGUE, NOT MEASURABLE**
H. **Ability to Perform Self-Care:**   **NONE**
I. **Ability to Converse:**   **INCONSISTENT**
25. May vocalize inconsistently to stimuli; but may be infrequent
26. May vocalize automatically with one- or two-word response or just make loud noises

J. **Ability to Learn New Information:**   **NONE**

LEVEL IV. CONFUSED-AGITATED

A. **Attention to the Environment:**   **BRIEF**
27. Demonstrates fleeting general attention to surroundings; unable to concentrate
28. Selective attention may be nonexistent or so brief that is not acted upon; easily distractible

B. **Response to Stimuli:**   **SPECIFIC, INAPPROPRIATE**
29. May respond consistently to a stimulus, but the response is inappropriate because of internal confusion
30. May become very agitated or yell in response to a mild stimulus and may sustain response after stimulus is removed; "sticks" in response; low tolerance for frustration or pain
31. Responds to presence of devices, attachments, or any confinement with strong, persistent, purposeful attempt to remove; impatient; demanding

C. **Behavior Status:**   **AGITATED, CONFUSED**
32. In a heightened state of activity related to internal agitation (independent of environment); restless; may engage in behaviors such as pacing, rocking, rubbing, moaning
33. May demonstrate aggressive, hostile behavior; has explosive or unpredictable anger; may be self-abusive in trying to free self
34. May show sudden changes in mood (e.g., crying, laughing, being angry, being quiet, or sleeping)

35. Performs overlearned motor activities automatically, but may resist commands to do these same activities, such as "sit up"

D. Ability to Process Information: **MINIMAL**

36. Unable to understand or cooperate with treatment efforts; may be combative; resistant to care; will leave area, if able

E. Ability to Follow Commands: **INCONSISTENT**

37. May respond briefly or inconsistently to simple commands when agitation is lessened

F. Awareness of Person (Self):   **ORIENTED X1**

38. Is oriented to own name; aware of own body

G. Awareness of Time (Present):   **NONE**

39. Unaware of present events; responds primarily to own state of severe confusion

H. Ability to Perform Self-Care: **MINIMAL**

40. Performs self-care activities for brief periods with maximum direction and cuing; cannot focus without redirection

I. Ability to Converse: **PRESENT, INAPPROPRIATE**

41. Verbalizes incoherently or with words unrelated to the current situation; talking may be rapid, loud, excessive
42. May confabulate (give incorrect answers to questions about the present from unrelated long-term memory stores); lacks short-term recall
43. Conversation reflects confusion and memory deficits

J. Ability to Learn New Information: **NONE**

LEVEL V. CONFUSED-INAPPROPRIATE, NONAGITATED

A. Attention to the Environment: **DISTRACTIBLE**

44. Demonstrates gross attention consistently
45. Has difficulty sustaining selective attention; highly distractible; limited concentration
46. Lacks ability to focus on a specific thing without frequent redirection

B. Response to Stimuli: **VARIABLE**

47. Responds readily to stimuli related to self, body comfort, family
48. Use of objects in environment often inappropriate, without direction

C. Behavior Status: **INAPPROPRIATE**

49. Unable to initiate functional tasks
50. May demonstrate frustration and negative, inappropriate behaviors in response to external stimuli, usually out of proportion to stimulus
51. Will tend to wander (on foot or in a wheelchair) from unit; will not remember a command to remain in a certain place; will not remember how to return from a strange area to a familiar place

D. Ability to Process Information: **LIMITED TO SELF**

52. May relate to conversation about own body comfort, personal needs, momentary concerns

E. Ability to Follow Commands: **CONSISTENT, IF SIMPLE**

53. Responds to single, simple commands consistently
54. Response to a complex command becomes fragmented, nonpurposeful, and unrelated to command; requires redirection to follow through

F. **Awareness of Person (Self):**   **ORIENTED X1**
   55. Oriented to self; knows name, special things about self, but not how the present self is different from past
G. **Awareness of Time (Present):**   **CONFUSED**
   56. Disoriented to time and place, confusing past and present; unaware of situation (what has happened to him/her)
   57. Demonstrates severe short-term memory deficit
H. **Ability to Perform Self-Care:**   **REQUIRES MAXIMUM ASSISTANCE**
   58. Performs overlearned tasks with maximum structure and cuing, but does not initiate the activity
I. **Ability to Converse:**   **SOCIAL-AUTOMATIC**
   59. May converse on a social-automatic level for short periods, as "I'm fine, how are you?" but responses are often unrelated to specific topics of conversation
   60. If not verbal, may use social-automatic gestures, as shoulder shrug, thumbs up
J. **Ability to Learn New Information:**   **NONE**
   61. Unable to learn new tasks; even though tries, listens, follows commands, outcome not achieved.

SUMMARY

Select a number from 1 to 5 that represents the *highest* Cognitive Level where most of the observed behaviors are checked at this time of observation.

---

* *BP*, Blood pressure; *P*, pulse; *R*, respiration; *NGT*, nasogastric tube.

Levels of Cognitive Functioning Assessment Scale Extended (LOCFASE): Using Levels 6-8 from the Rancho Los Amigos Scale

Jeanne Flannery

LEVEL VI. CONFUSED-APPROPRIATE

A. Attention to the Environment: **MODERATE, DISTRACTIBLE**

  62. Attends approximately 30 minutes, if activity is simple and there are no environmental distractions

B. Response to Stimuli: **VARIABLE**

  63. Response to familiar stimuli is consistent and generally appropriate

  64. Requires repeated explanation for new stimuli to gain appropriate response because of memory deficits

C. Behavior Status: **APPROPRIATE, IMPULSIVE**

  65. Still frequently requires cuing to initiate tasks

  66. Frequently requires cuing to continue a task, if prolonged

  67. Continues to act impulsively unless first cued to the process of thinking through the act carefully

D. Ability to Process Information: **APPROPRIATE, IF SIMPLE**

  68. Can follow a schedule with assistance

  69. Becomes confused by changes in the routine

  70. Becomes confused with details because of memory deficits

  71. Becomes frustrated when expected to make a decision (such as what to wear, which food to select, which activity to do first)

E. Ability to Follow Commands: **CONSISTENT, UNLESS MULTIPLE STEPS**

  72. Unable to do multiple acts at the same time (e.g., watch walk sign, traffic light, make sure no cars, step off curb, walk in crosswalk, and talk) due to lack of concentration

  73. Unable to follow multiple steps to a task in sequence (e.g., knock on bathroom door, open door, turn on light, close door, unfasten pants, take down, sit on commode, answer nurse, while maintaining balance) due to memory deficits

F. Awareness of Person (Self):   **ORIENTED X3**

  74. Knows who and where he/she is; may know he/she is in the hospital because of an injury, but relates to the physical injury rather than cognitive

75. Sees own problems as associated with being hospitalized and believes these problems will be gone when he/she goes home
76. Can relate superficially to the purpose of his/her rehabilitation program (e.g., to walk better, talk better)

G. Awareness of Time: **VAGUE**
77. Will usually know the month and year; may know it is time for lunch or visit
78. Will usually remember an event (such as a visitor this morning) but will not remember the details of the visit
79. Confuses details of events in his/her memory

H. Ability to Perform Self-Care: **MINIMAL ASSISTANCE**
80. Can do ADLs* with guidance (bathing, dressing, grooming)
81. Knows when he/she needs to toilet (continent)

I. Ability to Converse: **USUALLY APPROPRIATE, IMPULSIVE**
82. Speaks impulsively, without thinking first
83. Says what he/she thinks, without inhibition—may not be socially acceptable
84. Forgets or confuses details of conversation
85. May perseverate with a socially acceptable comment for the positive effect, rather than truly mean it (e.g., "Your dress is pretty," stated to each person in the room, and then around the same group again)

J. Ability to Learn New Information: **VERY LIMITED**
86. New learning still impaired by memory deficits
87. Requires repetition, separation of steps of a new task into small parts, with continued reinforcement and cuing

LEVEL VII. AUTOMATIC-APPROPRIATE

A. Attention to the Environment: **STABLE IN FAMILIAR SITUATIONS**
88. Able to do routine activities, but requires supervision because of decreased safety awareness

B. Response to Stimuli: **VARIABLE**
89. Response to routine stimuli is appropriate, but rigid and inflexible
90. Has trouble paying attention to stimuli when situation is stressful
91. Response is slower in stressful situations

C. Behavior Status: **APPROPRIATE, INFLEXIBLE; IMPULSIVE**
                                        IN NEW SITUATIONS
92. Will talk automatically about doing something, but will have problems actually doing it
93. Demonstrates difficulty planning, initiating, and following through with activities
94. May become frustrated in new situations and act without thinking
95. Highly distractible in situations with a number of people present (e.g., sports events, church, school)
96. Perceived as stubborn due to rigid, inflexible responses

D. Ability to Process Information: **APPROPRIATE IN STABLE SITUATIONS**
97. Can follow a set schedule independently
98. Usual processing is interrupted in stressful situations (unfamiliar or crowded)

99. Processing is slowed when stressed
100. Will require assistance (when usually independent) when he/she becomes frustrated
101. Demonstrates lack of judgment and insight; therefore requires supervision

E. **Ability to Follow Commands:**   **CONSISTENT, APPROPRIATE IN STABLE SITUATIONS**

102. Still requires assistance in initiating an activity that is not automatic (overlearned tasks)
103. Requires cuing to follow through with an unfamiliar activity

F. **Awareness of Person (Self):**   **ORIENTED X3**

104. Knows who and where he/she is
105. Can answer the question of why he/she is in the hospital ("I had a car wreck and injured my head") but does not understand the event's impact on the present cognitive deficits
106. May expect to return to the previous lifestyle activities, work, school; unrealistic future planning
107. Cannot connect his/her present memory problems with the required changes in future goals

G. **Awareness of Time:**   **APPROPRIATE, LIMITED**

108. Knows what day it is
109. Has shallow recall of recent past and timing of activities in the immediate future, but has limited memory for more global, abstract occurrences (course of events since injury)
110. Can discuss, automatically, distant past events, but may not relate present state to them
111. Can discuss, automatically, plans for future changes, with cuing, but does not really believe they will need to be done

H. **Ability to Perform Self-Care:**   **INDEPENDENT**

112. Can do ADLs independently, if physically able
113. Performs daily routine automatically, robot-like

I. **Ability to Converse:**   **APPROPRIATE, FLUENT**

114. Responds automatically to conversation with an appropriate answer or comment, within his/her cognitive capacity

J. **Ability to Learn New Information:**   **SLOWED**

115. Can learn new tasks, but at a slower rate than that of his/her pre-injury status

LEVEL VIII. PURPOSEFUL-APPROPRIATE

A. **Attention to the Environment:**   **ALERT, APPROPRIATE**

116. May function independently without supervision

B. **Responses to Stimuli:**   **FLEXIBLE, LIMITED**

117. Response to stimuli in stable situations is more flexible
118. May solve a problem with more than one solution
119. Becomes overloaded with difficult, stressful, or emergency situations

C. **Behavior Status:**   **APPROPRIATE IN STABLE SITUATIONS**

120. May demonstrate poor judgment in new situations and may require assistance
121. May demonstrate a low tolerance to stress

122. May have deficits in abstract reasoning
123. May demonstrate deficits in social, emotional behavior

D. Ability to Process Information: APPROPRIATE

124. Realizes he/she has a problem with thinking and memory
125. Is beginning to compensate for deficits (lists, reminders, calendar)
126. Thinking problems are subtle enough that they may not be noticeable to persons who didn't know his/her pre-injury abilities
127. Needs some guidance with decision making, especially large ones (e.g., moving, buying a car, going on vacation, job searching)

E. Ability to Follow Commands: APPROPRIATE, PURPOSEFUL

128. Follows written or oral directions appropriately, unless stressed

F. Awareness of Person (Self): ORIENTED X4

129. Able to recall and integrate past with present state

G. Awareness of Time: APPROPRIATE

130. Tells time accurately, can stay on schedule

H. Ability to Perform Self-Care: INDEPENDENT

131. Able to live alone and care for self

I. Ability to Converse: APPROPRIATE

132. Use of language is appropriate and fluent unless the situation creates stress
133. May demonstrate poor judgment in choice of phrases or be socially less than acceptable at times
134. May still be somewhat uninhibited in conversation, particularly during stress (e.g., tells people, who have no need to know, all the details of his/her deficits, as he/she understands them)

J. Ability to Learn New Information: GOOD

135. Can learn complex tasks and information, if not too difficult for his/her cognitive capacity, *and* if given enough time
136. May be ready to relearn driving
137. May be ready for job training evaluation
138. May still require assistance during emotional outbursts, stress responses, unusual situations, or when it is essential that responses must be accurate and fast

NOTE WELL: This level is **NOT NORMAL** cognitive functioning

SUMMARY

Select a number from 6 to 8 that represents the *highest* Cognitive Level where most of the observed behaviors are checked at this time of observation.

NO LEVEL APPLIED (PROVIDED FOR COMPARISONS TO LEVELS)
Normal

A. Attention to the Environment: ALERT, APPROPRIATE
B. Response to Stimuli: FLEXIBLE TO THE SITUATION
C. Behavior Status: APPROPRIATE TO THE SITUATION
D. Ability to Process Information: APPROPRIATE

- Can focus, concentrate, persevere, change approach until goal is met, in spite of the situation

E. **Ability to Follow Commands:**   **APPROPRIATE**
F. **Awareness of Person (Self):**   **ORIENTED X4**
   - Can compare one's perception to others' and grow from experience
   - Can adapt to one's own difficulties or compensate
G. **Awareness of Time:**   **APPROPRIATE**
H. **Ability to Perform Self-Care:**   **INDEPENDENT**
I. **Ability to Converse:**   **APPROPRIATE**
   - Degree of articulateness depends on education
J. **Ability to Learn New Information:**   **GOOD-EXCELLENT**
   - Degree of ability depends on intelligence

NOTE WELL: The degree of achievement at any level, including normal, is dependent to a certain degree upon upbringing, motivation, philosophy of life, personality, family relationships, social support, stress management, goal orientation, experiential learning, and sense of self.

---

* *ADLs*, Activities of daily living.

Nursing Management Care Plan for the Patient with Impaired Cognitive Functioning

Jeanne Flannery

LEVEL I. NO RESPONSE

Goals

Activate response and enhance well-being

Facilitation

Prevent physiological problems and complications such as
- bed sores/skin breakdown
- contractures
- muscle atrophy
- heterotopic ossifications
- bone atrophy/osteoporosis
- incontinence
- kidney stones
- urinary tract infection
- autonomic dysreflexia
- constipation/impaction
- diarrhea
- stress ulcers
- upper respiratory infection
- paralytic ileus
- hypostatic pneumonia
- aspiration
- sleep disorders
- anxiety
- sensory deprivation/overload
- malnutrition

Interventions*

Follow standards of care for the patient in coma using primary preventive measures to prevent complications.

Plan a program of coma stimulation (program is listed next) under the guidance of the health care team based on baseline cognitive level assignment. Start with 5 minutes every 2 hours, increasing up to a maximum of 20 minutes per session, as the patient progresses.

Tactile. *Pleasant:* Rubbing all over with terry cloth, bathing, stroking cheek (decreased abnormal responses). *Strong:* Rubbing brush bristles across skin (localizes to stimulated area). *Noxious:* Pin prick, nailbed pressure (grimace, phonation, withdrawal).

Auditory. *Pleasant:* Explaining simply, calling name, playing audiotape of family member, orienting with each encounter, your name, your task and purpose, information pertinent to patient's life (localizes, relaxes). *Strong:* Bell, loud radio on usual station (turns toward or away). *Noxious:* Clapping wood blocks or whistling at each ear (startle reflex, moves).

*Expected responses are noted in parentheses.

Continued

Goals *continued*

- fluid/electrolyte imbalance
- thermoregulation impairment
- physical injury

Elicit response to sensory input starting with *Pleasant*, progressing to *Strong*, and using *Noxious* only when response does not occur at other levels.

Prevent sensory deprivation.

Stimulate to move to the next developmental level of recovery.

Involve patient's family in sensory stimulation program.

Interventions* *continued*

Olfactory. *Pleasant:* Favorite food odor, perfume, or aftershave (phonation, increased respiration). *Strong:* Vanilla extract, peppermint (phonation; turns toward). *Noxious:* Moth balls, garlic (grimace, phonation).

Visual. *Pleasant:* Favorite television (TV) program, mobiles, family pictures, visitors, calendar, clock within visual field (relaxes, focuses). *Strong:* TV cartoons, bright moving objects with visual field (localizes, tracks). *Noxious:* Flashlight—may take 150 watts to elicit response through tightly closed lids (phonation, grimace, movement)

Gustatory. *Pleasant:* Orange sucker, popsicle (chewing, snouting reflex, increased respiration). *Strong:* Lemon juice, toothpaste (phonation, salivation). *Noxious:* Vinegar, horseradish (grimace, phonation).

Vestibular. *Pleasant:* Place on side, rock trunk back and forth (decreased tone, increased alertness). *Strong:* Trunk rotation, head turns (phonation, tracking). *Noxious:* Head of bed up, down, up (phonation, eye opening).

Proprioceptive/kinesthetic. *Pleasant:* Meaningful movements such as passively brushing hair, washing face, stroking (orienting, relaxing). *Strong:* Rolling, stretching limbs (phonation, decreased tone). *Noxious:* Moving spastic limbs against resistance (phonation, grimace, decreased tone).

*Expected responses are noted in parentheses.

LEVEL II. GENERALIZED RESPONSE

Goals	Interventions
Increase responsivity and maintain well-being *Facilitation* Continue as for Level I, adjusting for increased awareness and response to less than *Noxious* stimuli in some/most modalities.	Reduce environmental distracters. Remain calm and soothing in all verbal and physical contact.

Goals *continued*

Monitor stimulation program used by family and nonprofessionals so that too much stimulation does not occur, resulting in habituation (as in TV, radio, tapes, visitors) that produces reduced response.

If physiological response or reflex action (decerebration, decortication) is the only response, control length of stimulation to prevent exhaustion. Explain to family. Focus on bodily comfort, making frequent adjustments. Awareness of discomfort serves as a steady noxious stimulus and will exhaust the patient, reducing other responses.

Interventions *continued*

Assume everything said is understood, even if the patient does not respond. Implement coma stimulation: Limit interactions in which stimuli are presented to less than 15 minutes at a time, but establish a specific program of repetitions daily.

Assess for response to all sensory stimuli (tactile, auditory, olfactory, visual, gustatory, vestibular, proprioceptive).

Monitor pupil and eye movements in response to light.

Stand directly in front of the patient and call his/her name.

Always explain actions. Be certain not to continue the stimulation after the designated time (habituation reduces awareness).

Assess the time of day when the patient responds best, and schedule the best stimulation interaction at this time. Include a family member, teaching all the techniques and how to continue them.

Repeat name calling with each tactile, auditory, or visual stimulus; and repeat the same order of stimuli during an interaction period. Always continue to orient X4 and introduce yourself explaining what you are doing and for which purpose.

LEVEL III. LOCALIZED RESPONSE
General Behaviors

Inconsistent response to stimuli
Responses are related directly to stimuli
Vague awareness of body responding to discomfort, such as pulling at the nasogastric tube
May be responsive to family

Linguistic Behaviors

Inconsistent following of simple commands
Limited graphic processing
Automatic verbal responses (may be just sounds)
Single-word responses
Expression depends on elicitation by external stimulation

Goals	Interventions
Elicit specific responses and maintain well-being *Facilitation* Continue as for Levels I and II. Increase the frequency, rate, duration, variety, and quality of stimuli. Teach the family the same pattern of what words to say, what intervention to use. Familiar persons often can achieve much better response than strangers. Note to which family member the patient responds best and encourage interaction.	Consistently reorient to the environment: "You were in an accident" or "You had a stroke." Consistently explain the purpose of any intervention: "It's hard for you to ..." Control stimuli within a controlled environment: "Focus on ..." Reduce extraneous stimuli. Continue with tactile, auditory, visual, and kinetic stimuli (olfactory and gustatory in some instances); and record responses, up to 20 minutes per session. Allow extra response time because processing skills are slow.

LEVEL IV. CONFUSED-AGITATED
General Behaviors

Increased agitation
Patient responding to internal confusion
Decreased selective attending
Automatic motor activities present, but internally driven (sits, reaches, ambulates when "needs to," but not when asked)
Oriented to self (X1) generally, when able to assess

Linguistic Behaviors

Overall confusion; loud meaningless verbalization, not relevant to persons present
Decreased rate of processing
Decreased ability to retain, categorize, and associate information
Decreased attention for graphic processing
Lack of inhibition to internal stimuli: abusive or inappropriate language may occur

Goals	Interventions
Decrease agitation and increase awareness *Facilitation* Decrease intensity, duration, and frequency of agitation. Increase attention to the external environment. Decrease stimulation.	Be aware that safety precautions overshadow other measures while the patient is agitated. If the patient has tubes (feeding, intravenous, catheters), use mitten splints or elbow

Goals   *continued*

Prevent injury.

If possible, have a reliable family member present around the clock to soothe and protect the patient from himself, in order not to restrain (this increases agitation exponentially).

If family cannot stay at the time, see whether the family can afford a sitter (properly trained for Level IV behaviors). If sedatives can be avoided, the patient will progress more quickly out of this phase.

Spend adequate time with family to calm them with education about the meaning of the patient's progress through this level.

NOTE: Family members may be terrorized by their loved one's behaviors and believe the patient is worse. For the nurse to help them understand and elicit their help, if at all possible, is imperative. This level can be brief, depending on many factors.

Interventions   *continued*

restraints to prevent the patient from causing harm to self.

If the patient must be left in a regular hospital bed, raise side rails, but pad with pillows or bumpers to prevent the patient from bruising the body.

If no one can stay with the patient, keep a Posey belt on the patient to prevent the patient from climbing over the side rails or the ends of the bed. Keep bed alarm on. Respond quickly to alarm.

If one is available in the hospital, transfer patient to a *Craig bed*, a large padded cubicle with a two-mattress-width base resting on the floor. The padded sides are high enough to prevent the patient from climbing over them. The bottom is wide enough to allow rolling about without any harm. Nurses and other health team members provide care by crawling into the bed with the patient. Freedom from confusing restraints helps prevent added agitation. A net bed also may be used to prevent falling and eliminates the need for body restraints.

Continue reorientation X4, introduce yourself and explain all actions, with each encounter.

Allow "time out" from required measures when agitation is heightened.

Work on increasing selective attending: specific gross motor tasks, graphic tasks, games, naming of objects.

Tell the patient, "We are working on increasing your attention."

Modify the environment to decrease external stimuli (lowered lights, lowered noise level, no TV or radio, no unnecessary persons, low voice tones when talking to the patient).

When the patient's agitation becomes out of control, *DO NOT* try to reason with the patient; the patient cannot process at this time. *DO* reduce verbal interaction, and attempt to redirect attention (Distract with a noise or movement; present behavior may be forgotten.)

Continued

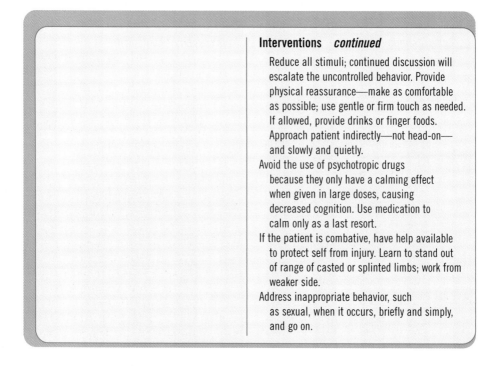

Interventions *continued*

Reduce all stimuli; continued discussion will escalate the uncontrolled behavior. Provide physical reassurance—make as comfortable as possible; use gentle or firm touch as needed. If allowed, provide drinks or finger foods. Approach patient indirectly—not head-on—and slowly and quietly.

Avoid the use of psychotropic drugs because they only have a calming effect when given in large doses, causing decreased cognition. Use medication to calm only as a last resort.

If the patient is combative, have help available to protect self from injury. Learn to stand out of range of casted or splinted limbs; work from weaker side.

Address inappropriate behavior, such as sexual, when it occurs, briefly and simply, and go on.

LEVEL V. CONFUSED-INAPPROPRIATE, NONAGITATED
General Behaviors

Oriented to self (X1) consistently

Consistent response to commands, with deterioration noted with increased length and complexity

Increased agitation following external stimulation (not internal)

Gross attention to environment, increased distractibility; needs redirection to task

Severe memory impairment, with confusion

Performs self-care activities with assistance

Wanders if left unattended

Linguistic Behaviors

Semantic or syntactic confusions

Responds with phrase or single sentence level

Processes verbal communication better than written communication

Responds to specific stimulus

Has word retrieval deficits

Social-automatic conversation frequently inappropriate, confabulatory

Verbal responses characterized by irrelevancies, tangential, incomplete, and circumlocutory expressions; confabulates

Goals	Interventions
Elicit appropriate responses and increase function	
Facilitation	
Decrease confusion precipitated by external environment.	Maintain constancy in environment (placement of belongings).
Increase frequency, rate, duration, and quality of appropriate interactions with environment.	Maintain consistency of routine (e.g., bath, medications, and therapy).
Stimulate development of cognitive abilities in a hierarchical sequence: mentally challenging, but not frustrating.	Provide memory aids (clock, schedule, calendar).
Incorporate cognitive abilities into functional activities, maintaining a consistent routine.	Remind patient verbally of written information (processes verbal better than written).
Correct incorrect responses with subtle, matter-of-fact statements without emphasis.	Try to maintain constancy in nurses assigned.
Set patient goals realistically; new information cannot yet be learned.	Orient the patient with your name, time, place, and activity with each interaction and why the patient is in the hospital (X4).
Teach the family how to assist the patient to relearn previously learned tasks (dressing, grooming, manners, toileting).	Increase awareness of condition and resulting deficit. "You have a brain injury" or "You need help to balance yourself."
An important part is not doing things for the patient until the patient shows limits in abilities. Family members must have a clear understanding of the purpose of cuing and prodding the patient to do tasks within the patient's capacity.	Identify confabulation with the patient and redirect: correct inaccurate responses with a nonthreatening restatement.
	Instruct with short, simple sentences.
	Maintain patient's attention; it will wander easily.
Teach family and nonprofessionals the importance of assisting/cuing to initiate tasks, but allow the patient then to continue independently until another cue is needed.	Teach strategies to achieve tasks; the purpose is to help the patient consciously process information in an organized sequence.
	Assist/cue patient to initiate tasks; this deficit in initiation still is strong.

LEVEL VI. CONFUSED-APPROPRIATE
General Behaviors

No longer wanders

Is inconsistently oriented to time and place (X3)

Shows increased awareness of deficits (states he/she does not know an answer)

Shows goal-directed behaviors but requires external structuring

Follows simple directions consistently and shows carryover for overlearned tasks (such as self-care)

Requires supervision only with old learning; has little or no carryover for new learning

Responses may be incorrect (because of memory deficits) but are appropriate to the situation

Past memory shows more depth and detail than recent memory
Has little anticipation or prediction of future events
Functional for common daily activities, but selective attention remains impaired
Has increased awareness of self, family; may have vague recognition of staff

Linguistic Behaviors

Receptive
Processing delayed; difficulty retaining, analyzing, synthesizing
Can process spoken word at compound sentence level
Can process graphically at short sentence level

Expressive
Appropriate to situation but reflects internal confusion, disorganization
Significantly reduced new learning capacity manifested
Confusion of time and place contexts demonstrated
Tangential, irrelevant responses emerge in complex open-ended discussions
No longer confabulates
Usually speaks briefly; stimulus bound
Speaks in monopitch, monoloudness

Goals	Interventions
Increase functional ability and decrease confusion	
Facilitation	
Provide respect to the patient as an adult in all interactions.	Teach strategies to achieve tasks (not just the task in isolation).
Remain calm and supportive.	Expand memory aids to keeping a notebook of events, tasks, and needs.
Provide mentally challenging, but not frustrating, activities.	Provide matter-of-fact feedback (or corrections) regarding use of melody, rhythm, or articulation of speech.
Maintain consistency in routines.	Maintain a consistent routine such as for activities of daily living, therapy, and meals.
Teach family that as the patient becomes more aware of deficits, withdrawal, irritability, or uncooperativeness may increase.	*Do not* persist if a challenge is too great for capacity (such as asking the patient to execute a complex task or process abstractly).
	Cue to maintain concentration and to complete a long task (do not do for the patient if patient is able to complete with cuing).
	Continue to explain relationship of deficits to original cause and requirements for therapy.
	Remind patient to think before acting; call attention to impulsive acts that created a less-than-positive outcome.

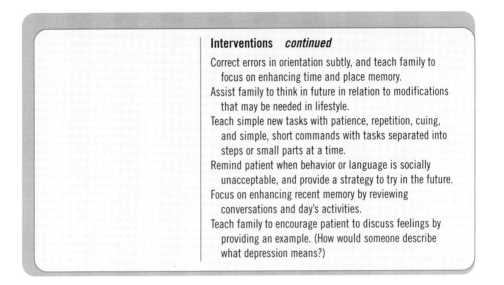

Interventions *continued*

Correct errors in orientation subtly, and teach family to focus on enhancing time and place memory.

Assist family to think in future in relation to modifications that may be needed in lifestyle.

Teach simple new tasks with patience, repetition, cuing, and simple, short commands with tasks separated into steps or small parts at a time.

Remind patient when behavior or language is socially unacceptable, and provide a strategy to try in the future.

Focus on enhancing recent memory by reviewing conversations and day's activities.

Teach family to encourage patient to discuss feelings by providing an example. (How would someone describe what depression means?)

LEVEL VII. AUTOMATIC-APPROPRIATE
General Behaviors

Appropriate but robotlike in familiar, routine activities

Demonstrates inflexibility

Still lacks initiation in activities that are not overlearned

Lacks insight, judgment, and ability to make realistic future plans

Requires supervision to maintain safety

Remains distractible, becomes frustrated, and processing is slowed in stressful situations

Can describe condition or deficits, but lacks insight in the impact

Orientation is intact, but limited (X3, plus)

Can learn new tasks, but still is impaired

Linguistic Behaviors

Most use of language in familiar environments is within normal limits.

Receptive
Slow in rate and quality with spoken words, related to length, complexity, and distractions

Can process graphically at a short paragraph level, but absence of detail and organization persists

Expressive
Occasional word retrieval errors persist

Can write a simple, short paragraph, but errors in syntax and organization are evident

Rhythm, melody, and articulation may still be aberrant

Goals	Interventions
Achieve independence in activities of daily living	
Facilitation	
Increase initiation	Focus on strategies to improve, based on self-report of needs, as well as observation.
Increase responsibility in executing tasks	Teach family how to support, praise, and correct social interactions.
Implement functional tasks that can be applied at home (straighten up bathroom, hang up clothes).	Review diary and cue memory on overlooked entries.
Encourage social interaction with family and visitors.	Praise accomplishments in both functional and social situations.
Encourage to keep a diary of feelings, conversations, events, activities, required responsibilities.	Encourage verbal reasoning and specificity.
Encourage family (and patient) to participate in support groups.	Continue to facilitate awareness of deficits and how they may create a need for changes in life.
	Continue to cue when situation is stressful or new.
	Reduce distractions when performing any task.
	Assist with new learning at patient's capacity with no limit on time.
	Help family to discuss concerns for future in support groups and with health care providers.
	Encourage family to express feelings in support groups.

LEVEL VIII. PURPOSEFUL-APPROPRIATE
General Behaviors

Alert and oriented X4

Relates current problems with past events and uses strategies to compensate

Functions independently within capabilities

Social, emotional, and intellectual capabilities may remain less than premorbid status, but functional levels are acceptable for society

Rate and quality of processing, stress tolerance, abstract reasoning, and judgment remain less than premorbid capacity

Can learn new roles, information, and tasks if deemed important to the patient's future

Linguistic Behaviors

Use of language falls within normal limits

Receptive

Rate of processing auditory and graphic input is slowed

Retention span remains at paragraph level, but compensatory strategies are used to help

Analysis, organization, and integration are reduced in rate and quality

Expressive

Syntax and semantics are within normal limits, but verbal reasoning and abstractions
  are reduced
Graphic expression remains below premorbid capacity
Verbal rhythm, melody, and articulation are within normal limits

Goals	Interventions
Achieve capacity to function independently at home, work, school, and in the community	
Facilitation	
Teach family areas that will require assistance (major decisions, difficult or stressful situations, driving, emergencies, complex problems).	Encourage continued use of memory aids.
	Suggest membership in organizations (such as Brain Injury Association) where new information, equipment, and strategies are discussed at conferences and help is available through a hotline.
Encourage family to support attempts to create a new lifestyle (training for a new job, college, vocational education).	Encourage continued use of a daily log with reflections of feelings, self-evaluation, and goals.
	Allow the patient to assume responsibility for decisions about his/her own care; allowing control may reduce denial response.
Encourage to continue work to increase capacity in areas of deficits.	Increase responsibility of the patient by providing less supervision and expecting the patient to ask for assistance when needed.
Encourage family and patient to attend support groups to discuss problems as they arise.	Focus on increasing initiation and task completion (but within patient's own time frame).
	Provide feedback related to behaviors resulting from stress intolerance; evaluate acceptance and discuss strategies to improve.
	Correct socially inappropriate conversation or behavior and discuss strategies to improve.
	Work with family members to assist the patient with deficits by having them discuss "real" home problems with the patient for the patient to practice solving.

Index

A

AAMR Adaptive Behavior Scale, 336t
Abdominal catheters
  for continuous ambulatory peritoneal dialysis (CAPD), 139-140
Ablative procedures
  to relieve chronic pain, 310t
Abuse
  alcohol
    common among brain injured patients, 212
    as risk factor for strokes, 215b
  child
    osteogenesis imperfecta mistaken for, 344
  drug
    common among TBI patients, 212
  geriatric, 351, 352b
Active theory of sleep
  reticular activating system (RAS)
    diagram illustrating, 95f
Activities of daily living (ADLs)
  assessment scales, 114-115
  in end-stage renal disease (ESRD) patients, 139-144
  following kidney transplants, 146
  functional mobility, 113-119
  guidelines
    for Parkinson's disease patient rehabilitation, 282-283
  levels in spinal cord injury cases, 242t
  rehabilitation needed by burn patients, 177
  rehabilitation nursing goals for
    in multiple sclerosis (MS) patients, 267
Activity tolerance
  assessing
    in pulmonary rehabilitation patients, 159-160
Acupressure
  for chronic pain, 312t
Acupuncture
  for phantom limb pain, 181
  to relieve chronic pain, 310t
  uses of, 122, 124

Acute confusion
  definition of
    in older adults, 354b
Acute pain
  versus chronic pain, 303
Acute transverse myelitis
  symptom of multiple sclerosis (MS), 265
Addiction
  versus drug tolerance, 328
  fears by older adults, 359
Advance directives
  and rehabilitation nursing, 327
Advance practice nurse (APN)
  competencies of, 44
  important role of
    in rehabilitation nursing, 44
African Americans
  cultural considerations concerning, 133
  diabetes prevalence in, 191
  issues with aging, 350
Aging; *See* older adults
Alcohol
  abuse
    common among brain injured patients, 212
    as risk factor for strokes, 215b
  affecting sleep quality, 102
Allograft, 318
Alteplase therapy
  to treat acute strokes, 217-218
Alternative medicine
  government oversight of, 121
  history of, 121
  realms of approach, 123-124
  versus Western medicine, 122-123
Alveolar hyperventilation
  definition of, 166
Alveolar hypoventilation
  definition of, 166
Alzheimer's disease
  available treatment for, 275
  definition and warning signs
    in older adults, 360-361